'This wonderful and utterly unique book i
scholarly examples showing how concept
and play in new ways can help vulnerable ch
clear and concise chapters that highlight how the rhythms of relating are a
fundamental feature of human existence. A "must read" for anybody interested in
therapies for children.'

— *Professor Raymond MacDonald, Professor of Music Psychology and
Improvisation, University of Edinburgh, co-founder of the Glasgow Improvisers
Orchestra, co-editor of* The Handbook of Musical Identities

'This is an extraordinary book that gives innovative insight, understanding and
practical intervention on the importance of rhythm in therapy. Written by diverse
and cross-cultural therapists, artistes and clinicians, it invites us into the internal
world of a child's musicality, rhythmic reciprocity and communication. Simply, it
inspires wonder!'

— *Professor Sue Jennings, Professor of Play, European Dramatherapy Federation,
author of* Healthy Attachments and Neuro-Dramatic-Play

'Each chapter in this international collection brings a unique perspective with
depthful insights and rich wisdom. Written in clear, engaging and embodied
language by dedicated and passionate educators, therapists and artists, *Rhythms of
Relating in Children's Therapies* will profoundly inspire anyone who works or lives
with children.'

— *Bonnie Bainbridge Cohen, founder and Educational Director of the School
for Body-Mind Centering®, author of* Sensing, Feeling and Action

'Having no idea what to expect, this book was a surprising delight. Like therapy
itself, it is a journey; it is filled with opportunities to reflect and grow. Its very title
says it all, as "rhythms" and "relating" are the most core and healing qualities of
psychotherapy. The relevant and engaging *Rhythms of Relating in Children's Therapies*
should be in the library of all child therapists. Highly recommended!'

— *Daniel Sweeney, Professor of Counseling, Director of Northwest Center for Play
Therapy Studies, Director of Clinical Mental Health Counseling program at George Fox
University [Portland, OR], co-author of* Group Play Therapy: A Dynamic Approach

'This is an important book. It addresses a subject which has long been neglected.
It offers the means towards devising more effective ways of dealing with the effect
of trauma. Although the book is concerned with the therapeutic significance of
rhythm and the notion of "communicative musicality" in children, it has major
implications for adult therapy. It is an engaging "read" — scholarly, well-written,
and even enjoyable.'

— *Russell Meares, Emeritus Professor of Psychiatry, Sydney University,
author of* The Poet's Voice in the Making of Mind

'Starting with the communicative musicality of mum and baby's loving embodied dance, these international innovative contributors from the arts, research and trauma invite us on a journey into the essential and transformative power of the rhythms of human connection. From harnessing dragons to evolving into butterflies, be delighted and inspired.'

– Suzi Tortora, author of The Dancing Dialogue: Using the Communicative Power of Movement with Young Children

'Contributors from around the world have come together to make this book a huge inspiration on the rare and essential subject of shared life rhythms in children's psychotherapy. A sense of fun radiates from the text and offers the reader both insights and joyful now-moments.'

– Susan Hart, Psychologist, editor of Inclusion, Play and Empathy

'This fascinating volume is rich with varied perspectives and descriptions about working with children. The premise of rhythm as the music of communication is presented compellingly in early chapters, grounded in science and a brief history of infant–adult interaction research. Expert illustrations from a wide range of specialists, including creative arts therapists, make this comprehensive collection a valuable and engaging resource for both professionals and the public.'

– Robyn Flaum Cruz, Professor, Lesley University [Cambridge, MA], Past-President, American Dance Therapy Association, co-editor of Dance/Movement Therapists in Action

'Rhythm is at the core of all relationships; it is also the basis for effective therapeutic attunement. This valuable contribution articulately explains the importance of rhythm in work with children and generously provides practical and "attuned" strategies for helping professionals to immediately apply in treatment.'

– Cathy Malchiodi, Director, Trauma-Informed Practices and Expressive Arts Therapy Institute, author of The Art Therapy Sourcebook

'I was entranced by the premise of this book – that rhythmic experiences are powerful means of connecting with and relating to others without words – and enthralled by the wide range of therapeutic contexts where such an approach is clearly so potent.'

– Dorothy Miell, Professor of Social Psychology, University of Edinburgh, co-author of Musical Communication

'Trevarthen's generous and inclusive history of communicative musicality provides a powerful segue into this riveting collection. Trust and attunement are prominent threads in these stories, which transcend the notion of an expert who attempts to fix a needy child. Instead they teach us how children can actively participate in their own growth when met with creativity and emotional sensitivity.'

– Katrina McFerran, Professor and Head of Music Therapy, The University of Melbourne, Australia, author of Music, Music Therapy and Adolescents

RHYTHMS OF RELATING IN CHILDREN'S THERAPIES

RHYTHMS OF RELATING IN CHILDREN'S THERAPIES

CONNECTING CREATIVELY WITH VULNERABLE CHILDREN

Edited by **Stuart Daniel** and **Colwyn Trevarthen**

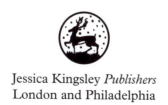

Jessica Kingsley *Publishers*
London and Philadelphia

The epigraph on page 172 has been reproduced with kind permission of Bonnie Bainbridge Cohen.

Figure 21.1 on page 342 has been modified from Figure 11b in *Moving Ourselves, Moving Others* by Lüdtke 2012, p.330 (A. Foolen, U. Lüdtke, T. Racine and J. Zlatev (eds)) with kind permission from Johns Benjamins Publishing Company.

First published in 2017
by Jessica Kingsley Publishers
73 Collier Street
London N1 9BE, UK
and
400 Market Street, Suite 400
Philadelphia, PA 19106, USA

www.jkp.com

Copyright © Jessica Kingsley Publishers 2017

Front cover image source: Tim Webb and the Oily Cart team. The cover image is for illustrative purposes only, and any person featuring is a model.

Library of Congress Cataloging in Publication Data
A CIP catalog record for this book is available from the Library of Congress

British Library Cataloguing in Publication Data
A CIP catalogue record for this book is available from the British Library

ISBN 978 1 78592 035 6
eISBN 978 1 78450 284 3

Printed and bound in Great Britain

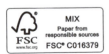

In memory of Dan Stern

Note on client confidentiality and pronoun use

Throughout the book you will find many case stories involving children, parents, carers and therapists. These stories use various methods – changed names, composite characters and cases, altered details – to protect the identities of those involved. On the occasions where these alterations have not been made, full and written permission has been given to publish by those concerned.

Please note that contributors have sometimes used alternating pronouns to reflect client balance (and also, in some instances, 'they/their/them' in the singular). Hence inconsistency in pronoun use is intentional on behalf of the contributors.

Donation of royalties

All author and editor royalties from this book will be donated to the National Society for Prevention of Cruelty to Children – a UK based children's charity.

CONTENTS

INTRODUCTION

Rhythm from the Beginning

STUART DANIEL AND COLWYN TREVARTHEN

Time is an odd thing. It's hard to catch. For most of us, most of the time, it seems to flow fairly consistently in a particular stream, a particular direction. On any regular day in our regular lives, our personal story of time is made standard – just information from a clock. But then again, every so often that story goes a little strange.

On a Wednesday, in 2005 at 2.30 p.m., a particular zoo-keeper of Darjeeling Zoo (North East India) was preparing the meat to feed a snow leopard. The snow leopard was pacing a well-worn path along the edge of her large basin-style enclosure. She was frustrated and violently angry. The zoo-keeper's slow, noisy and smelly approach to meat preparation was clearly taunting her. Her movement was raw potential. I was captivated.[1] I was kneeling down at the edge of the basin, at the top where, in addition to the steep slope of the basin wall, there was a wire fence. The basin wall was high. High enough, I figured. From the moment she caught my eye time definitely went a bit wobbly. The snow leopard turned in her tracks, kind of folded in on herself, getting positioned to run. She took just a few soft steps and then somehow was face to face with me. I didn't understand the jump. I couldn't perceive how she was there. The wire fence between us was absolutely invisible to my mind. The detail of her cold eyes was flawless. And so was the concrete body-knowledge that her teeth were on an inevitable trajectory to my neck. Time did the long, drawn-out stretchy thing. I experienced too much, took in too many details for that moment to be part of my usual story of time. Fortunately for me, cold hard Newtonian physics kicked in and the snow leopard crashed off the invisible fence. I shuffled off, as my time re-regulated, and spent many of those standard minutes shaking with shock.

---

1   Here, this is Stuart's personal recollection.

Our stories of time (based on the changeable qualities of our time perception) are dependent on the nature of our neuro-psychological individuality, on culture, on age, on mood (for instance, what we ate for lunch, or a need for sleep) and on the entire context of every single experience we have (Hammond 2013). When we begin to examine these stories, we start to question the solidity (even the logical possibility) of the basic narrative ingredients. For instance, the 'now' – something usually considered to be the instantaneous present. Playing with a simplified version of a Buddhist practice called 'the one or many reasoning' (Burbea 2014) consider the logic of an instantaneous 'now'. If a 'now' has duration over time, then it of course has temporal component parts: a 'past', a 'present', a 'future'. If it has these things then it cannot be an instantaneous 'now'. And if it has no duration, the other possibility, then in any common sense view of time it cannot inherently exist – there is literally no time for it to arise. From this perspective, being in 'the here and now', as they say, just doesn't make any sense. From this impossible place, we can then ask ourselves – without a 'now' how would we get our bearings on a 'past' or a 'future'? From where would our sense of structured time arise? If a 'now' is impossible, would our story of time (the narrative of our entire life) simply fall away?

So what tools do we use to build our personal stories? We rely on the experience of having temporal structures wrapped up with our experience of being alive. But given that structure is not inherent in time, where does it come from?

Here, in this book, we are interested in the idea that we impute structures (like directionality, regularily, chunks of time and the 'now') on to the flow of time. These structures are felt through the internal and external rhythms of our bodies in motion (Goodrich 2010; Stern 2010). This felt-sense being integral to a fabrication process resulting in prospective and remembered psychological experience.

In our first chapter, Nigel Osborne takes us on a tour of the many chronobiologies (rhythms) of our human bodies. They are the sometimes hidden, sometimes felt, sometimes conscious rhythms that regulate us. We can play with the possibility of different 'times', each a derived sense from a different chronobiological rhythm: different pulses giving us different experiences of the passing of time; different frequencies of pulse giving us a sense of varied expectation and different durations of 'now' (Stern 2004).

But most of all, here we are interested in how our rhythms of life are shared, how they sync up, how they can enable two or more people to connect and feel connected. We are interested in social rhythm. In Chapter 2, I (Colwyn) explore the innately 'musical' essence of human communication – 'communicative musicality'. This thread of exploration is returned to again and again throughout the different chapters of the book. My chapter seeks to identify the passionate qualities of time in early communication between infant and carer. And then, on to the potential for these qualities to bring health and happiness into relating with vulnerable children – we move into the 'rhythms of relating in children's therapies'.

The life of this book began with this title offered as an open inspiration for many contributors from across the globe: music therapists, trauma specialists, dance movement therapists, psychobiologists, dramatherapists, explorers in music education, counsellors, play therapists, somatic therapists, specialist theatre and arts-project pioneers, composer–therapists, teachers and researchers. The editors wish to thank everyone involved for their insight, passion and patience. Each contributor was invited to have fun exploring their own interpretation of our title – their particular ways to phase in-sync with children who otherwise find communication and depth challenging. The results form this collection. We hope you have fun reading it.

References

Burbea, R. (2014) *Seeing That Frees: Meditations on Emptiness and Dependent Arising*. West Ogwell, Devon: Hermes Amara Publications.

Goodrich, B.G. (2010) 'We do, therefore we think: time, motility, and consciousness.' *Reviews in the Neurosciences 21*, 331–361.

Hammond, C. (2013) *Time Warped*. Edinburgh: Canongate Books.

Stern, D.N. (2004) *The Present Moment in Psychotherapy and Everyday Life*. New York: W.W. Norton.

Stern, D.N. (2010) *Forms of Vitality: Exploring Dynamic Experience In Psychology, the Arts, Psychotheraphy, and Development*. Oxford: Oxford University Press.

PART 1

THE MUSICAL ESSENCE OF HUMAN CONNECTION

1

LOVE, RHYTHM AND CHRONOBIOLOGY

NIGEL OSBORNE

The origins of chronobiology: Hearts and flowers

Today, Highgate Hill is a busy thoroughfare, with public buildings, Victorian terraces and leafy spaces. In the late 17th century, however, it was largely rural, with a country mansion or two nearby, like the timber-framed Lauderdale House, and for the rest, rolling fields, copses, hedgerows and gardens. It was where the metaphysical poet, satirist and politician Andrew Marvell had a cottage and spent the latter years of his life.

It was perhaps the relative rural peace of Highgate Hill that inspired Marvell to write one of the most significant English-language poems of the 17th century, 'The Garden' (Marvell 2006). The garden of the poem is a metaphysical conceit: a Restoration Garden of Eden of tranquility, music, luminosity and abundance, graced with the power of beauty, quietude and reflection; but it is also the garden of the Fall, and the last verse is an extraordinary description of nature and time – culminating, or ultimately gloriously blooming, in the image of a clock made of flowers.

> *How well the skilful Gardner drew*
> *Of flow'rs and herbs this dial new;*
> *Where from above the milder Sun*
> *Does through a fragrant Zodiack run;*
> *And, as it works, th' industrious Bee*
> *Computes its time as well as we.*
> *How could such sweet and wholsome Hours*
> *Be reckon'd but with herbs and flow'rs!*

Carl Linnaeus, the father of modern taxonomy, was born in Sweden some 30 years after Marvell had written 'The Garden'. Linnaeus' motto was *omnia*

14

mirari etiam tritissima – 'wonder at all things, even the humblest'. He spent considerable time collecting and classifying specimens of nature in the fields and forests of Uppland and Västmanland. 1751 was the year of publication of *Philosophia Botanicae* (Linnaeus 2005), a complete review of the classifications, or taxonomies, Linnaeus had developed to date. We do not know if Linnaeus ever read Marvell's poem, but Linnaeus' treatise also included a design for a 'flower clock' uncannily like the garden of time that Marvell had imagined. It is not known whether Linnaeus ever 'planted' his clock, but it was based on the principle of flowers opening and closing at different times of day – for example, Morning Glory or Convolvulus tricolor opening at 5 a.m., Hawkweed or Hieracium umbellatum at 6 a.m., White Waterlily or Nymphaea alba at 7 a.m., and so on. Of course Linnaeus' choices of plants and their opening times were dependent on seasons and climate zones.

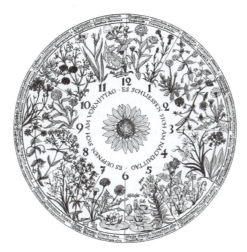

FIGURE 1.1 CARL LINNAEUS' 'FLOWER CLOCK'

Linnaeus had observed patterns in the opening of flowers and knew that these were connected to daylight and times of day, and in turn to the production and dissemination of seeds. But he did not know how plants sensed the time of day – in other words, how they 'knew' when to open and close. It was not until 1959 that biophysicist Warren Butler and biochemist Harold Siegelman, using powerful spectrophotometry, discovered the secret (Butler *et al.* 1959). Butler called it phytochrome, a pigment existing in some form in most flowers, which reacts to red light. When the sun is shining, phytochrome molecules in the cytoplasm (that is to say, in the surface of a plant's cells) absorb red photons. Red photons are quanta of the electromagnetic energy of the red-colour part of the spectrum of light. This absorbed energy triggers changes in the phytochrome molecule. The molecule then descends to the nucleus of the cell where it initiates gene regulation, with a number of effects, including the opening of petals. Far-red light, which is of frequencies between red and infra-red, causes the molecule to return to the cytoplasm, reversing the genetic activations, and the petals to close. So beneath Linnaeus' clock of flowers there lies a complex biological timepiece: a photosensory, cellular, molecular and genetic clock.

This process, replicated in cells across surfaces of the plant, allows the plant to sense not only the presence of light but also its intensity, direction, duration and spectral quality, in other words the presence of different colours. This in turn allows the plant to regulate germination, growth direction, growth rate, chloroplast development (the control of photosynthesis), pigmentation, flowering and senescence. These processes are collectively known as photomorphogenesis. The line which leads from Marvell's poetic imagination to Linnaeus' observations and creativity, and further on to the discoveries of scientists such as Butler and Siegelman is one of the lines along which the science of chronobiology evolved. It is the science of biological clocks, the rhythms of life, how they are regulated and how they relate to external forces like the sun or the moon.

The rhythms of darkness and sunlight and of night and day are of course crucial to human beings, most evidently because of their relationship with sleeping and waking. We are rationally aware of times of day and night, but as anyone who has suffered from jet lag knows, our patterns of sleep are regulated by forces beyond the control of conscious thought. In fact, human beings have a system for sensing light not unlike plants, even though the respective biologies are separated by hundreds of millions of years of evolution. The human equivalent of the phytochrome is a pigment called melanopsin (Provencio et al. 1998). Melanopsin is present in photosensitive ganglion cells, or clusters of cells, very near to the surface of the retina of the eye. Unlike phytochrome, melanopsin absorbs photons from the blue and violet area of light. This intake of energy depolarizes the ganglion cells; continuing exposure increases the rate of firing of the cell. These rhythmic impulses travel along the retinohypothalamic tract, as messengers of the presence of light, to the Suprachiasmatic Nuclei (SCN) in the hypothalamus. The SCN is the command centre of the body's reaction to day and night (Bernard et al. 2007).

Like the nuclei of plant cells, the cells of the SCN generate the equivalent of a 24-hour clock. The SCN does this through cycles of expression of genes, using the migration of molecules between the cytoplasm and the nucleus to turn on and off their transcriptions. What is important is that this is a largely autonomous DNA-regulated clock. When we physically change time zone, it continues regardless and operates as before. The flow of neural messengers of light from the retina to the SCN will ultimately 're-set' our clock, but it can take several days, hence the sensation of jet lag. There is also a direct pathway between the photosensitive ganglion cells of the retina and the pineal gland at the joining point of the thalamus. When the pineal gland receives signals of reduced light directly from the retina – usually described as 'dim-light onset' – it secretes melatonin, related to the neurotransmitter serotonin, and associated with preparation for sleep. This may explain the challenging combination of sensations of drowsiness and wakefulness – melanopsin and melatonin versus the SCN – so often experienced after journeys across time zones. It also reminds us that our chronobiology can trigger powerful responses of arousal and counterarousal, and even more complex bio-chemical emotional changes. This becomes particularly important for the chronobiology of musical rhythm.

These 24-hour cycles are the basis of 'circadian rhythms' (from the Latin *circa diem*, 'around the day') a term originally coined by Franz Halberg in his Chronobiology Laboratories at the University of Minnesota in the 1950s. Circadian rhythms in humans embrace far more than sleep–wake cycles (Ahlgren and Halberg 1990). They include cycles of change in body temperature through the day and night, and cycles of hormonal change (for example in plasma cortisol, the glucocorticoid steroid hormone associated with stress and readiness for action). These bodily circadian rhythms are important for pharmacology: for establishing the most effective means, and the optimal time of day, to intervene in the body's biochemistry. Indian classical musicians would argue that specific times of day and night are important for responses to music too.

The lives of human beings fall into many different cycles: the cycles of birth and death, various cycles of cellular renewal (red blood cells live for about four months, for example, while white cells live for over a year), of the seasons (where body weight may change to prepare for different temperatures and conditions of life), menstrual cycles, the 24-hour circadian rhythms we have described, and then shorter cycles, like gamma-wave parasympathetic and EEG fluctuations, beta-wave thermoregulatory Mayer waves, breathing, the heart, basic movements like walking, tongue articulations, eye saccades and the neurological clocks that support them (Osborne 2009a).

The chronobiology of musical rhythm: Minds and bodies

There is a particularly important window in our human chronobiology. I call it the 'window of rhythm' (Osborne 2009a). Only within this window lies our ability to perceive regular patterned pulses, to associate beats and to perform them meaningfully as musical rhythm. It is within this window that we are able to connect with one another without words, to potentiate movement for health, and to co-regulate each other via entrainment through rhythmical experience.

In what follows, we shall explore the many ways this window enables therapeutic connection.

There is no perceived *rhythm* outside the window. There is, of course, audible sound – which is characterized not by individually perceivable pulses, but instead by pitch. Pitch is a measure of the periodic vibrations (cycles) in sound energy, recorded in hertz (Hz) – the number of cycles per second. Our human audible range is 20Hz (the lowest audible pitch) to 20,000Hz (the highest, brilliant and nebulous sounds). Interestingly, the window of rhythm opens, at its upper threshold, at roughly the point where pitched notes become inaudible to us – at 20Hz. It is here, at 20Hz and slower, that vibrations become perceivable to humans as regular patterned pulses. Below 20Hz we can feel our own physical motion as rhythmical, sense patterns within our body's regulatory functions, and feel the rhythm of another's touch. Within mechanical sound energy, although we can no longer hear pitched notes below 20Hz, we can sometimes 'feel' pressure waves at high amplitudes, and hear low frequency resultant tones or 'beats' in the space between notes heard close together. It is only in the window of rhythm that we have the possibility of taking these low-frequency felt pulses and making them audible to each other through 'enacting' (or playing) them as musical rhythm (Osborne 2009a). The boundary marking the frequency of the lowest imaginable note also marks the fastest perceivable and playable rhythm. An expert Hindustani tabla player, for example, can play coordinated pulses up to around 18Hz, in other words 18 finger movements or 'beats' per second. A skilled Western violinist can play a fast, measured tremolo at the tip of the bow up to around same speed, but no faster. The performance closest to the upper threshold of the window of rhythm recorded to date is by Ukrainian pianist Lubomyr Melnyk, who can play up to 19.5 notes per second.

Further into the window of rhythm, and therefore at slower rhythmic frequencies, we enter more familiar territories of music. The fastest typical classical tempi, for example Presto or Prestissimo, are in the area of three to four cycles per second, with subdivisions, or individual notes, around eight and possibly as high as 12 cycles per second. At 12Hz, this is in fact near to the limits of what is straightforward and comfortable, as opposed to literally possible, to play. The slowest, lowest frequency classical tempi, for example Grave or Larghissimo, may be as slow as 0.5 cycles per second, in other words, a beat every two seconds. It is difficult to establish precisely where the window of rhythm closes at its lower frequency, or slowest beat, threshold. It is theoretically at the point where the tempo is so slow that human beings can no longer associate one beat with another. It is at this point that the mind and body can no longer 'lock on' – either actively through playing, or passively through listening – to the rhythm as a pulse (see discussion of the brain stem, auditory and motor cortices below). The current consensus in music psychology and cognitive neuroscience is that the ability to associate beats or perform them meaningfully as a pulse stops at around six seconds or 0.16Hz. For our purposes then, the 'window of rhythm' opens at 20Hz and closes at 0.16Hz (Osborne 2009a).

All common voluntary and involuntary human movement falls within the window of rhythm: eye saccades and tongue articulations (10–20Hz); physiological tremor (8–12Hz); speech, hand and finger gesture (up to 10Hz); Parkinsonian resting tremor (3–5Hz), heartbeat, walking and sexual intercourse (1–3Hz); body sway (0.5–1Hz); normal breathing (0.16–3Hz) and of course the whole of human musical rhythm of all cultures (0.16–18Hz). The principal frequencies relating to 'regulated' consciousness and thought also occupy the window. Taking examples from within the range of entrained firing of neurons, we observe: alpha rhythms (8–12 Hz) associated with calm wakefulness; frontal and sensory-motor beta rhythms (12–20 Hz) linked to high activation or intent concentration; and the delta and theta rhythms of drowsiness or sleep (4–7Hz and 4Hz respectively) (Osborne 2009a). Beta 3 waves (18–40Hz) fall outside the window of rhythm but interestingly, these are associated with stress, paranoia, high arousal and dysregulation. I argue that what occurs in the window of rhythm is as significant for human chronobiology (and as transformative of our bodies) as circadian cycles are for our autonomic and endocrine systems, and diurnal cycles are for Linnaeus' flowers.

The window of rhythm defines the only section of our human chronobiology where the cycles and pulses that regulate the body fall within the possibility of being 'enacted' or 'embodied'. This enactment or embodiment may of course take many forms. In the act of walking for instance, we embody the chronobiology of motor neural programmes for human movement. We enact similar chronobiologies when we wield an axe or hammer a nail. But these activities operate within limited segments of the window of rhythm – in this case, as we have noted above, between approximately 1 and 3Hz. The performance of musical rhythm is the only activity where human beings explore the whole of the window of rhythm, from the fastest finger movements of the tabla player to the slowest cello Adagio. In this sense, musical rhythm may be seen as an embodiment or externalization of the rhythms of human chronobiology. Musicians can literally 'play', and therefore embody or re-embody (in the case of chronobiologies of human movement) the pulses and rhythms of all natural human physical and mental activity – from tongue movements to tremor, from blinking to brainwaves. It is interesting, however, and perhaps encouraging to musicians, that they cannot 'enact' the brainwave frequencies of stress and paranoia (18–40Hz).

In registers beyond the window of rhythm, rhythms remain silent and hidden. For example, we cannot see, hear or 'play' circadian rhythms or the cycle of the seasons, but we can play the rhythms of the heart, walking, talking or making love. The window of rhythm is the only register where our chronobiology may be shared, moment by moment, with others. It is the only circumstance where one person may entrain the chronobiology of another. Only in very rare and special circumstances may we share aspects of our circadian cycles with another person, and occasionally women living in close proximity may unconsciously entrain one another's menstrual cycles. But we may all walk or dance to the rhythm of a drum spontaneously, consciously or unconsciously, with ease. Furthermore, the rhythm of the drum may support, regulate and potentiate us in our bodily movement – the almost irresistible force of one chronobiology, in this case the chronobiology of the drummer, entraining another. This potential for sharing and regulating chronobiology is of course a key part of the usefulness of musical rhythm in educational and therapeutic work.

The experience of rhythm, communicated initially and primarily through the ear, provokes powerful responses in the mind and body. Rhythmic events (i.e. cyclic sound events below 20Hz made audible by musicians enacting them) are detected as 'surges'. Such surges are initially detected by the auditory brain stem. The Inferior Colliculus (IC) appears to be an important collecting point for such information in the ascending sensory pathway for sound (Jorris, Schreiner and Rees 2004). The IC generates powerful neuronal responses to significant changes in sound intensity, regulated by the neurotransmitter GABA A (Sivaramakrishnan et al. 2013). There is clear evidence of pathways ascending from the IC to emotional systems, as well as a descending, emotional 'feedback' pathway from the amygdala (a key centre for processing prime emotions) linked directly to the autonomic nervous system and endocrine systems such as cortisol release. In other words, the manner of articulation of a single pulse may already evoke an 'emotional' response in the brain with immediate feedback to primitive neural systems. Our musical chronobiology is linked to autonomic arousal and emotion from the first moment of the first beat we play or hear.

The sensing of sequences of pulses as 'rhythms' appears to depend on cortical as well as brainstem processing. There is evidence that the right anterior secondary auditory cortex has a specific role in the retention of rhythmic patterns (Penhune, Zatorre and Feindel 1999; Peretz 1993). In the transformation of combined cortical and subcortical activity into rhythmic movement, however, a complex loop is involved which recruits many levels of the brain. This loop involves the premotor cortex, and the basal ganglia and cerebellum, which respectively 'smooth' voluntary movement and fine-tune motor activity (Osborne 2009a). Mirror neurons – the neural systems through which we experience the sensations we observe in other people in our own bodies – appear to play a role in sensing rhythm; they may well enable the listener to absorb rhythmic cues and states of mind and body from live music performers or from a recording

(Ferrari *et al.* 2003; Rizzolati, Fogassi and Gallese 2001). It is important to note that musical rhythm may also entrain autonomically controlled periodic movement inside the visceral mechanisms of the body, such as heartbeat and breathing (Bernardi. Porta and Sleight 2006). And it may trigger neurotransmitter activity including dopamine release (connected to motivation and reward) (Salimpoor *et al.* 2011), and further endocrine release including epinephrine (at fast, arousing tempi), and oxytocin (at more relaxing frequencies) (Grape *et al.* 2003). There is also evidence for brainwave entrainment in both humans and rats, in particular in association with the regulation of frequencies related to epileptic seizures (Lin and Yang 2015). So musical rhythm not only entrains physical movement in the window of rhythm, but also autonomic, endocrine, neurotransmitter and brainwave activity.

The phenomena described above make rhythm-based educational and therapeutic processes particularly life enhancing – they are the 'window of rhythm' in therapeutic action. Musical rhythm may entrain, extend and potentiate human movement. It may increase the range of movement of people with cerebral palsy (Kim *et al.* 2011) and other physical challenges (for example, in recovery from orthopaedic surgery, Hsu *et al.* 2016). It may help people in certain phases of Parkinson's Disease to walk (probably a combination of cueing, potentiating and dopamine release). It may enliven or relax, stimulate or motivate, and in general help everyone to think, talk, move, work, synchronize and relate to one another in time and emotion. It is therefore particularly effective in work with children who have been traumatized by war (Osborne 2009b; Osborne 2012).

Chronobiology, love and war

The SAWA school in Bar Elias is a small paradise. Bar Elias is a town in the east of the Beqaa Valley in Lebanon, just a few kilometres from the Syrian border. The school is an informal school for Syrian refugee children from among the half million people living in tents (made of fragile wood, flimsy tarpaulin and cardboard) scattered throughout the valley amongst piles of garbage and plastic refuse. Some refugees have been there since the beginning of the war. It is extraordinary how they have maintained their dignity and civility, and taken care of their mental and personal hygiene.

I have worked with SAWA for Development and Aid, a Lebanese–Syrian NGO, since Spring 2015. SAWA means 'together' in Arabic. At the invitation of its founder, Rouba Mhaissen, I worked with visionary philosopher Driss Ben Brahim to set up a programme of creative workshops for children, led by music, and designed to offer therapeutic activities as well as educational support in arts, science, technology and sports. I recruited and trained a number of animateurs from among Syrian refugees in Lebanon, including: Abeer, a former air hostess from Homs, highly emotionally intelligent and with a passion for creative arts; Ghiath (pronounced Riyaz), a wonderful freelance musician from Aleppo with a Samurai pony tail; Omar, a tall and genial former sports professional; Amar, a sensitive visual artist and writer; Mahmoud, a singer, Jack-of-all-trades and inspiration in everything; Maxim, a brilliant Sufi oud player and singer; and Sali, a gentle-spirited Lebanese girl from Bar Elias, gifted photographer and media technologist. In the first phase of the project I also had three excellent animateurs from Ma'lula in Syria whose native tongue was Aramaic – the language of Christ. The school day is split into two halves. In the morning there is the Syrian curriculum, taught by professionally qualified teachers recruited from among the refugees, and in the afternoon, the workshop programme led by the animateurs.

In the atrium of the school, Abeer has planted a garden of flowers. They not only count the hours, but also measure the seasons. There are begonias (some of which flower all year round and some just in summer), multi-coloured Mirabilis Jalapa which open at night, Jasmine (the symbol of Damascus) which flowers in the two Mediterranean springs, Orange Flowers, and Camellias named by Linnaeus after the Jesuit botanist Georg Joseph Kamel. The theme of chronobiology continues throughout the school. Abeer has named classrooms after the flowers, each with the image of its flower on its door, and we study the cell life of the plants with magnifying camera lenses in our arts-led science and technology workshops.

The atmosphere in the atrium and classrooms is a mixture of calm attention, gentle 'work noise', the sounds of singing and percussion, and bursts of enthusiastic laughter and applause. This was not the case when we began the workshops. The Diagnostic and Statistical Manual of Mental Disorders (DSM-V) identifies four symptom clusters for Post Traumatic Stress Disorder (including childhood PTSD): re-experiencing, avoidance, negative cognitions and mood, and arousal. In the early days of our project, the children were both hyperactive and sluggish (often lacking in focus and concentration) and sometimes quite destructive. The improvement has been dramatic. Individual children who were struggling in their morning studies, and even sent back to their tents by their teachers, are now top of their classes. I attribute this to our team, to the quality of their work – and to music and art. I shall attempt to explain why I think this is the case as the last part of the chapter unfolds.

Those familiar with the Arab world, and in particular with the world of the Levant, will be aware of the strong social bonds in day-to-day life among families, extended families, friends and whole communities. There is a capacity for love, in its best and most simple human sense, at all of these levels. It is something that much of our Western media, with its prejudices and phobias, fails to register or communicate. I was conscious that I needed to help create the right space for this love in our work, both in the ethos of the community and within our creative activities. It needed to be done the 'Syrian way'. But I made mistakes during the journey. I began my musical work with the children imagining that I would have the same response as I had had in other parts of the Middle East. But it was surprisingly different. In the camps of the West Bank – for example Balata, Askar and Al Ein, a mere 150 miles away – the children relished journeys through the music of the world, including African rhythms and children's songs and dances from all four continents. But the Syrian children wanted to sing Syrian songs. The difference is of course that although the Palestinian children are internally displaced, they are 'home' and eager to explore the outside world. The Syrian refugee children yearn for their culture and want to go home. So we switched focus to traditional Syrian music from all regions of Syria. Fortunately Ghiath has a comprehensive knowledge of the relevant percussion repertoire, and Maxim and Mahmoud of the songs. For good measure I invited Anas Abu Qaws, son of the distinguished Syrian singer Sabah Fakhri, to be our Syrian music advisor.

I began the training of our animateurs with simple musical exercises based on sharing pulses and inventing rhythms, as well as explorations of sound in space and of musical emotion. This helped the non-musically experienced animateurs gain skill and confidence, and it offered the children enjoyable exercises in listening, concentration, patience, motor skills, response, memory, coordination and creativity, as well as trust and the processing of emotion. We progressed through these exercises to Syrian music very quickly.

We join Ghiath and a group of 25 children, mid-afternoon some time in late October 2015. The Beqaa Valley is 1000 metres above sea level, so the air is beginning to cool now, but the sun is still strong, and dazzling light floods through the classroom window. The focus for the session will be the Baladi rhythm, which alongside Maksum is one of the simplest and most popular rhythms of Arabic classical and folk music. As such it is a useful starting point for beginners. Ghiath starts the session by revising the rhythm of Baladi. Arab musicians use syllabic mnemonics to remember rhythmic patterns and percussion articulations. The two most important syllables for Baladi are Dum and Tak. Dum is a slap using the whole hand in the middle of the drum (in this case the Darabukka) and Tak is a slap with the fingers at the edge of the skin. The children rehearse chanting vocally the rhythm (see Figure 1.2).

beats (= quavers @ mm90)	1	2	3	4	5	6	7	8
	Dum	Dum	-	Tak	Dum	-	Tak	-

FIGURE 1.2 THE RHYTHM OF BALADI

Then the children clap the rhythm together. Here, Dum is a clap, Tak is a slap on the knee. When these two exercises have been repeated many times – maintaining high motivation, full engagement and real enjoyment – Ghiath revises percussion techniques. He works hard on sound quality and resonance, teaching the children to listen carefully and take pride in decisive, clean actions and strong, vibrant colours. Then the group play the full Baladi – half of the group on instruments, the other half clapping, slapping their knees and stamping. As they play, the children sing a song they have composed in the rhythm – Suria hob hari hayat aman – 'Syria, love, the colours of life and peace' (see Figure 1.3).

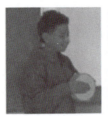 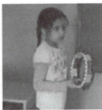 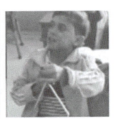

Hassan plays Dum Dum -- Dum --- on the darabukka

Marian plays --- Tak -- Tak - on the tambourine

Omar plays Dum -------- on the triangle every four cycles

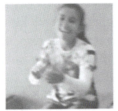 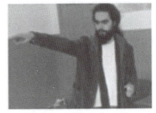

Safar claps, slaps and stamps Dum Dum - Tak Dum - Tak -

Giath cues entries

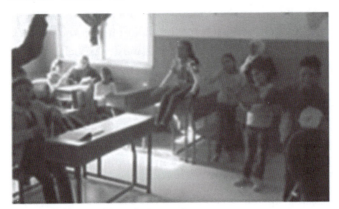

The end of the performance.

FIGURE 1.3 PLAYING BALADI AND SINGING

Note: The dashes count out silent, unplayed beat counts in the rhythm.

The Baladi chronobiogram (see Figure 1.4) offers a chronobiological perspective of what is happening.

Marian									
Tambourine	**fingers**					**Tak**		**Tak**	
Omar									
Darabukka,	**hand**	**Dum**	**Dum**			**Dum**			
Hasan									
Triangle,	**arm**	**Dum**							
Safar and group									
slap,	**fingers, knee**					**Tak**		**Tak**	
clap,	**two hands**	**Dum**	**Dum**			**Dum**			
stamp,	**leg, foot**	**Dum**							
3Hz	**fingers**	•	•	•	•	•	•	•	•
0.75 Hz	**hands**	•				•			
0.375 Hz	**feet, lets, arms**	•							

FIGURE 1.4 THE BALADI CHRONOBIOGRAM

The rhythm evolves in nested cycles: of 0.375Hz for the gestures that mark the beginning of the 'bar' or eight-beat primary cycle (these are strong actions from the centre of the body, involving legs, feet and arms); of 0.75Hz (the cycle of hand slaps); moving outwards through the body to finger slaps articulating within a 3Hz cycle. The rhythm in effect maps itself on to the body, moving from the centre to the extremities. What is significant is that the children are sharing a rhythm normally played by one person. Together, they are using multiple fingers, hands, arms and legs to enact what would normally be achieved by a single body. It is a small triumph of concentration, listening, motor control, coordination and synchronization – some of the very qualities that traumatic experiences so often deprive children of.

Musical experience is a safe way for children to re-engage with their emotions. There need be no words. The simple chronobiology of musical rhythm offers children healthy cycles of immersion in the primal neurology and biochemistry of the underlying substrates of emotion – like arousal, relaxation, stimulation, motivation. The same kind of engagement offers children an innocent, non-referential release from negativity. The 'arousal' symptom cluster (DSM-V, PTSD algorithm) often manifests itself in children as chronic hypervigilance and hyperactivity. There is no better way of dealing with hyperactivity than offering children high-activity experiences in musical rhythm – for example a fast, loud Maksum. The rhythm itself will naturally attract, absorb and regulate restlessness and hyperactivity, and then may be used to entrain the children to gentler expressions and tempi – a flow which occurs naturally in the formal structures of Arabic music.

While working with Ghiath and the children, and indeed with all of the animateurs, I am constantly reminded of the importance of 'communicative musicality' (Malloch and Trevarthen 2009) as a means not only of understanding our work as it is, but also of helping it to grow. The natural, complete and powerful way in which children relate to one another through musical rhythm suggests inherent, temporally organized motives to interact from birth, and beyond specific culture (Malloch and Trevarthen 2009; Trevarthen 1999). It seems to me that the 'musical' communication, that flows so naturally between mothers and babies, activates many of the human processes that we make use of with traumatized children. It is in some ways the 'love' I seek the space for in our creative activities. The idea of the sharing of time, pulse, movement and sympathy through an intimate communication well practised since our earliest childhood makes sense of our work. It makes even more sense when we consider the way that sounds may attract movement in mother–infant communication, and how neural systems associated with, for example, arousal and relaxation may be activated.

I think of this when I see the children leaving the afternoon music session. They are happy, relaxed, clapping the rhythms they have learnt and singing their songs. It is 4 o'clock. The buses are waiting to take the children back to the tents. In Abeer's garden the Mirabiis Jalapa plant opens its petals.

References

Ahlgren, A. and Halberg, F. (1990) *Cycles of Nature: An Introduction to Biological Rhythms.* Washington DC: National Science Teachers Association.

Bernard, S., Gonze, D., Cajavec, B., Herzel, H. and Kramer, A. (2007) 'Synchronization-induced rhythmicity of circadian oscillators in the suprachiasmatic nucleus.' *PLoS Computational Biology 3,* 4, e68. DOI: 10.1371/journal.pcbi.0030068

Bernardi, L., Porta, C. and Sleight, P. (2006) 'Cardiovascular, cerebrovascular and respiratory changes induced by different types of music in musicians and non-musicians: the importance of silence.' *Heart 92,* 4, 445–452.

Butler, W.L., Norris, K.H., Siegelman, H.W. and Hendricks, S.B. (1959) 'Detection, assay, and preliminary purification of the pigment controlling photoresponsive development of plants.' *Proceedings of the National Academy of Sciences of the United States of America 45,* 12, 1703–1708.

Ferrari, P.F., Gallese, V., Rizzolatti, G. and Fogassi, L. (2003) 'Mirror neurons responding to the observation of ingestive and communicative mouth actions in the monkey ventral premotor cortex.' *European Journal of Neuroscience 17,* 8, 1703–1714.

Grape, C., Sandgren, M., Hansson, L.O., Ericson, M. and Theorell, T. (2003) 'Does singing promote well-being? An empirical study of professional and amateur singers during a singing lesson.' *Integrative Physiological and Behavioral Science 38*, 1, 65–74.

Hsu, C.C., Chen, W.M., Chen, S.R., Tseng, Y.T. and Lin, P.C. (2016) 'Effectiveness of music listening in patients with total knee replacement during CPM rehabilitation.' *Biological Research for Nursing 18*, 1, 68–75.

Jorris, P.X., Schreiner, C.E. and Rees, A. (2004) 'Neural processing of amplitude-modulated sounds.' *Physiological Reviews 84*, 2, 541–577.

Kim, S.J., Kwak, E.E., Park, E.S., Lee, D.S., Kim, K.J., Song J.E. and Cho, S.R. (2011) 'Changes in gait patterns with rhythmic auditory stimulation in adults with cerebral palsy.' *NeuroRehabilitation 29*, 3, 233–241.

Lin, Lung-Chang and Yang, Rei-Chang (2015) 'Mozart's music in children with epilepsy.' *Translational Pediatrics 4*, 4, 323–326.

Linnaeus, C. (2005 [1751]) *Linnaeus' Philosophia Botanica*. Translated by S. Freer. Oxford: Oxford University Press.

Malloch, S. and Trevarthen, C. (2009) 'Musicality: Communicating the Vitality and Interests of Life.' In S. Malloch and C.Trevarthen (eds) *Communicative Musicality: Exploring the Basis of Human Companionship*. Oxford: Oxford University Press.

Marvell, A. (2006) 'The Garden.' In N. Smith (ed.) *The Poems of Andrew Marvell*. Abingdon, Oxon.: Routledge.

Osborne, N. (2009a) 'Towards a Chronobiology of Musical Rhythm.' In S. Malloch and C. Trevarthen (eds) *Communicative Musicality: Exploring the Basis of Human Companionship*. Oxford: Oxford University Press.

Osborne, N. (2009b) 'Music for Children in Zones of Conflict and Post-conflict: A Psychobiological Approach.' In S. Malloch and C. Trevarthen (eds) *Communicative Musicality: Exploring the Basis of Human Companionship*. Oxford: Oxford University Press.

Osborne, N. (2012) 'Neuroscience and "real world" practice: music as a therapeutic resource for children in zones of conflict.' *Annals of the New York Academy of Sciences 1252*, April, 69–76.

Penhune, V.B., Zatorre, R.J., Feindel, W.H. (1999) 'The role of auditory cortex in retention of rhythmic patterns inpatients with temporal-lobe removals including Heschl's gyrus.' *Neuropsychologia 37*, 315–333.

Peretz, I. (1993) 'Auditory atonalia for melodies.' *Cognitive Neuropsychology 10*, 21–56.

Provencio, I., Jiang, G., De Grip, W.J., Hayes, W.P. and Rollag, M.D. (1998) 'Melanopsin: an opsin in melanophores, brain, and eye.' *Proceedings of the National Academy of Sciences of the United States of America 95*, 1, 340–345.

Rizzolatti, G., Fogassi, L. and Gallese, V. (2001) 'Neurophysiological mechanisms underlying the understanding and imitation of action.' *National Review of Neuroscience 2*, 9, 661–670.

Salimpoor, V., Benovoy, M., Larcher, K., Dagher, A. and Zatorre, R.J. (2011) 'Anatomically distinct dopamine release during anticipation and experience of peak emotion to music.' *Nature Neuroscience 14*, 257–262.

Sivaramakrishnan, S., Sterbino-D'Angelo, S.J., Filipovic, B., D'Angelo, W.R., Oliver, D.L. and Kuwada, S. (2004) 'GABA (A) synapses shape neuronal responses to sound intensity in the inferior colliculus.' *Journal of Neuroscience 24*, 21, 5031–5043.

Trevarthen, C. (1999) 'Musicality and the intrinsic motive pulse: evidence from human psychobiology and infant communication.' *Musicae Scientiae* (Special Issue 1999–2000), 155–215.

2

HEALTH AND HAPPINESS GROW IN PLAY

Caring for Intimate, Musical Vitality from Birth

COLWYN TREVARTHEN

Introduction: The newborn companion

I am not a therapist, but I have long been interested in the creativity and hopefulness of communication with infants and young children. I admire and learn from the natural ways in which they enjoy life with companions they know and love. Innate gifts for playful companionship are the foundation for school learning, and also for therapy when life has betrayed childish optimism. I am glad to present an update on a detailed vision of early human communication – an exploration of the motives for life in expressive movement. A life that begins before birth.

In the past 50 years a new vision of education and childcare has emerged – a vision which attends to the innate human impulses of consciousness and memories of how it feels to be alive in body movement and to share moving. In this vision each new human being is an inherently creative communicator, reaching out to learn from the world with their intelligent body. This is a change from the theory of the young mind as a space to store facts, and from teaching practice that ignores the active body of the learner and its feelings. New evidence reveals how a child learns in affectionate and playful communication with parents before school, and before speech (Donaldson 1978; Trevarthen, Gratier and Osborne 2014). As my colleague and teacher Dr T. Berry Brazelton showed parents, a newborn is not 'helpless and ready to be shaped by his environment' (Brazelton 1979, p. 79). The baby has an imaginative human mind that knows affectionate company and enjoys adventurous learning with companions. The infant has 'primary intersubjectivity', which means a gift for meeting other minds by direct engagement of expressive movements (Trevarthen 1979).

My work on early intelligence and learning began with Jerome Bruner, a leader in child-centred educational psychology. In 1967 I began work on infant learning at Harvard University's Center for Cognitive Studies. Here, Bruner was directing research towards a study of intelligent awareness in infancy and the development of skilful use of tools, searching for the source of human cognition before words. This was a science of observation, not experiment:

> As the joint efforts within the Center have turned more toward infancy, there has occurred a gradual change toward the viewpoint of a naturalist exploring a new species, and away from an exclusive emphasis on the testing of specific hypotheses derived from a general theory of infant development. (Bruner 1968, p.ii)

In his book *The Culture of Education* (1996) Bruner described human beings as 'story-making creatures'. He distinguished two motives for telling stories – discovering meaning for oneself, and presenting oneself to others as a messenger.

> Storytelling performs the dual cultural functions of making the strange familiar and ourselves private and distinctive. If pupils are encouraged to think about the different outcomes that could have resulted from a set of circumstances, they are demonstrating useability of knowledge about a subject. Rather than just retaining knowledge and facts, they...use their imaginations to think about other outcomes... This helps them to think about facing the future, and it stimulates the teacher too. (Bruner 1996, pp.39–40)

The idea that human consciousness is for story-telling (the active creation and sharing of 'meaning') was brought to life with descriptive work showing how a child creates, and feels self-satisfaction in movement. Together, these insights invited attention to the intuitive dynamics of how an infant moves to explore and manipulate objects and how she learns how to share her interests. Bruner was redefining 'cognitive studies' as a science of playful invention in activity. Young babies are not learning with the logic of static, bodiless computers. They move with precisely controlled rhythms that feel their efficiency, exercising a predictive control of the sensations of moving in a body-related space. Most importantly, they have an innate sensitivity for the rhythms of a companion moving and how the other person responds to events and chooses actions in a shared world. That is how the comedy of human knowledge begins in play and builds friendships. And it is a means for comfort and support given to a person in distress, of any age.

Discovering how the human mind expresses its hopes, fears and need for company

At Harvard I recorded how a baby's eyes and head move in precise synchrony to look at, or track, an object of interest. In looking, a baby's measured steps or saccades made consistent rhythms which were the same as those of an adult scanning a picture. By six months the infants had efficient binocular depth perception, and they could track a slowly moving object smoothly, without saccades, which requires prediction of the object's path and its velocity. Tracings I made of infants, one or two months old, reaching out to touch or grasp objects were regulated in rhythms that were close to an adult reach-and-grasp (Trevarthen 1974). There were innate rules of vitality in human beings who were very different in size and knowledge.

This 'motor intelligence' of the baby for engaging with things in the world was astonishing. But even more remarkable were the body movements of communication with attention directed to an interested mother. These were creative, prosocial and mutually regulated. They included delicate face expressions of emotion, like a smile or a scowl, deliberate eye-to-eye contact, 'prespeech' movements of the lips and dramatic gestures of the hands (Trevarthen 1979). These movements can only have an effect if they are sensed by another human being. And, the baby could take the lead in the 'dialogue'. They were not simply imitating the expressions of their mothers.

We made films at 16 frames per second, week by week, with five infants and their mothers from two to six months of age. We compared how each infant behaved towards the mother herself, and to a suspended toy presented by her. The room was a quiet studio surrounded by heavy curtains, with subdued lighting. A camera was aimed to take a full-face view of the whole baby, and a front-surface mirror placed behind the baby gave a head and shoulders view of the mother. We filmed the mother and infant enjoying intimate chat, undisturbed.

A 'conversation' between 12-week-old Jody and his mother, in which the baby clearly led the engagement, was an eye-opener (Figure 2.1).

This leading by the baby was confirmed by further micro-analysis of the body movements of infants of the same age when they were communicating with their delighted mothers. Infants rarely imitated the mother in these 'proto-conversations'. They had their own stories to tell, and the mothers followed the plot with confirming and encouraging expressions.

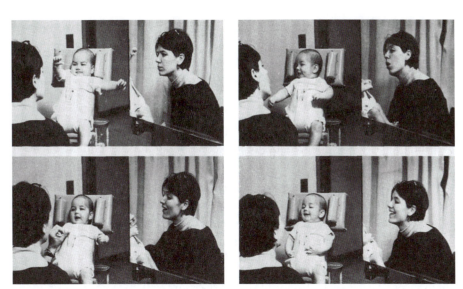

FIGURE 2.1 JODY, 12 WEEKS OLD, AND HIS ATTENTIVE MOTHER

The mother's expressions follow and reflect the infant's shifts of attention and expressive movements with a delay of about one quarter of a second. She imitates the emotional signs, calls and hand waving of the baby, behaving like an interested and appreciative 'audience' as he spoke his part. She is accepting his 'story'. (From a film made at the Harvard Center for Cognitive Studies in 1967, Trevarthen 1974)

A new psychology of infants: Celebrating their intentions to communicate

Our project at Harvard was just one, of many, in which micro-analysis of films was used to discover the energy-in-movement of the infant mind and its conscious eagerness for attentive company. Working in different fields, researchers were inspired by Charles Darwin's natural history of emotions, by the brain science of Charles Sherrington, by the neurophysiologist of movement Nicolai Bernstein, and by translations of observations made (several decades earlier in Moscow) by the cultural–historical psychologist Lev Vygotsky. The anthropologist Ray Birdwhistell studied 'body language' in different cultures. He concluded that a large proportion of the meaning in any human 'dialogue', including its references to a shared context, is actually 'non-verbal' and expressive of universal human impulses for sharing. He established a science of 'kinesics' to describe these behaviours. His term was derived from an ancient word for moving or acting with intentional reference, as in 'cite' or 'excite' (Birdwhistell 1970). In every cultural group, changing attitudes and gestures of the whole body convey information of a speaker's intentions and feelings, with and beyond what words can say. This kind of expressive communication is possible for a young baby too.

A young anthropologist and linguist Mary Catherine Bateson, working on her PhD at Massachusetts Institute of Technology (MIT) while expecting the birth of her child, reported a study of films of an infant (at 7 and 14 months old) communicating with the mother. Bateson described the behaviours she perceived as 'proto-conversation':

> The study of timing and sequencing showed that certainly the mother and probably the infant, in addition to conforming in general to a regular pattern, were acting to sustain it or to restore it when it faltered, waiting for the expected vocalization from the other and then after a pause resuming vocalization, as if to elicit a response that had not been forthcoming. These interactions were characterized by a sort of delighted, ritualized courtesy and more or less sustained attention and mutual gaze. (Bateson 1979, p.65)

Study of the prosodic patterns of mothers' speech, when interacting with their infants, confirmed a special mode of vocal expression, called 'motherese' or 'infant directed speech' (Fernald 1992). Infants are born attracted to the higher range of the female voice and its affectionate modulations, and they soon appreciate the sounds of music. They prefer harmonious chords and melodic phrases to those that are dissonant or mechanical. Papoušek and Papoušek (1981) described the mother's 'intuitive parenting' speech as showing 'musicality'. They concluded, with Bateson, that intimate sharing of musical expressions establishes trust and guides the infant to learn language. This is confirmed by the patterned timing of prelinguistic vocalizations of infants (which have the same patterns of syllables, utterances and phrasing as in adult speech in any language), and by universal measures of song and music. The psychologist of infancy and music, Maya Gratier, describes the rhythmic impulses and playful rituals with which a baby reaches out for company as 'the improvised musicality of belonging' (Gratier and Apter-Danon 2009, p.301). Gratier sees this rhythmical play as 'the shaping of the infant's utterances in willing engagement with culture' (Gratier and Trevarthen, 2007, p.169), establishing the baby as an active member of a human family. Her cross-cultural studies show that this shared musical way of life is the framework in which an infant learns the habits and language of a particular human world, and how this learning may be affected by migration of the family to a different world (Gratier 1999, 2003).

From language to emotion and back

The first studies of infant communication in the 1970s concerned the development of speech and language. But rhythms of relating are not only important for learning to talk. Their musicality also transmits feelings. *The way we move together is how we share emotions.* This idea was picked up by medical doctors and therapists as a significant tool in the ongoing attempt to improve diagnosis of emotional disorders and to find more effective therapies within mental health. They were supported in this exploration by Brazelton's therapeutic method, a method emerging from his observations and understanding of the natural intuitions of a newborn baby for sharing feelings (Brazelton 1979). Brazelton developed a method of guiding the emotional maturation of the child in intimate relations at specially sensitive stages, which he later called 'touch points' (Brazelton 1993).

William Condon collaborated with pediatrician Lou Sander at the Boston University School of Medicine in a study of infant kinesics. They showed that on the first day of life hand gestures of an infant may synchronize with the prosodic rhythm of an adult voice (Condon and Sander 1974). This 'inter-synchrony' of expressions, and its importance for language acquisition, has been confirmed by subsequent studies. From birth, the rhythm of life, and the stories of human vitality made up of serially ordered expressions in ways of moving, are shared to make life meaningful (Trevarthen and Delafield-Butt 2015; Trevarthen, Gratier and Osborne 2014).

In New York, Daniel Stern, a psychiatrist training in psychoanalysis, followed Birdwhistell's 'kinesics' and the work of Condon to focus on the natural dynamics of communication before language. Studying a film of playful communication of a mother with three-and-a-half-month-old twins, he observed that the infants were directing their mother by precisely timed movements (Stern 1971). This discovery led Stern away from psychoanalytic child psychiatry and on to path-finding studies of the need for positive, life-enriching joy, which he reported in *The Interpersonal World of the Infant* (Stern 2000 [1985]) and *The First Relationship: Infant and Mother* (Stern 2002). He built a new foundation for appreciating the therapeutic potential of non-verbal or 'implicit' communication with infants, without resorting to 'explicit' linguistic accounts (relied upon heavily in psychoanalytical models) to recollect distressing events (Stern 1993).

With colleagues at Columbia University, Stern defined constructive dynamic principles of 'affect attunement' (Stern *et al.* 1985). He later developed these in a practice of psychotherapy that sought to derive emotional benefit from intimate 'moments of meeting'. Here, these shared moments are used as invitations to deepen understanding in dialogues between therapist and patient as they explore their 'implicit knowledge' of subjective experiences, both immediate and recalled (Boston Process Change Study Group 2010; Stern *et al.* 1999).

Daniel Stern's work on communication of feelings has also contributed to the science of aesthetics and artful creations. With an interest in dance and choreography, he presented a comprehensive science of 'vitality dynamics' (Stern 2010). Stern related findings from research on the expressive movements of foetuses, infants and their mothers to the principles studied by performing artists. His encompassing concept 'Vitality' (of self-generated life in movement) enriches our understanding of the nature of well-being and learning for human beings of all ages, as well as the appreciation of graphic arts, dance and music as natural communication.

The above research on infant communication established a new appreciation of gestural and vocal meaning making in concordant company. A skilled musician, Stephen Malloch, using acoustic analysis of the sounds exchanged between mothers and young infants in proto-conversations, songs and action games, has defined this human skill precisely as the 'pulse', 'quality' and 'narrative' of 'communicative musicality' (Malloch 1999; Malloch and Trevarthen 2009).

Musicality to share vitality, story-telling and comedy

Stephen Malloch created the science of communicative musicality by studying the behaviour of a baby girl and her mother.

In 1979 I made a recording of six-week-old Laura, chatting with her mother in a recording room at the Psychology Department of Edinburgh University. They were recruited for a project on *Prespeech in Communication of Infants with Adults* based on studies done by my graduate students Lynne Murray, Ben Sylvester-Bradley and Penelope Hubley (Hubley and Trevarthen 1979; Murray and Trevarthen 1985; Sylvester-Bradley and Trevarthen 1978).

In intimate dialogue with Laura, the mother greeted her daughter's signs of attention, and encouraged her to express herself by asking questions with a clear rhythm (Trevarthen 1980). At appropriate moments Laura gestured and vocalized expressions of interest and pleasure, and her mother spoke about these as if the baby were talking to her. They were sharing a proto-conversation as described by Bateson, with the 'mutual attunement' of feelings that impressed Stern.

In 1996, Dr Murray Campbell (a physicist and expert on musical acoustics) and Professor of Music, Nigel Osborne, treated this recording to a refined micro-analysis. We considered the vocal expression in mother–infant communication as a form of song and wanted to make a thorough examination of the evidence. Stephen Malloch worked as a post-doctoral researcher on this task. Listening to Laura and her mother, he found himself responding to the sounds as music:

> It suddenly dawned on me that I was tapping my foot to human speech – not something I had ever done before, or even thought possible. I replayed the tape, and again, I could sense a distinct rhythmicity and melodious give and take to the gentle promptings of Laura's mother and the pitched vocal replies from Laura... A few weeks later...the words 'communicative

musicality' came into my mind as a way of describing what I had heard. (Malloch and Trevarthen 2009, pp.2 and 4)

To illustrate the melodic and rhythmic co-creativity of the sounds, Stephen made spectrograms and pitch plots with precise measurements of the onset and offset times of the vocalizations of both mother and baby (Trevarthen and Malloch forthcoming). He made a precise formulation of the theory of communicative musicality in three parameters, *pulse, quality* and *narrative*, as follows (please refer to Figure 2.2):

> *Pulse* is the regular succession of discrete behavioural events through time, vocal or gestural, the production and perception of these behaviours being the process through which two or more people may coordinate their communications… *Quality* refers to the modulated contours of expression moving through time. These contours can consist of psychoacoustic attributes of vocalizations – timbre, pitch, volume – or attributes of direction and intensity of the moving body… Daniel Stern *et al.* (1985) have written on this in terms of 'vitality contours'. Pulse and quality combine to form *Narratives* of expression and intention… From vocalizations centred on C4 at the start of the exchange, the mother takes her cue from Laura's upward moving vocalization by abruptly moving her pitch to C5. This sudden upwards movement is 'reprised' by the mother during the rising pitch 'swoop' of utterance number 9. From here till the end, the pitch level slowly descends back to C4, reflected in the downwards pitch movement of Laura (utterance 11). It is also suggested that the narrative structure may be thought of in a 'classical' four-part evolution of a story, through *Introduction, Development, Climax* and *Resolution.* (Malloch and Trevarthen 2009, p.4)

Figure 2.2 shows photographs illustrating the postures and gestures of Laura, and her mother's responsive face expressions. It also shows the pitch plot Stephen made of their short narrative, with a transcription of the speech and inarticulate sounds made by baby and mother.

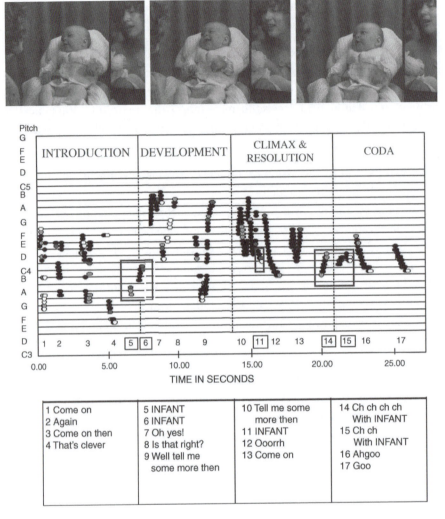

FIGURE 2.2 SIX-WEEK-OLD LAURA SHARES A
PROTO-CONVERSATION WITH HER MOTHER

Laura is in dialogue with her mother who delivers her message at first in words, and at the end in non-verbal sounds that attune with Laura's expressions. Their utterances are numbered. Above, Laura pays attention, smiles and makes a 'coo' sound, with small gestures of her hands. (Figure adapted from Malloch and Trevarthen 2009, p.5; further adapted from Malloch 1999, where a more detailed explanation and analysis will be found.)

This version (Trevarthen and Malloch forthcoming) proposes that the final 'thoughtful' sounds made by the mother and infant may best be considered as a *coda*. This word, from the Latin word *cauda* for a 'tail of an animal', refers to an 'extra' concluding passage of a piece of music, which carries recollections of previous passages and a sense of peaceful appraisal. They seem to be recollecting the pleasure of their exchange. The last sound the infant makes, number 15, has a slight downturn. She was anticipating the two sounds her mother would make to end this dialogue. As in the proto-conversation with Jody (Figure 2.1), the infant leads the way at critical 'moments of contact'.

> We clarified the meaning of 'musicality', to distinguish it from the artful productions of 'music': 'When we talk of musicality we are pointing to the innate human abilities that make music production and appreciation possible. And not only music, also dance and any other human endeavour that could be considered one of the temporal arts, such as religious ceremonies or theatre – all instances of 'the human seriousness of play' (Turner 1982). (Malloch and Trevarthen 2009, p.4)

Every conversation we share, and any creative task we undertake, will seek to have the pulse, quality and narrative of musicality felt in body movement.

A blind baby reveals an intrinsic body consciousness for sharing actions in sound

Gunilla Preisler studies deaf and blind children at Stockholm University. She recorded a video of a five-month-old baby girl, Maria, who was born totally blind, listening to her mother's singing. Maria was lying down feeding from a bottle held by her mother who sang a famous Swedish baby song 'Mors lilla Olle'. Watching the film, Maria's mother and Dr Preisler noticed that Maria, who had never seen her own or any other human hand, was 'conducting' her mother's singing. Maria was using her left hand, marking phrases, shifts of melody and closure of a verse: pointing up for a high note, gracefully circling her hand to describe a melodic line, then closing the verse with a drop of her hand, moving her hand up and down the axis of her body to represent the pitch and 'vitality dynamics' of the sounds.

Professor of Music Nigel Osborne, viewing Preisler's video, confirmed that Maria was sharing her mother's song with gestures as a trained conductor would do. Nigel noted that at certain moments Maria's hand led the mother's melody by a fraction of a second, or she synchronized her hand perfectly with a sound she heard as 'punctuation' in the story. This precise interactive timing was confirmed by graphs we made to compare the mother's voice and the movements of the tip of Maria's index finger (Trevarthen 1999). At significant moments the hand moved 300 milliseconds ahead of the mother's voice, and at other times they moved in perfect synchrony. Maria's 'performance' with her mother shows the same flexible synchrony as two skilled jazz musicians improvising the story of a duet (Schögler and Trevarthen 2007).

Trans-modal sympathy of hand gestures for the melody of speech or song is not a rare skill unique to this blind child, though she may have developed it as a habit to help her hear. In the films I have of babies from a few weeks old to one year, there are frequent cases where subtle gestures are made in spontaneous inter-synchrony with rhythms (of vocal or instrumental sounds), or with the observed movements of other people (see Figure 2.4 for examples). I have called this innate time coordinator demonstrated by newborns to adults the 'Intrinsic Motive Pulse' (Trevarthen 1999, 2016).

The imitating neonate

The two most influential authorities in psychological theory of infantile intelligence of the 20th century, Sigmund Freud and Jean Piaget, insisted that a newborn could not imitate an adult, and certainly not any movements requiring responses of their own mouth, which the newborn cannot see. Olga Maratos made a fresh examination of the issue in her PhD thesis on 'The origin and development of imitation in the first six months of life'. This was completed in 1973 and presented to Piaget at the University of Geneva. He accepted her evidence but said he could not understand it. Her findings were confirmed by Andrew Meltzoff, Giannis Kugiumutzakis and others using a wide range of expressive movements to test the infant's interest and impulse to respond (Kugiumutzakis and Trevarthen 2015).

The fact that newborns do imitate was given a richer reinterpretation by Emese Nagy, who changed her testing so that the nature of the infant's intention became clearer. Waiting with attention after the baby had made an imitation, she witnessed 'provocations' by newborns. By her 'polite' waiting she showed that the neonate's expectation was for a dialogue or game requiring exchange of signs. The newborns were not just learning a new behaviour. They deliberately repeated the imitation to receive a response from her (Nagy 2006). Thus begins the search for intimate agreement about actions to achieve a common understanding, which must be the way any cooperative awareness of a shared reality develops. Jacqueline Nadel (2014) has shown how imitation flourishes among toddlers without speech, expanding their shared experience and helping learning of language, and how it can be used to help an autistic child communicate.

Musical sounds can calm the distress of a newborn, giving rhythm to delicate life (Malloch *et al.* 2012). Newborns are sensitive to the pulse and expressive energy of human movements and can join in a simple improvised interaction or 'game' less than an hour after birth (see Figure 2.4, A).

The sympathetic foetus

Recently the knowledge we gained a few decades ago about the young infant's imagination in communicative movement has been enriched by films of foetuses inside their mother's body. Their behaviours can be recorded accurately on film with ultra-sound radiation to reveal the development of human feelings and sensitivities. In addition to an integrated self-awareness explored actively by touching their own body parts, and a sensitivity for 'other-awareness' demonstrated by more 'careful' movements directed to a twin (Piontelli 2002), the foetus shows facial expressions of emotion related to the well-being or distress of the mother, as well as to tastes of substances in the amniotic fluid, reacts to the sound of speech with movements of the mouth and clearly identifies the mother's voice (Reissland and Kisilevsky 2015). This new descriptive science proves that by 25 weeks of gestation a human being behaves as an emotional person, intimately sharing life in movement with the mother while being protected and nourished by her vitality (Reissland and Kisilevsky 2015).

A musical and playful dialogue with an affectionate father at 32 weeks gestational age

Naseera, born three months premature in a hospital Intensive Care Unit (ICU) in Holland, was recorded one month later by Saskia van Rees, a film-maker who is expert at intimate documentation of the births of infants and their neonatal care. This work was done in close collaboration with the paediatrician in charge, Richard de Leeuw, who encourages use of the 'kangaroo' method to support the life of very premature newborns (van Rees and de Leeuw, 1993). Immediately after her birth, Naseera was placed against her mother's chest in 'kangarooing' several times a day. Then her mother had to have an operation and could not continue that care. The father took over and held Naseera every day, offering his body as a vital resource for her. When Naseera was 32 weeks gestational age, the video made by van Rees recorded a spontaneous 'conversation' between a gentle and attentive father who is proud to be his daughter's companion.

Naseera and her father made a rhythmic exchange, the father closely imitating the baby's simple sounds (Figure 2.3). A spectrograph showed they alternated sounds on an *andante* pulse, composing a musical phrase together of 3.6 seconds (Malloch 1999). An important detail is that in a group of six sounds made with the timing of syllables in normal adult speech, the interval between Naseera's sound and her father's response is longer. This corresponds to what a phonetician recognizes as 'final lengthening' – the last syllable of an utterance is longer. After that the baby called her father with three short cries at four-second intervals when his attention had wandered. This period corresponds with a spoken phrase or a single breath cycle. Naseera was able not only to converse with her father making a well-formed phrase, but to wait for him to join her over a time period of three phrases.

Naseera's smile is a 'comical' response in an affectionate encounter. A kind of joke. Their interaction is accepted as a game.

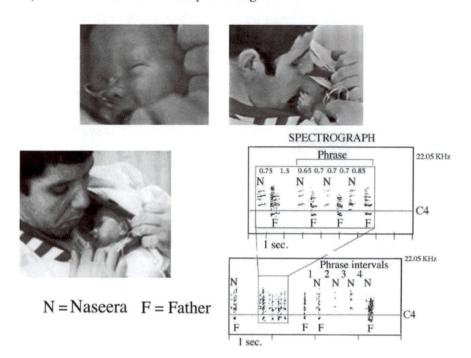

N = Naseera   F = Father

FIGURE 2.3 NASEERA

Here a two-month preterm baby communicates with her father in an ICU in Amsterdam.

Top left: With her eyes closed, Naseera smiles in response to her father's touch and speech.

Below: She participates in a well-phrased 'conversation' with him by alternating simple 'coo' sounds pitched a little above middle C (C4) (N, Naseera; F, father). The upper spectrograph, over nine seconds, shows that they alternated with a pulse of andante, c. 0.7 seconds, with the final interval being longer, 0.85 seconds. The lower 40-second graph records calls by Naseera at four-second intervals when her father was not responding. She called softly, then louder and her father spoke to her after the third call.

Top right: After their dialogue is finished Naseera makes a gesture with her free left hand, pointing her index finger and thumb as if reflecting on what they had 'discussed'.

What shall we play next? Development of companionship and meaning in the first year

All social animals play, especially when they are young and exploring how they can move. We enjoy playful actions of pets on the beach or birds flitting about or hopping in the garden. Their play is expressed in the enjoyable rhythmic way the muscles of sensuous bodies are excited. Its periodic impulse and the narrative patterns are richer in species with more complex bodies of many parts. Play for the individual actor is imaginative and hopeful, to test the unknown with the pleasures of self-directed awareness. And movements in play have evolved for communication, and are especially rich in the social behaviour of animals that act cooperatively in families and larger social groups.

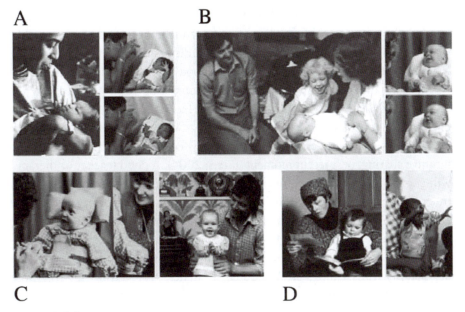

FIGURE 2.4 STAGES IN THE DEVELOPMENT OF INFANT SOCIABILITY IN THE FIRST YEAR

A. A newborn infant, in the first day, imitates tongue protrusion, and another about one hour after birth tries to imitate hand movements.

B. Laura at home at three months, chats with her mother Kay. Her three-year-old sister wants to talk with her too. Father proudly watches them.

C. Leanne at five months enjoys her mother's recitation of 'Round and Round the Garden', with actions. Emma at six months, sitting on her father's knee, is proud she knows 'Clappa-Clappa-Handies' when her mother asks her to show it. This smile of pride is important for her learning.

D. Basilie, a one-year-old in Edinburgh, Scotland, reads her book as her mother reads the telephone bill. In a home with lots of books, they both know what reading is. In the very different world of Lagos, Nigeria, Adegbenro, also one year old, sitting on his mother's lap, is proud of his rattle. After asking someone in the compound to hand it to him, he shows it to everybody.

In research to trace the development of infant play, it is clear that there are 'age-related changes' that prove we are born with an innate project of actions-with-awareness-and-feelings to be developed with companions (Stern 2000, Introduction). Changes through the first year are illustrated in Figure 2.4.

These changes encompass developments in knowledge and moral emotions, such as pride, that mark important transitions on the way to more independence in knowledge and skills (Trevarthen 1998). Children retain and build on the talents they were born with to relate with other people, sharing the rhythms and values of experience, demonstrating both aesthetic and moral feelings that guide learning (Trevarthen 2005; Trevarthen and Malloch 2002, forthcoming).

In conclusion: Playful pleasure in learning and therapy

Sharing the essence of Jerome Bruner's 'story-making', play serves to 'mak(e) the strange familiar, and ourselves private and distinctive' (Bruner, 1996, p.39). Play has a self-nurturing vitality that 'feels good', using life in movement well. At the same time, playing is attractive and nourishing for a playmate. By the mysterious feeling of sympathy – acting and feeling 'as if' being in the body of another individual – the playmate is truly 'with' the player. This is not a conscious 'mentalizing' estimation of another's emotions by 'empathy'. It is an intuitive sharing, or 'present moment' (Stern 2004). A good teacher or therapist will engage with, value and foster these moments of meeting. It is here where true creativity emerges and finds new directions. Guidance from a teacher must allow and facilitate discovery by the child who is developing talents for action with imagination (Bruner 1974). Teaching, and therapy too, require more than coercive 'instruction' or 'treatment' according to prescribed rules. They require negotiation with feelings in 'relational awareness' (Trevarthen 1998). Both depend on sharing 'the human seriousness of play' (Turner 1982).

References

Bateson, M.C. (1979) 'The Epigenesis of Conversational Interaction: A Personal Account of Research Development.' In M. Bullowa (ed.) *Before Speech: The Beginning of Human Communication.* London: Cambridge University Press.

Birdwhistell, R. (1970) *Kinesics and Context.* Philadelphia, PA: University of Pennsylvania Press.

Boston Process Change Study Group (2010) *Change in Psychotherapy: Unifying Paradigm.* New York: Norton.

Brazelton, T.B. (1979) 'Evidence of Communication during Neonatal Behavioural Assessment.' In M. Bullowa (ed.) *Before Speech: The Beginning of Human Communication.* London: Cambridge University Press.

Brazelton, T.B. (1993) *Touchpoints: Your Child's Emotional and Behavioral Development.* New York: Viking.

Bruner, J.S. (1968) *Processes of Cognitive Growth: Infancy.* (Center for Cognitive Studies, Eighth Annual Report 1967–1968). Cambridge, MA: Harvard University.

Bruner, J.S. (1974) *Toward a Theory of Instruction.* Cambridge, MA: Harvard University Press.

Bruner, J.S. (1996) *The Culture of Education.* Cambridge, MA: Harvard University Press.

Condon, W.S. and Sander, L.S. (1974) 'Neonate movement is synchronized with adult speech: interactional participation and language acquisition.' *Science 183,* 99–101.

Donaldson, M. (1978) *Children's Minds.* Glasgow: Fontana/Collins.

Fernald, A. (1992) 'Meaningful Melodies in Mothers' Speech to Infants.' In H. Papoušek, U. Jürgens and M. Papoušek (eds) *Nonverbal Vocal Communication: Comparative and Developmental Aspects.* Cambridge: Cambridge University Press.

Gratier, M. (1999) 'Expression of belonging: the effect of acculturation on the rhythm and harmony of mother–infant vocal interaction.' *Musicae Scientiae* (Special Issue 1999–2000), 93–122.

Gratier, M. (2003) 'Expressive timing and interactional synchrony between mothers and infants: cultural similarities, cultural differences, and the immigration experience.' *Cognitive Development 18*, 533–554.

Gratier, M. and Apter-Danon, G. (2009) 'The Improvised Musicality of Belonging: Repetition and Variation in Mother–Infant Vocal Interaction.' In S. Malloch and C. Trevarthen (eds) *Communicative Musicality: Exploring the Basis of Human Companionship.* Oxford: Oxford University Press.

Gratier, M. and Trevarthen, C. (2007) 'Voice, vitality, and meaning: on the shaping of the infant's utterances in willing engagement with culture.' *International Journal for Dialogical Science 2*, 169–81.

Hubley, P. and Trevarthen C. (1979) 'Sharing a Task in Infancy.' In I. Uzgiris (ed.) *Social Interaction During Infancy: New Directions for Child Development* (Vol. 4). San Francisco, CA: Jossey-Bass.

Kugiumutzakis, G. and Trevarthen, C. (2015) 'Neonatal Imitation.' In: J.D. Wright (editor-in-chief) *International Encyclopedia of the Social & Behavioral Sciences* (2nd edition, Vol. 16). Oxford: Elsevier.

Malloch, S. (1999) 'Mother and Infants and Communicative Musicality.' In I. Deliège (ed.) *Rhythms, Musical Narrative, and the Origins of Human Communication. Musicae Scientiae,* Special Issue, 1999–2000, 29–57. Liège, Belgium: European Society for the Cognitive Sciences of Music.

Malloch, S. and Trevarthen, C. (eds) (2009) *Communicative Musicality: Exploring the Basis of Human Companionship.* Oxford: Oxford University Press.

Malloch, S., Shoemark, H., Črnčec, R., Newnham, C., Paul, C., Prior, M., *et al.* (2012) 'Music therapy with hospitalized infants – the art and science of communicative musicality.' *Infant Mental Health Journal 33*, 4, 386–399. DOI: 10.1002/imhj.21346

Murray, L. and Trevarthen, C. (1985) 'Emotional Regulation of Interactions between Two-month-olds and Their Mothers.' In T.M. Field and N.A. Fox (eds) *Social Perception in Infants.* Norwood, NJ: Ablex.

Nadel, J. (2014) *How Imitation Boosts Development in Infancy and Autism Spectrum Disorder.* Oxford: Oxford University Press.

Nagy, E. (2006) 'From imitation to conversation: the first dialogues with human neonates.' *Infant and Child Development 15*, 223–232.

Papoušek, M. and Papoušek, H. (1981) 'Musical Elements in the Infant's Vocalization: Their Significance for Communication, Cognition, and Creativity.' In L.P. Lipsitt and C.K. Rovee-Collier (eds) *Advances in Infancy Research* (Vol. 1). Norwood, NJ: Ablex.

Piontelli, A. (2002) *Twins: From Fetus to Child.* London: Routledge.

Reissland, N. and Kisilevsky, B. (eds) (2015) *Fetal Development: Research on Brain and Behavior, Environmental Influences, and Emerging Technologies.* London: Springer Verlag.

Schögler, B. and Trevarthen, C. (2007) 'To Sing and Dance Together.' In S. Bråten (ed.) *On Being Moved: From Mirror Neurons to Empathy.* Amsterdam/Philadelphia: John Benjamins.

Stern, D.N. (1971) 'A micro-analysis of mother–infant interaction: behaviors regulating social contact between a mother and her three-and-a-half-month-old twins.' *Journal of the American Academy of Child and Adolescent Psychiatry 10*, 501–517.

Stern, D.N. (1993) 'The Role of Feelings for an Interpersonal Self.' In U. Neisser (ed.) *The Perceived Self: Ecological and Interpersonal Sources of Self-Knowledge.* New York: Cambridge University Press.

Stern, D.N. (2000 [1985]) *The Interpersonal World of the Infant: A View from Psychoanalysis and Development Psychology* (2nd edition). New York: Basic Books.

Stern, D.N. (2002 [1977]) *The First Relationship: Infant and Mother.* Cambridge, MA: Harvard University Press.

Stern, D.N. (2004) *The Present Moment: In Psychotherapy and Everyday Life.* New York: Norton.

Stern, D.N. (2010) *Forms of Vitality: Exploring Dynamic Experience in Psychology, the Arts, Psychotherapy and Development.* Oxford: Oxford University Press.

Stern, D.N., Bruschweiler-Stern, N., Harrison, A.M., Lyons-Ruth, K., Morgan, A.C., Nahum, J. P., *et al.* (1999) 'The process of therapeutic change involving implicit knowledge: some implications of developmental observations for adult psychotherapy.' *Infant Mental Health Journal 19*, 3, 300–308.

Stern, D.N., Hofer, L., Haft, W. and Dore, J. (1985) 'Affect Attunement: The Sharing of Feeling States between Mother and Infant by Means of Inter-modal Fluency.' In T.M. Field and N.A. Fox (eds) *Social Perception in Infants.* Norwood, N.J.: Ablex.

Sylvester-Bradley, B. and Trevarthen, C. (1978) '"Baby Talk" as an Adaptation to the Infant's Communication.' In N. Waterson and K. Snow (eds) *The Development of Communication.* London: Wiley.

Trevarthen, C. (1974) 'Conversations with a two-month-old.' *New Scientist,* 2 May, 230–235.

Trevarthen, C. (1979) 'Communication and Cooperation in Early Infancy. A Description of Primary Intersubjectivity.' In M. Bullowa (ed.) *Before Speech: The Beginning of Human Communication.* London: Cambridge University Press.

Trevarthen, C. (1980) 'The Foundations of Intersubjectivity: Development of Interpersonal and Cooperative Understanding of Infants.' In D. Olson (ed.) *The Social Foundations of Language and Thought: Essays in Honor of J.S. Bruner.* New York: W.W. Norton.

Trevarthen, C. (1998) 'The Child's Need to Learn a Culture.' In M. Woodhead, D. Faulkner and K. Littleton (eds) *Cultural Worlds of Early Childhood.* New York: Routledge.

Trevarthen, C. (1999) 'Musicality and the intrinsic motive pulse: evidence from human psychobiology and infant communication.' *Musicae Scientiae* (Special Issue 1999–2000), 155–215.

Trevarthen, C. (2005) 'Stepping away from the Mirror: Pride and Shame in Adventures of Companionship. Reflections on the Nature and Emotional Needs of Infant Intersubjectivity.' In C.S. Carter, L. Ahnert, K.E. Grossman, S.B. Hrdy, M.E. Lamb, S.W. Porges and N. Sachser (eds) *Attachment and Bonding: A New Synthesis.* Dahlem Workshop Report 92. Cambridge, MA: The MIT Press.

Trevarthen, C. (2016) 'From the Intrinsic Motive Pulse of Infant Actions, to the Life Time of Cultural Meanings.' In B. Mölder, V. Arstila and P. Øhrstrom (eds) *Philosophy and Psychology of Time.* Dordrecht: Springer International.

Trevarthen, C. and Delafield-Butt, J. (2015) 'The Infant's Creative Vitality, in Projects of Self-discovery and Shared Meaning: How They Anticipate School, and Make it Fruitful.' In S. Robson and S.F. Quinn (eds) *The Routledge International Handbook of Young Children's Thinking and Understanding.* Abingdon: Routledge.

Trevarthen, C. and Malloch, S. (2000) 'The dance of wellbeing: defining the musical therapeutic effect.' *The Nordic Journal of Music Therapy 9*, 2, 3–17.

Trevarthen, C. and Malloch, S. (2002) 'Musicality and music before three: human vitality and invention shared with pride.' *Zero to Three 23*, 1, 10–18.

Trevarthen, C. and Malloch, S. (forthcoming) 'Grace in Moving and Joy in Sharing: The Intrinsic Beauty of Communicative Musicality from Birth.' In S. Bunn (ed.) *Anthropology and Beauty: From Aesthetics to Creativity.* Abingdon: Routledge.

Trevarthen, C., Gratier, M. and Osborne, N. (2014) 'The human nature of culture and education.' *Wiley Interdisciplinary Reviews: Cognitive Science 5*, 173–192. DOI:10.1002/wcs.1276

Turner, V.W. (1982) *From Ritual to Theatre: The Human Seriousness of Play.* New York: Performing Arts Journal Publications.

van Rees, S. and de Leeuw, R. (1993) *Born Too Early: The Kangaroo Method with Premature Babies.* Video by Stichting Lichaamstaal, Scheyvenhofweg 12, 6093 PR, Heythuysen, The Netherlands.

PART 2

RHYTHMS OF RELATING IN CHILDREN'S THERAPIES

3

'I'M RIGHT HERE, LITTLE ONE'

A New Mother's Reflections on Dance Movement Psychotherapy

CAROLYN FRESQUEZ

It is blue in the early morning light, the sun still east of the mountains. I am awake, though I would rather not be. Everyone else is audibly sleeping, my sweetheart, my little baby, and the cat, breathing in their own times, a trio of gentle snores. I feel the blanket's warmth, protecting against the bedroom's cool air. My thoughts are shifting like clouds above me, taking one shape and then another as they float by. When I look at my daughter Fiona, asleep in her crib, I am filled with wonder.

I have never known someone so deeply, been so remarkably connected in the most bodily way. I feel like I know her in my cells, in my blood and in my bones. I sense a pulsing energy in my arms and the space in front of me when I am not holding her, a sense that wanes as she grows and becomes more mobile. My internal clock has reset to match her two-hourly cycle of eating, diapering, sleeping, and playing. I believe I know her preferences and inclinations, her temperament and humor, even as her ways of being fluctuate with development. But there is so much I do not know. I think that she is not an entity to be entirely known, that none of us are.

When I was pregnant, I didn't want to have anticipations, expectations, or preconceived ideas about who my baby might be. (Incidentally, we did not yet know she was a she.) But I yearned for the context to shape my thoughts and memories. I couldn't wait to meet this tumbling, kicking, seemingly curious being.

I felt occasional little flutters really early on in my pregnancy, but I had nothing to compare them to, and I didn't know if it was you. Then the movement was stronger and seemed to happen all the time. You liked laughing, music, singing, and dancing. You moved for the sake of moving. I could see you wiggling around, and it seemed like you were doing somersaults in there. Often when I had someone put their hand on my belly, you would stop, knowing something had changed. We shared a private communion. I joked that you were my imaginary friend.

When she arrived I felt a calm excitement, happy in the gratitude of a safe and healthy birth. I was immensely relieved the labor was over. I held her for the first time, my husband and I creating in that moment her immediate world. Things were moving fast around us, but my sense of time transformed. Perhaps it felt slower, maybe expansive, encompassing this gentle meeting full of curiosity and care. I was wide eyed, watchful, looking to see every little thing: the flow of expressions across her face, her dark eyes, her hungry rooting, her strong legs! She was so tiny, and paradoxically so big. I sensed the expanse of the unknown and understood her as unfolding, becoming, constantly changing. I realized that I would never meet her as complete, but rather each time afresh in every interaction.

Like all living systems, humans are autopoietic, or continuously self-creating (Maturana 1978): while undergoing constant change as a result of the environmental interaction necessary to sustain life, every living system maintains and realizes the organization of its composite parts and boundaries. Autopoietic systems are closed systems, bounded and distinct entities whose structural dynamics create and maintain those boundaries and distinctions. An autopoietic system is also, necessarily, in dynamic relationship with its environment, which includes other organisms. Environmental interaction triggers living systems to adapt in ways that perpetuate self-creation. A powerful example of the protection autopoiesis affords is the human immune system. It is the dynamics of autopoiesis, and not some inherent mechanism of detection, which drives the immune response; external influences such as bacteria or parasites simply do not fit within functional organization and are destroyed, adapted to, or expelled, all through continuous self-creation. Through structural coupling with aspects of its environment, an autopoietic system provokes and responds to stimuli, thus initiating, learning, and cognizing even at the most basic level.

This process is repetitive. Let's consider a single cell. It has a boundary and organelles inside that serve different functions – converting fuel to energy, controlling movement in and out of the cell, protecting the cell, reproducing the cell, etc. The process of creating and maintaining repeats in a circular manner. As the cell interacts with others around it, we are able to observe a new system, for example a nervous system, with all of the nerve cells and neurotransmitters working dynamically to create and maintain the system. The interactive process displaces the repetitive process, and a new level or domain of repetitive process is created. This is recursion (Maturana, Mpodozis and Letelier 1995), and it also repeats, creating new phenomenal domains that extend outwards from the metabolic, to the behavioral, to the psychological, to the relational. Recursion explains how autopoiesis can be used to understand dynamic systems at different levels of human life. For example, in the cellular domain, autopoiesis begins with fertilization and the first cell divisions, then in cell specialization during development, and in cell reproduction throughout life (Sherrington 1955). In the psycho-motoric domain, autopoiesis occurs as the embodied mind imaginatively anticipates the consequences of interacting in the world and creates the organized potential to carry out a dynamic interaction (Llinás 2001; Trevarthen 2012; Varela, Thompson and Rosch 1991). The concept of autopoiesis is also applicable in understanding the domains of the psychological self and social dynamics, as a process *and* a metaphor central to the development of individual and collective life narratives. Autopoiesis is a central driving force within human development, movement, empathy, play, and learning (Trevarthen *et al.* 2006).

Let us look at a process that impacts the development of the human immune system: breastfeeding. This process encompasses a reciprocal, dynamic, structural coupling that supports autopoiesis across different domains. This is to say, breastfeeding impacts both mother and baby, biologically and socially, in ways that contribute to continual, adaptive, self-creation. It is outwith the scope of this chapter to provide a detailed discussion on the astonishing attributes of breastmilk, but the 'messages' it carries between mother and baby are remarkable (Garbes 2015) and underscore the multi-leveled complexity of interaction.

I liked thinking about autopoiesis when I was pregnant. It helped me understand the experience and shape my intentions as a parent. Through our mysterious interaction, my baby was undertaking the impressive act of creating herself, along with developing a sense of that self, and both were happening in no small part through movement (Piontelli 2010). How astonishing! How exciting! Here she was, kicking the inside of my ribs, and in so doing she was beginning to understand that she was a being with autonomy and agency, separate from other beings and things (Sheets-Johnstone 2010; Trevarthen and Fresquez 2015). My baby was growing connections between those powerful, expressive legs and the rest of her body and mind. Before she was born, while I was still imagining what it might be like, I thought a lot about how I would nurture my baby and love and support and help regulate and guide her and a million other things. I thought about how I wanted to do all this in service of her self-actualization (Maslow 1999). For this to happen, I feel I have to be deeply committed to truly seeing Fiona and myself, seeing our dynamic dance and the profound ways we impact one another.

The concept of autopoiesis also helps frame my understanding of the potential within different forms of social interaction. I see autopoiesis as recognizing the agency people have, not just as responsible parties, but as imaginative, artistic creators. It describes continual dynamic interaction with the total environment as a generative force in self-creation. For me, autopoiesis infuses interactions with the potential – through imaginative, adaptive movement – to influence organic structure, ways of being, life stories, and relationships.

Autopoiesis is similar, but adds an extra dimension, to concepts within therapeutic approaches. The social constructionist standpoint posits that the therapeutic relationship is defined by the mutual search for understanding (Anderson and Goolishian 1992). This jives with infancy research that examines our intrinsic motivation to use expressive movement for sharing in the discovery of meaning with good companions (Trevarthen 2012). Indeed there is ample evidence for an innate intersubjectivity (Trevarthen 1979): that we are born ready to engage actively in social interactions, dynamically communicating attention, intention, thoughts, and feelings. The processes for understanding someone else's experience, as well as communicating our own, are expressed in our biology through an integrated nervous system and the complex regulation of movement (Berrol 2006; Chodrow 2009; Fischman 2009; Homann 2010; Porges 1993; Trevarthen and Fresquez 2015). This foundation is present before we are born, and develops in infancy and early childhood from reciprocal imitation, to protoconversation, to play, all in an effort to learn and share companionship, meaning, and knowledge. I believe when people come together all parties will be impacted, and there is potential for meaning-making in the dynamic exchange. From this perspective, in therapy, each unfolding moment requires the therapist's responsivity to the client (Sheila McNamee in Guanaes and Rasera 2006). We are able to sense what someone else is experiencing, and we respond.

Michael walked into the room with the others, but this was his first time. He was suspicious. His arms were crossed, and he was letting everyone know he thought this dance thing was stupid, that he didn't want to be there. Underneath his words, however, his eyes surveyed with curiosity, and a tilt to his head betrayed just a little excitement. He had a quickness to him, a bouncy energy, and he couldn't maintain his tough demeanor. It was porous.

I was kneeling as the boys formed the usual circle. I often kneeled to begin, not wanting to come across as authoritarian, opening the space for them to fill. I got the sense that Michael needed to enter on his own terms, that the more explanation I included in an introduction, the more he would feel compelled to stand against it. I thought it would be helpful for him to see the group begin.

'Hi Michael, it's nice to meet you.'

'Whatever.' He looked away.

When the music started, Michael smiled and sang along, following the other boys in a warm-up.

There is a rhythm to meeting someone, whether it is for the first time or every time you meet them. The tempo is laid down, listened to, collaborated on, shaped. When I meet a child I try to let them know that I am safe, that I respect them. I want to meet them in a way that allows them to be and to become. I want to give someone space for themselves, show them I'm responsive.

Responsivity, for me, is based on perceiving and moving from a very central place within myself, as though I am looking from the backs of my eyes, responding with my whole nervous system. I use 'kinesthetic empathy' (Fischman 2009): perceiving, experiencing, and responding to emotionally contoured expressions on a bodily level. It includes information and action, which manifest as a phenomenal understanding of someone else's experience in relation to one's own.

I let the child's movements guide me. Are they shy, keeping to the edge of the room or behind their mother's leg? Are they ricocheting around the room, changing topic with rapid fire? Do they face you straight on and boldly explore the space? What is the rhythm they bring? I play with 'mirroring': reflecting someone's non-verbal communications, including their actions and the meaning carried within (Levy 1992). I get on their level. I might match their shape or the angle of their body, maybe echo a gesture, or have someone teach me a movement they create, refining the nuances until they are satisfied I am repeating it faithfully.

I play with 'attuning': 'matching and sharing dynamic forms of vitality, but across different modalities' (Stern 2010, p.42). I might make a sound, 'Schoooopppp!' – the contours of which match the motion of a swinging arm, or, after someone sighs in exasperation, I might fall to the floor and spread out, taking the same amount of time and following the downward emphasis present in their breath.

I also use 'resonating': allowing my body 'to be moved by the experience of others' (Fischman 2009, p.43). I understand this to include a more physiological process, what I sense in my own body while being with another. The resonance of someone's experience is present in changes to my heartbeat or breathing, in fluctuations in my temperature, and in traces of tension or relaxation. The whole time I am also paying attention to how I feel – an essential aspect of multi-sensory information gathering about self, other, and relationship (Tortora 2009). Kinesthetic empathy, mirroring, attuning, and resonating are some of many therapeutic principles that are extensions of the natural dynamics of healthy early interaction and companionship.

We were working on a dance. The boys wanted to incorporate a drill from football practice. This was incredibly important. Football was one of the few instances they felt included, skilled, and valued. It held positive aspects they were trying to integrate into the formation of new identities.

'How does it go?' I asked. 'Like this?'

'You've got to get your knees up higher.' Daniel always had some helpful criticism.

'Okay, like this?'

'Yeah, that's better.'

'I feel like I'm missing something.' I was trying to get him to pay attention to the intention behind the movement. 'What's my face supposed to be doing?'

'It's beast mode, Miss!' We roared with laughter!

We all tried the movement together, mirroring the action and the intention. Sam added arm movements that reflected what our feet were doing and he exaggerated the vocalization of his breath in rhythm.

We incorporated these elements, everyone adding their own flair, matching and attuning, as we practiced this way of being, associated with power and competency. I felt energized and sensed the flow of play within the group.

In order to be responsive, I place great importance on meeting someone newly in each and every encounter. I do this for a couple of reasons. One has to do with creating space for the other's autopoiesis, allowing changes to be a part of our shared reality during sessions so that they can try them out and integrate them. The other has to do with curiosity. Obviously, the way you meet someone changes over time as you get to know them. But we can fall into the trap of assumption that sometimes comes with familiarity. It is important to maintain curiosity at every step. This attitude can be difficult to hold onto.

When I was a dance movement psychotherapy student, during an experiential group I was drawn to the movement in my right foot. I recognized the habit and immediately assumed it was telling me the story it had told me in the past. So I began to react to that, getting upset over what I thought I knew. Though I was wrapped up in my own quiet experiencing, the facilitator must have noticed, because she said something to the effect of 'our movement might not be what it was before', it might be telling us something new this time. I don't remember the words exactly, but I do remember surprise at how easily I had slipped out of a curious state of mind, and relief at being able to drop the narrative and look anew. This lesson has stayed with me.

What a practice, to see with new, curious eyes, something you have seen before! I practice finding and maintaining a state of curiosity through

Feldenkrais, improvisational theatre, Authentic Movement, dance, and play, but nowhere is it more available than in my daughter's constant manifestation of curiosity and exploration. She can explore the same four-page fabric book for hours a day, days on end: each crinkly whale flipper and kelp, each shiny fish, the finger puppet aquanaut. The textures, shapes, sounds – they always offer something exciting for her. Her whole environment is ripe with excitement, all the people and things fascinating, intriguing and, apparently, delicious!

A SONG FOR BABY FRESQUEZ

There's a baby here

There's a baby coming this year

I've waited for you for so long

I've waited for you to come along

We're excited to welcome you

We can't wait to show you how much we love you

We're ready to play, we're ready to sing, we're ready to dance and dream

We're excited to learn new things

Baby, sweet Baby

The first weeks of motherhood were swathed in a fog of exhaustion and postpartum discomforts. I was surprised to find myself entrusted with this vulnerable little life. I had never been around infants before. Who had hidden all the mothers and babies? I can only imagine how useful it would have been to have seen it done before! All the things I had read about infants' amazing abilities did nothing to assuage my fears. 'Is this normal?' I would ask myself about everything from the strange breathing pattern to the jerky movements to the amount of crying. Yes, she was brilliantly alert and engaging, but I was embarrassingly surprised to discover how infrequently newborns' eyes are open in the first days, how many of their systems are still coming online.

It deepened my understanding of human needs and human interaction. All of our needs begin with the body in relation with another or others, and are understood, expressed, perceived, and met through dynamic, meaningful, interpersonal moving (Trevarthen and Fresquez 2015). This goes for protection, nourishment, sleep, and hygiene, as well as comfort, companionship, and learning. I was reminded that, even in the best-case scenario, it can be hard to grow up.

It's been four months since your birth. Today you had a very hard time taking a nap – you never got a good one. You were so sleepy it hurt! We would play, and walk, bouncing and shhshhing, swaying and singing, holding and trying to lay you down. You cried and screamed, but you also laughed and smiled and worked so hard on your baby business. It was a long day. The whole time my heart was full of love for you, I felt entirely devoted to you. We looked at the roses, and the wind made you catch your breath.

There is no shortage of information on the impact a mother's actions and ways of being may have on her children. The way she touches and carries, holds and contains, supports and comforts, plays with and provides boundaries, all contribute to the way her infant develops. Of course, the absence of healthy maternal care likewise has significant implications across the span of one's lifetime. But it is in the *how* of relating, the vitality dynamics of movement, time, force, space, and intention or directionality that the dyadic interaction is shaped (Stern 2010). It is through these contours that we communicate our thoughts, beliefs, and experiences. The dynamics serve to regulate the dyad and initiate development of the infant's relational patterns (Fischman 2009).

Fiona offers instant amplified feedback. If my mind wanders, she calls me back. If, in conversation with my husband, my voice reveals tension or concern, her voice raises and picks up tempo. She can sense the tiniest shifts in energy and intensity and she reacts to that. Her response magnifies what is happening between us, like one of those goofy make-up mirrors. I have to constantly reflect on and regulate my own stuff – fatigue, grief, anger, my shoulders rising towards my ears as she tries to roll over, stand up, and walk off the diaper changing table. I feel as though our nervous systems are like sponges, and I work to see what I'm picking up and what I'm dropping off.

The infant experiences vitality dynamics with all of her senses and, through the primary relationship with her caregiver, begins to 'make sense' of the world and the established ways of relating to and moving within it. This is part of how we make sense and share meaning in all relationships. It underscores my belief that it is essential to acknowledge movement and the body as contributors to the new meaning co-created in therapeutic relationship. In dance movement psychotherapy, this acknowledgment is primary: 'Dance movement therapy focuses on the experience of movement sensing and how movement makes sense. The dance therapist gets empathically involved in an intersubjective experience that is rooted in the body' (Fischman 2009, p.34). Fiona and I have a common vocabulary of dynamic movements through which we share our experiences. We move in concert together. I see in action Sheets-Johnstone's

(2010) assertion that, 'thinking in movement is at the core of our sense-making lives' (p.12).

It was autumn, and you were about nine months old.

'What is the sound the wind makes?'

'Whoooooooo.' You pursed your lips and tried to blow.

'The leaves fall down to the ground.'

'Dowwwwwwwwwwwn', you said, as you put your arms up and slowly moved them down. You twisted around to look out the window, to see if the wind was blowing leaves. Then you looked at the page in your book where the bunny watches the leaves fall.

We were at a restaurant and you were excited. You wanted everything on the table, pointing and kicking your legs and squeaking. You hadn't taken a nap yet and your eyes looked tired. You were getting worked up!

'Eh! EH! EHH!'

Grandpa slowly said, 'Bring it down, and level it out,' moving his arms to match his words.

'Dowwwwwwwwwwwn.' Your movement condensed, your arms coordinated in a focused motion downwards, your legs still for a moment. Your voice was quiet and clear. This game was fun for all of us!

A few nights later you were having a hard time falling asleep. This was not unusual. Through tears, you reached your arms up, unprompted, and brought them 'dowwwwwwwwwwwn.' How very clever, to soothe yourself this way!

My friend Heather stopped by for a visit not that long after Fiona was born.

'What's it like being a mom? What do you do all day? Is it hard?' she asked.

'I guess I just play and make up songs. I don't know. It's kind of hard to describe. I don't feel like I do anything, but I feel exhausted. I mean, it's amazing, but also hard, but not bad hard.'

It occurred to me later that this experience was directly related to being present. All the time. Or at least attempting to be. No amount of mindfulness practice could have prepared me for the non-stop presence a baby requires, indeed deserves. It takes a lot of energy. I find it much more difficult than being present for the length of a therapeutic session.

Fiona has the most amazing capacity for presence. We speak of mindfulness or being present in the moment as an intentional act, a practice, a chosen approach. I know I have to do something different inside of myself in order to be truly and wholly present. I orient my awareness to face both outward and inward. I turn on the 'witnessing' so central to Authentic Movement (Payne 2006), attending to myself and other in resonant experience. Payne (2006) describes it like this: 'The witness…is not a watcher or an observer of the mover, but an empathic conscious and receptive participant' (pp.166–167). I extend this intention and attention to all my time with Fiona, as much as I am able. In this way I am learning and growing, an apprentice to her mastery of presence.

Bhanu Joy Harrison, a clinical social worker practicing somatic psychotherapy, described to me her children continually calling, 'Watch me, Mommy, watch me,' as they went up and down the playground slide. She came to understand that only by feeling 'seen' by another again and again would they be able to grow the 'capacity to see oneself'. Again, this resonates with Authentic Movement: 'After repeatedly being seen clearly by a witness…the mover begins to see herself with the result that her own inner witness develops further' (Payne 2006, p.169). I see Fiona with tender, curious, non-judgment, and I let her know this through my presence, my interactions, and my words. It echoes the person-centered approach of building a strong relationship through the therapist's unconditional positive regard, genuineness, and empathy (Rogers 1951).

In parenthood and as therapists, we offer gifts of ourselves in a creative exchange that includes a sense of self, safety, joy, pain, rest, play. Stephen Levine (2009) describes a particularly poignant interplay between creative arts therapists and their clients that is relevant here:

> We often speak of the therapist as the witness to the work of the client, but it is important to conceive of witnessing not as detached observation but as aesthetic response. Art aims to become effective, to have an effect on others. For therapists to fulfil their role as witness, they must be open to the 'effective reality' of the work (Knill 2004), to its impact upon them, and they must be able to respond in a manner that is itself effective. This response can take the immediate form of words or gestures but it can also be fashioned aesthetically, so that there is a circle of meaning made manifest through the exchange of gifts, of what is given freely to the other. The work comes to the client as a gift and the response by the therapist is part of the process of gift exchange that binds us to each other. (Levine 2009, p.46)

Within the context of Authentic Movement, Payne (2006) describes a unifying phenomenon of the witness experiencing, with profound empathy, as though she herself were moving. In tension with this, she must contain her own projections, interpretations, and impulses to move as 'it is experienced as unhelpful when the witness does project or interpret rather than owning their own story in their witnessing' (Payne 2006, p.170). I likewise wish to hold a similar tension of knowing and not knowing. Through being conscious of my own inner experiences while witnessing Fiona, I am able to sense her thoughts and intentions. And I must differentiate and 'own' my story in order for her to continue to define and refine the understanding of her own experience. Tortora (2009) also stresses the significance of this vantage point, emphasizing that one cannot *truly* know someone else's experience.

You are so busy. You never stop learning and growing, wiggling and exploring. And all day I am with you, paying attention to the movements and sounds you make, to each shift of interest in your small but exciting world. I follow your lead. Your movements are all authentic, congruent within yourself, and arising organically. You follow your impulse to move without restraint. Sometimes it seems like you are motivated to do something, and you move to accomplish your goal. Sometimes it seems like you are motivated to move for the sake of it, or in hopes that something will appear tantalizing enough to form a goal – like that piece of fluff on the floor. We sing together the whole day, back and forth, an opera of la las, bop bops, da das. We play games with each other and with the things around us.

Sometimes we are not in sync. Maybe Fiona isn't feeling right or settled. It's not smooth sailing. Sometimes there is even the quality of an internal conflict, like when she's committed to staying awake but is so tired, or when she is nursing and at the same time swinging her leg and twisting her body, or when she is sleeping but tossing and turning. She is clearly uncomfortable, but the source of discomfort is not evident.

You hate going to sleep. You fight the good fight, and almost a year on we are not able to lay you down before you are asleep. It isn't as hard as it used to be, but some nights remind me of when you were very little. You would cry and fuss, and nothing would soothe you. We would try to figure out what you needed to calm down, how to connect in order to regulate. But a good trick doesn't work every time.

Well fed, check. Clean diaper, check. Not sick, good temperature, check. Okay. Change positions. Side hold. Belly hold. Upright again. Do you want to lie down? Nope. Hold close. Hold less close. Shhshhing in threes. Shhshhhing in fours. Singing a lullaby. Singing a song made up of noises you're making. Singing the blues. Patting your back. Rubbing your back in a downward motion. Rubbing your back in circles. Turning in circles. Bouncing. Walking. Shuffling. Swaying. Sighing. Breathing deeply. Laying you down and moving a silk scarf above you. Match your rhythm. Contrast your rhythm. Match your rhythm and try to gradually slow it down. Provide resistance when you push. Hand you to your dad.

This feeling out of sync is also present when we have different agendas, for example when Fiona wants to do something we can't let her do, like explore the trash bin or turn her books into paper pulp for consumption. She gets frustrated or mad, and who wouldn't?

'One finger, Fiona. You can touch the lamp with one finger.' This is a trick my husband's aunt showed us. It has a slightly higher success rate than 'gently' or 'softly'. With impressive dexterity, you used one finger to start pulling the floor lamp towards you. Since I didn't want my baby crushed by metal and glass, I intervened. 'Urgh!' you shrieked, as tension seized your face and neck, arms and hands. You were very upset that I moved you away from the lamp. You reached out and grabbed my face. I was stunned! You were crying.

'Oh! You're so upset! You wanted to play with that lamp so badly! It seems very unfair that I took you away. Are you mad at Mommy? Are you frustrated? I know how much you wanted that, but don't grab Mommy's face, that hurts. Let's see if we can find something to play with that's not dangerous.'

I stumble through this. I don't know how I'm doing, but I have no other ideas regarding how to discipline a ten-month-old.

There is a difference in the quality of being out of sync when the cause is a conflict of agendas vs discomfort. When it is discomfort, I am more vigilant, but I also try to just be with the unknown. When we have different agendas, I focus more on a process of communication. But there is something in my internal reaction that is similar in both instances. I feel agitation, not towards Fiona, but in my body. I have to be conscious about it, pull it into my awareness. I have to work extra hard to ground or center myself, try different things to lessen both my own and her agitation. I use breath, and here also I use mirroring and attuning. I play with rhythm, slowing down, speeding up, or keeping steady. At any rate, I seek to express compassion, to validate her experience, and to maintain my stance as it relates to safety or collective wellbeing.

On some level, parenting and therapy is filtered through a lens of, 'Am I doing this right?' And, honestly, I cannot be sure. I do not feel like I know what I am doing. I know that I have some skills, a clear, strong intention to hold the other's best interest at heart, and a deep commitment to reflexivity. I feel like, at the base of it, I know how to be with someone else, to hold and to contain.

I also reassure myself that though I should inevitably fall short of being perfect, I might still be 'good enough' (Winnicott 1974).

I let the boys rough-and-tumble play. They are in a highly structured setting, and they hardly ever get the chance to move freely, to play and to feel joy and pride in their actions. They all have issues with impulsivity and attention, amongst other things, and there is important research to support my decision to allow this (Panksepp 2006). But the boys also have difficult personal histories, most of which include violence, and it is easy for them to shift from rambunctious play to play-fighting. Once they start throwing punches and swinging kicks and rushing tackles, I ask them to stop. There is an ongoing discussion about the distinction I draw between energetic, physical play and play-fighting, as well as why that is not allowed. There are also many different ways I intervene and redirect their play, with more or less success in any given scenario. But on one particular day, my usual attempts were not working.

'Tony, I need you to stop play-fighting. It's not safe.'

'That's stupid! I wasn't even doing anything!' Anger spread throughout his body. He was flushed and his fists were clenched. His eyes narrowed, and he shoved his chin forward. He shifted his weight from side to side. He was ready for a real fight.

I centered myself, sensing my core and my feet on the ground. I made my movements soft and clear.

'You are not in trouble, Tony.'

With all of his restraint, he walked towards the edge of the room.

I waited a few moments, then walked slowly and indirectly over to him. In a smooth motion, I got closer to the ground and ended kneeling, sitting on my heels, hands in my lap, about four feet away from him. I could tell he was still angry, his heart rate quick. I sat there, trying my best to emanate calm and acceptance, staying present with my intention, sensations, and perceptions. After a few minutes, the tension in his body started to dissipate. His shoulders relaxed and his eyes eased up. I sensed a growing calm. He got down on the ground, too. We were parallel.

'I'm not mad at you, Tony. You're not in trouble. I know you were playing. I just need to make sure that you and everyone else stay safe in here.'

I metered what I was saying, keeping a slow rhythm. He didn't say anything in response, though he was generally very quiet. I do not know what he made of the interaction, but afterwards he was less ambivalent about the group. There were fewer times he started play-fighting, and I never again had to ask more than once for him to stop.

Amongst the difficulties of conflicting agendas, I find connection. This experience, whether with Fiona or a client or someone else, feels free flowing and happens in a shared rhythm. It is playful, curious, coordinated. When I am connected with someone, there is a turning towards each other, or a turning towards a shared focus. Together we follow a collaborative, creative impulse, a vital, creative–artistic process often at the heart of dance movement psychotherapy (Meekums 2002; Wengrower 2009). We are able to explore our sensing, feeling, moving, and imagining – each mode its own access point to creative change. Because these modes are deeply integrated within the human nervous system, exploring one impacts the others, which can lead to new, integrated understanding, expressions, and ways of being (Trevarthen and Fresquez 2015).

There's an activity that I like to use in groups, I call it 'imagine a bubble'. It begins with a body awareness exercise, paying attention first to breathing, then other visceral sensations, moving along to successive body parts. After assessing a sense of the inside, including qualities of weight, tension, and temperature, I ask participants to bring their attention to their skin, to the boundary between themselves and the environment around them. From here we return to the breath, and I offer the suggestion that they begin to imagine a bubble forming around them. I ask them to get really specific in their imagination about shape, texture, smells, sounds, colors, whether there is anyone or anything inside or outside their bubble. Before 'returning' to the room, I ask them to notice any changes in their body or the way they feel. Afterwards, I ask if they would like to write, draw, or move their bubble. The point is to see what arises in the imagination that describes their boundary.

Two of the boys decided to draw their bubbles. Billy decided to move, but it quickly became clear that he wasn't sure where to begin.

'I don't really get what to do.'

'Do you want me to figure it out with you?'

'Yeah.'

'Okay. So tell me about your bubble. How did it feel?'

'It feels awful!' He's speaking in the present tense.

'Awful! Oh, no! What feels awful?'

'I'm stuck inside the bubble with all my problems.'

'Oh! No wonder you feel awful! Maybe we should start by changing that. What do you want to do?'

'I want to get out of the bubble!'

We started by paying attention to how it felt in the bubble, and how he imagined he could get out. He felt heavy and tense and sick to his stomach, but he thought his arms might be strong.

'Really do it, even if you think it's silly!' I exaggerated my movements so that he knew what I meant and so that he didn't feel embarrassed. He laughed. We used our strong arms, activated our muscles, pushed with our feet, to break open a hole in the bubble. He climbed out.

'How do you feel now?'

'I'm sweating! But I feel a little better.'

'We still have this bubble full of all your problems here, huh?'

The room had only one door to the outside, and the bubble was too big to fit through. We set to work shrinking the bubble, pushing on it with all our might. We pushed and pushed and squeezed it out the door! It floated off and disappeared. Billy was so excited. He gave me a high five.

'What do you notice now?' I thought I sounded kind of silly, but he got what I was asking, and didn't hesitate to answer.

'My arms are tingling! I feel great, lighter! That's crazy. I can't believe it.'

The lightness showed in his posture, his playful bounce returned with the color in his cheeks. He left the session with his singing voice echoing down the hallway.

It is clear that my values, significantly informed by dance movement psychotherapy, shape my views on parenting. I value body awareness and connectivity, emotional literacy, regulation through movement, a non-judgmental curiosity towards self and others, kinaesthetic empathy, the ability to follow creative impulse, and autopoiesis. My baby nourishes all of these values. Through my experience of mothering, my capacity for being present and connecting deepens every day. There is a multi-directional dialogue between familial and therapeutic experiences that will no doubt continue. As we pay attention to mother–infant interactions, we reveal and more deeply understand the dynamic (and naturally therapeutic) aspects present in the relationship:

[A]dapting the ways a healthy, attentive mother connects with and receives her baby as a person, the rhythmic musicality of its dynamic emotions and the stories or performances they compose together, sharing joy and comforting pain or loneliness or supporting fatigue, will help create the safe and supportive conditions necessary for companionship and play within the therapeutic relationship (Tortora 2009; Stern 2010). Having positive, emotionally rich and authentic experiences of connecting to another therapeutically through being seen and responded to in...[dance movement psychotherapy], can build a capacity for, or expand an ability for, attuning to and connecting more self-confidently with others outside a therapeutic context. (Trevarthen and Fresquez 2015, p.206)

When I think about being connected to you, Fiona, I feel a series of internal changes. Like sunlight, there is warmth spreading. There is condensing and expanding happening simultaneously. I feel contained, and I feel open. I feel a downward, inward direction, grounding and centering, while also feeling a gentle unfurling around my heart and in my arms, in my face.

I was sitting on the ground next to you while you were playing and chewing on a rubber duckie. My back was sore, so I lay down. You noticed and clambered onto my belly.

'Da!' You said.

'Da!' I said.

You chewed on my shirt and smiled. You chewed on your duckie and pushed through your legs. I smiled and said sweet little things to you. You rested your head on my chest, your arm draped on top of me. It was the sweetest thing.

'Can you hear mommy's heartbeat, Fiona?'

'Bum, bum,' you whispered.

References

Anderson, H. and Goolishian, H. (1992) 'The Client is the Expert: A Not-Knowing Approach to Therapy.' In S. McNamee and K.J. Gergen (eds) *Therapy as Social Construction*. London: Sage.

Berrol, C. (2006) 'Neuroscience meets dance/movement therapy: mirror neurons, the therapeutic process and empathy.' *The Arts in Psychotherapy 33*, 302–315.

Chodrow, J. (2009) 'Dance Therapy, Motion and Emotion.' In S. Chaiklin and H. Wengrower (eds) *The Art and Science of Dance/Movement Therapy: Life is Dance*. New York: Routledge.

Fischman, D. (2009) 'Therapeutic Relationships and Kinesthetic Empathy.' In S. Chaiklin and H. Wengrower (eds) *The Art and Science of Dance/Movement Therapy: Life is Dance*. New York: Routledge.

Garbes, A. (2015) 'The More I Learn About Breast Milk, the More Amazed I Am.' *The Stranger*, 26 August. Seattle: Index Newspapers LLC. Available at www.thestranger.com/features/feature/2015/08/26/22755273/the-more-i-learn-about-breast-milk-the-more-amazed-i-am, accessed on 28 August 2015.

Guanaes, C. and Rasera, E.F. (2006) 'Therapy as social construction: An interview with Sheila McNamee.' *Interamerican Journal of Psychology 40*, 1, 127–136.

Homann, K.B. (2010) 'Embodied concepts of neurobiology in dance/movement therapy practice.' *American Journal of Dance Therapy 32*, 80–99.

Levine, S. (2009) *Trauma, Tragedy, Therapy: The Arts and Human Suffering*. London: Jessica Kingsley Publishers.

Levy, F. J. (1992) *Dance Movement Therapy: A Healing Art*. Reston, VA: National Dance Association, American Alliance for Health, Physical Education, Recreation and Dance.

Llinás, R. (2001) *I of the Vortex: From Neurons to Self*. Cambridge, MA: MIT Press.

Maslow, A. (1999) *Toward a Psychology of Being* (3rd edition). Chichester: Wiley.

Maturana, H.R. (1978) 'Biology of Language: The Epistemology of Reality.' In G.A. Miller and E. Lennenberg (eds) *Psychology and Biology of Language and Thought: Essays in Honor of Eric Lennenberg.* New York, NY: Academic Press.

Maturana, H., Mpodozis, J. and Letelier, J.C. (1995) 'Brain, language and the origin of human mental functions.' *Biological Research 28,* 15–26.

Meekums, B. (2002) *Dance Movement Therapy: A Creative Psychotherapeutic Approach.* London: Sage.

Panksepp, J. (2006) 'Examples of Application of the Affective Neuroscience Strategy to Clinical Issues.' In J. Corrigall, H. Payne and H. Wilkinson (eds) *About a Body: Working with the Embodied Mind in Psychotherapy.* London: Routledge.

Payne, H. (2006) 'The Body as Container and Expresser: Authentic Movement Groups in the Development of Wellbeing in Our Bodymindspirit.' In J. Corrigall, H. Payne, and H. Wilkinson (eds) *About a Body: Working with the Embodied Mind in Psychotherapy.* London: Routledge.

Piontelli, A. (2010) *Development of Normal Fetal Movements: The First 25 Weeks of Gestation.* Milan: Springer.

Porges, S.W. (1993) 'The infant's sixth sense: awareness and regulation of bodily processes.' *Zero to Three: Bulletin of the National Center for Clinical Infant Programs 14,* 12–16.

Rogers, C. (1951) *Client-Centered Therapy.* London: Constable.

Sheets-Johnstone, M. (2010) 'Why is movement therapeutic? Keynote address, 44th American Dance Therapy Association Conference, October 9, 2009, Portland, OR.' *American Journal of Dance Therapy 32,* 2–15.

Sherrington, C.S. (1955) *Man on His Nature.* Harmondsworth: Penguin Books.

Stern, D.N. (2010) *Forms of Vitality: Exploring Dynamic Experience in Psychology, the Arts, Psychotherapy and Development.* Oxford: Oxford University Press.

Tortora, S. (2009) 'Dance/Movement Psychotherapy in Early Childhood Treatment.' In S. Chaiklin and H. Wengrower (eds) *The Art and Science of Dance/Movement Therapy: Life is Dance.* New York: Routledge.

Trevarthen, C. (1979) 'Communication and Cooperation in Early Infancy: A Description of Primary Intersubjectivity.' In M. Bullowa (ed.) *Before Speech: The Beginning of Human Communication.* London: Cambridge University Press.

Trevarthen, C. (2012) 'Embodied human intersubjectivity: imaginative agency, to share meaning.' *Journal of Cognitive Semiotics 4,* 1, 6–56.

Trevarthen, C., Aitken, K.J., Vandekerckhove, M., Delafield-Butt, J. and Nagy, E. (2006) 'Collaborative Regulations of Vitality in Early Childhood: Stress in Intimate Relationships and Postnatal Psychopathology.' In D. Cicchetti and D.J. Cohen (eds) *Developmental Psychopathology, Volume 2, Developmental Neuroscience* (2nd edn). New York: John Wiley and Sons.

Trevarthen, C. and Fresquez, C. (2015) 'Sharing human movement for well-being: research on communication in infancy and applications in dance movement psychotherapy.' *Body, Movement and Dance in Psychotherapy 10,* 4, 194–210.

Varela, F. J., Thompson, E. and Rosch, E. (1991) *The Embodied Mind.* Cambridge, MA: MIT Press.

Wengrower, H. (2009) 'The Creative-Artistic Process in Dance/Movement Therapy.' In S. Chaiklin and H. Wengrower (eds) *The Art and Science of Dance/Movement Therapy: Life is Dance.* New York: Routledge.

Winnicott, D.W. (1974) *Playing and Reality.* Harmondsworth: Pelican Books.

4

ESTABLISHING A THERAPY OF MUSICALITY

The Embodied Narratives of Myself with Others

STEPHEN MALLOCH

Dedicated to the memory of my friend in the dharma Ani Lodro Maverika

Introduction

Beethoven's 'Große Fuge' (the Great Fugue), Op.133, is a movement of a string quartet composed towards the end of the composer's life when he was almost completely deaf. It struggles and writhes, with sharp edges and angular melodic lines. It is a difficult piece to listen to, as well as to play, and it is also beautiful and at times tender. With all its angularity and harshness it seems to strive to break out of the limitations of its own structure. Yet this is the vitality of the music – the dynamic push and pull of structure and expressive movement.

As a psychotherapist and coach (executive coach and life-coach) I hear stories from my clients that at first remind me of Beethoven's fugue. People tell stories of making expressive moves that reach towards the limits of their life structures, but then they find themselves wanting – they are left tired, angry, frustrated, dissatisfied, not sure what to do next. My task is to assist them to re-find their creativity, to keep the piece unfolding so that it may flow to the next melody, which will be all the richer for what has gone before. This chapter is my story of how I have explored the foundations of the therapeutic relationship – the 'musicality' of the shared gestural narratives of Self and Other – and woven my discoveries into a model of therapy with both adults and children.

An introduction to Communicative Musicality

Communicative Musicality emerged out of the work I did with my friend and colleague Colwyn Trevarthen during my post-doctoral research at the University of Edinburgh in the mid-1990s. Colwyn is an authority on child psychology and psychobiology, I had just received my PhD in music and psychoacoustics, and together we investigated the musicality of infancy.

The model of Communicative Musicality has its roots in the observed abilities of infants – humans without speech who create with those who love them the most sensitive and intimate relationships. The 'musical' and 'dance-like' gestures of these relationships – *non-verbal expressions of thought and feeling carried by the infant's and caregiver's voice and body* – are harnessed to the intention to reach out to and companion with others (Malloch 1999; Malloch and Trevarthen 2009a; Papoušek and Papoušek 1981; Stern 2000, 2010; Trevarthen 1999). Our musicality (and our 'dancicality') is with us through the lifespan (Bjørkvold 1992; Blacking 1976; Jusczyk and Krumhansl 1993; Osborne 2009; Trevarthen and Fresquez 2015; Trevarthen and Malloch 2000; Wittmann and Pöppel 1999). It serves our need for companionship just as language serves our need to share facts and coordinate practical actions with others using objects in our environment (Cross and Morley 2009).

Until the late 1960s, mainstream medical and psychological research rarely credited infants with complex skills or creative mental abilities, and certainly not with any active sympathy for other persons' thoughts and feelings. In addition, the mother's role was not seen to extend much beyond being a provider of basic physiological protection and nourishment. This began to change as researchers paid closer attention to infant behaviour with caring, loving adults. Babies were observed to have a strong attraction and curiosity for other humans. This attraction, expressed with responsive smiles, vocalizations and gestures, delighted their mothers and drew them into the flow of the present moment of the exchange (Stern 2004). This was communication before speech (Bullowa 1979) grounded in the baby's innate intersubjectivity (Trevarthen 1998). Infants' and adults' communicative gestures arise out of the combination of an infant's innate communicative competence coupled with a shared rhythm for turn-taking between infant and caring adult. These gestures share in-the-moment embodied meaning.

The model of Communicative Musicality (Malloch 1999; Malloch and Trevarthen 2009b) is built on the understanding that human beings develop consciousness in intimate companionship. The emotional Self gives shape to these 'dancing' and 'musical' narratives of imaginative communication, and is in turn shaped by them (Bjørkvold 1992). Both infant and caregiver are motivated to connect, share and develop the vitality of their selves in patterns of communicative movement (Stern 2010).

This motivated movement has certain attributes that can be measured. In the Communicative Musicality model, three components are identified – *pulse, quality* and *narrative*. They are defined as follows:

- *Pulse* is the regular succession of discrete behavioural steps through time, representing the 'future-creating' process by which a person may anticipate what might happen and when.

- *Quality* consists of the contours of expressive vocal and body gesture, shaping time in movement. These contours can consist of psychoacoustic attributes of vocalizations – timbre, pitch, volume – or attributes of direction and intensity of the moving body perceived in any modality.

- *Narratives* of individual experience and of companionship are built from sequences of co-created gestures, which have particular attributes of pulse and quality. These 'musical' narratives allow adult and infant, and adult and adult, to share a sense of sympathy and situated meaning in a shared sense of passing time (Malloch 1999; Malloch and Trevarthen 2009a).

As we grow and develop, our innate musicality – our 'muse within' (Bjørkvold 1992) – underpins our creation and appreciation of the arts (temporal and non-temporal). Narrative gestures of the body create dance and song, narrative gestures with an instrument create instrumental music, and the physical objects produced from body gestures create paintings and sculptures. Intricate formulations of gestures create ceremonies (Dissanayake 2000; Trevarthen and Malloch forthcoming). These same narrative gestures can also be therapeutic – they are a direct way of engaging the human need to be sympathized with, to have what is going on inside appreciated by another who may also assist, encourage or console (Berrol 2006; Trevarthen and Fresquez 2015; Trevarthen and Malloch 2000). It is our common musicality that makes it possible for us to share meaningful actions as we plan and work together on projects, and to communicate and share the vitality and interests of life as we tell our stories. Our learning, anticipating and remembering, our infinite varieties of communication including spoken and written language are all given life and vitality by our innate Communicative Musicality.

My approach to therapy: Narratives of the Self

The therapeutic relationship is one of companionship

Many years ago I read these words by Thich Nhat Hanh (a Vietnamese Zen Master): 'The greatest gift we can offer anyone is our true presence' (Thich Nhat Hanh 1998, p.182). In my work as a psychotherapist and coach, I sit with people and talk with them, and sit in silence with them. Having trained as a musician, and researched and written about Communicative Musicality, my approach to being-with-another has strong strands of my curiosity about our innate musicality. Let's begin by looking at the opening of a coaching conversation.

Elizabeth, a single woman in her mid-40s, previously married, came to see me for career coaching. She was in a mainly administrative role, and told me she felt stuck and bored and wanted so much more from her work, but didn't know in which direction to turn. She wanted a role helping others and to live her career from, in her words, her 'authentic self'. In her marriage she had felt she couldn't speak up, and speaking up for her wants and needs was still a challenge for her, in work and out of it. During the course of our coaching I had introduced a model around letting go the old and letting come the new (Scharmer 2007). In sessions prior to the one I'm about to describe we had spent time looking at her desire at work to 'keep busy' and 'smile and be happy', which she wished to let go of, and we had been exploring her uncertainty of what might come in its place. In this session, her eighth, she enters the room with her usual anticipation for what might emerge.

After exchanging some remarks around how her week had been ('quite good'), she tells me a short story about how she has felt relaxed and spacious staying for the week in a friend's house by herself (she usually lived in a small apartment). But now it is 'back to the real world – it wouldn't be sustainable me living like that'. I smile slightly, not sensing any particular direction as yet, and feel the conversation starting to lose energy. My mind goes to what we had discussed the previous week, her wish to speak up for herself, and I mention it. She says she has thought about it, but nothing in particular had happened where she felt she had spoken up more for herself than usual. The conversation once more starts to fade. I ask if there is anything in particular she wants to bring to the session, and she replies no.

In the moment of silence that follows I notice the feeling of the lack of vitality between us. Our relationship feels calm, but rudderless. In our relationship's musicality, our emotional Selves are calmly drifting.

As infants we communicate with others through our shared gestural narratives, and as we grow our languaging develops 'on top of' these narratives, enabling us to share facts and coordinate practical actions with others. Meaning is created intrapersonally and interpersonally out of the interacting streams of gestural, body narratives and language.[1]

The aim of psychotherapy for me is to create a shared experience that heals. And while clearly I do not ignore the linguistic narratives that are occurring, a

---

1   See the work of Ray Birdwhistell who was pivotal in establishing the study of non-verbal behaviour (which he called 'kinesics') as a central part of human communication (e.g. Birdwhistell 1970). His writings influenced the work Daniel Stern towards the study of 'vitality contours'.

vital focus of my therapeutic attention, and the focus of this chapter, is the flow of our co-creating gestural narratives.[2]

In the session with Elizabeth, clearly words are being exchanged, but the affective meaning of the relationship is not to be found in those words. It is in the feeling of lack of direction, felt by me as calm drifting and acknowledged (and almost certainly felt) by Elizabeth, that our embodied Selves are meeting. I believe it is here, in the felt sense of shared vitality that 'therapeutic leverage' within the relationship can be found.

There are two layers of therapeutic intention in the way I conceptualize the relationship between myself and a client.

The first and deeper layer is my overall twofold intention for the relationship: to be present to the client, receiving and appreciating non-judgementally whatever the client offers me; and to be congruent and authentic in a manner that is tuned to what will enable the client to be more congruent and authentic with me (and thus more congruent and authentic within themselves). This approach is influenced by Carl Rogers' client-centred approach (Rogers 1951), the humanistic psychology movement, and my many years practice of mindfulness (e.g. Ram Dass 1978 [1971]; Thich Naht Hanh 1991 [1975]). It is also deeply informed by my many years' observations of the dynamics of healthy, loving caregiver–infant interactions. In the words of Carl Rogers, 'The curious paradox is that when I accept myself just as I am, then I change' (Rogers 1961, p.17).

The second layer adds a dimension of therapeutic intention – I aim to 'conduct' the session, both non-verbally and verbally, in such a way to encourage 'balance' in the companionable interactions between myself and the client, and so also balance *within* the Self of the client. This is what I am about to do in the session with Elizabeth.

'This space between us feels quite calm to me', I say to Elizabeth, 'but I don't know where this conversation is going, and you've said you don't have any particular topic you want to bring up. I wonder if you are wanting me to take responsibility for its direction?' She looks away, and seems thoughtful, and then looks back towards me, and with a slight nod, indicates she wants me to continue.

Our 'piece of music', if we are to be moved by it, needs something else, as yet unsounded. I sense our musicality is seeking a balance to the drifting state we are currently creating, so I go searching for what that element might be. When I search, I start by describing what is in front of me (which

---

2   See Norcross and Lambert (2011) on the centrality of the therapeutic relationship for therapeutic outcome.

in itself is an act of searching). We can't know how to move unless we know our current environment.

'I want to hand responsibility back to you for this session. I wonder if this lack of direction I feel is part of why you said the time in your friend's house was unsustainable. Relaxing and calm, yes, but also lacking a sense of direction. Part of what you are wanting in your career is a sense of direction. Maybe we are right now sitting in the energy that is blocking that forward movement?'

Her posture has changed, and she is sitting upright and leaning towards me, an expression of focused curiosity on her face. I discover I also have changed position, and am sitting more upright, and leaning towards her. My voice is louder and clearer, my hand gestures are larger. A new element has been introduced, and the piece is moving. I feel awake!

The therapeutic relationship is underpinned by the manner of our gestural exchanges. In terms of the model of Communicative Musicality it is about the sharing of human vitality. An understanding of the vehicle for this exchange of affective meaning through the externalization of an aspect of one's inner world is provided by Daniel Stern's theory of vitality contours (Stern 2010) and affect attunement (Stern 2000). Affect attunement is the mechanism by which vocal and body gestures carry meaning in parent–infant communication – it is 'the performance of behaviours that express the quality of feeling of a shared affect state, but without imitating the exact behavioural expression of the inner state' (Stern et al. 1985, p.142). This unfolding quality of feeling expressed in a behaviour Stern calls a 'vitality contour'. Affect attunement is a multi-modal or trans-modal phenomenon, where the affect of a vocal and/or bodily gesture is attuned to by another and expressed in a different form from the original. According to Stern, this largely unconscious 'recasting' of events is necessary to 'shift the focus of attention to what is behind the behaviour, to the quality of feeling that is being shared' (Stern et al. 1985, p.142).

This is much more than mimicking. Mimicking implies we are attentive to a person's behaviour (an important factor in building a relationship) but it tells the other person very little, if anything, about the inner state of the person who mimics. However, to abstract a component from those movements, and relay it back to the initiator in a changed yet recognizable form, says we are creating with something that has been given to us by the other. I am externalizing some of my own inner life while in relationship. The relationship is now one of companionship (from the Latin meaning 'to break bread with', and defined here as the wish to be with an other for a mutually beneficial 'inner' purpose, apart from reasons of immediate survival, procreation or material gain). Companionship involves exchanging affect through sharing impulses of motivation (Trevarthen 2001).

In the session with Elizabeth, I have just started to co-create with her, through affect attunement, a much more vital experience. The impetus for my upright body, firmer voice, more expansive hand gestures, is the sharing of our innate musicality. And through bringing my attention to what is usually a largely intuitive process I am building on these 'raw materials' of companionship so that the inner affective life is amplified. Within our song and dance my companioning gestures will be more vitally focused with the other, and I will at times verbally name and reflect upon the gestural narrative that is present – as I am about to do with Elizabeth. But also words must be used wisely, and at times withheld. We may 'agree' with ourselves and others in the affective shared embodied space of our musicality, but disagree in the shared objective space of verbal discussion (Cross and Morley 2009). This is also about to happen in the session.

'Look, both of us are suddenly leaning in and sitting up. What is this?'

Elizabeth starts to talk about the eager part of her that so often starts enthusiastically but then nothing really happens. She starts arguing with herself whether it is useful energy or not. I gently interrupt…

'Words are usually about this or that, black or white. I'm curious what would happen if you just continued to lean into whatever is occurring here. Something seems to be happening in the space between us (I indicate with my hand the space above the table that is between us). Just feel it.'

After a moment Elizabeth's eyes start to mist over with a hint of tears. 'What's that?' I ask gently, sensing she is now much nearer to the new musical element that is emerging. 'Relief,' she replies.

It was relief that she didn't need to 'keep busy' and always be smiling. She was experiencing the letting go that was allowing the letting come. As our session continued the letting come turned out to be 'playfulness' – a musical element that beautifully balanced the initial melody of calm meandering.

The therapeutic relationship is a piece of music, experienced in the unfolding present

How do I approach the question of balance? I do not arrive at it through analysis. The beginning point is always a felt sense of the state of the whole. I do not wish to reduce my client to a set of behaviours.[3] In the session with

---

3   See McGilchrist (2009) on the right hemisphere of the brain and its attitude which this approach to the therapeutic relationship epitomizes. Also see Martin Buber who wrote of the 'is-ness' and inherent companionable respect of an *Ich-Du* relationship (Buber 1970 [1923]).

Elizabeth I did not begin by *thinking about* the conversation and its parts, I *felt* its imbalance and its quality of seeking a balancing movement into the future.

Daniel Stern captures this beautifully in his book *The Present Moment in Psychotherapy and Everyday Life*, where he discusses our experience of the flow of music:

> The mind imposes a form on the [musical] phrase as it unfolds. In fact, its possible endings are intuited before the phrase is completed, while it is still passing by. That is to say, the future is implied at each instant of the phrase's journey through the present moment. (Stern 2004, p.26)

Note that Daniel Stern says a phrase has possible endings – *plural*. In the opening of the conversation with Elizabeth its calm and directionless musicality initially implied different possible futures to her and to me. The client seemed to want to impose a familiar future – the music would loop back on itself, its vitality remain low, and she would continue to look to others to set her direction. I sensed the possibility of a future as yet untested – Elizabeth could move forward into a different, more creative melody, still implied by the first, but one that might bring greater balance to the unfolding 'piece' as a whole. This new melody Elizabeth discovered to be 'playfulness' – she began to explore possibilities for her career with energy and creativity, and with much greater self-direction.

So, in terms of the therapeutic relationship based in a model of Communicative Musicality, attention is given to the shaping of the interpersonal musical narrative, and the sense of 'balance' in this interaction as it moves through time. This sense of balance is intuited in the moment. A therapy session for me is like a piece of music unfolding, and an unbalanced piece of music is unsatisfying. The role of the therapist utilizing the model of Communicative Musicality is to be sensitive to and foster a more creative, more balancing, longer-term musicality.

What might be the sensory mechanism through which we sense this unsatisfactoriness of unbalanced movement through time? Colwyn Trevarthen proposes our appreciation of balanced, graceful movement and our ability to produce it is based in a system in the brain called the Intrinsic Motive Formation (IMF). The IMF, which is also intimately involved in the neurochemical system of emotions, is based in the brain stem, basal ganglia and limbic structures. It enables us to navigate our way physically and imaginatively into the future with energetic efficiency and graceful vitality (Trevarthen and Aitken 1994). From the IMF comes the Intrinsic Motive Pulse (IMP) of our musicality. The IMP acts as a central timekeeper and helps orchestrate the temporal regulation of brain/body-wide systems, both mental activity and physical moving (Trevarthen 1999). It is one of the factors underpinning our conscious embodied experience of time (Osborne 2009). As Colwyn Trevarthen explains, 'Neural energy flows as a consciousness of inner time that structures and regulates thoughts, images, memories, emotions and movements' (Trevarthen and Fresquez 2015, p.199).

Within the flow of Communicative Musicality, produced by the IMP within the moving, feeling, vocalizing body, we can sense a balanced and responsive vitality in ourselves and others. And when that balance is lacking, we sense a state which is unpredictable, lethargic or overly energized. Balance is created through moving between different states, and within each state is the implication of a movement to come. A tense body longs to move towards relaxation, a relaxed body is fulfilled in action; a discord in music reaches towards resolution in concord, and musical harmony seeks activity through disharmony. Unbalanced movement is 'stuck' but is felt to want to resolve into a greater balance through a flow of movement. A balanced flow of communicative movement comes about through creative expression (as with Elizabeth 'letting come' her playfulness).

The philosopher Alan Watts, writing on Taoism, says:

> Wu-wei is the lifestyle of one who follows the Tao, and must be understood primarily as a form of intelligence... This intelligence is not simply intellectual; it is also the unconscious intelligence of the whole organism and, in particular, the innate wisdom of the nervous system. (Watts and Huang 1975, p.76)

It is this innate wisdom that I aim to harness in creating therapeutic movement, leading to balance and wellbeing.

Different melodies

'My wife thinks I'm depressed – what do you think?' Mark asked me about half way into our first session. In his early 40s, married for 16 years, he told me his wife wanted him to have more energy, to take more responsibility, even to hang out the washing in a different way. He felt uncomfortable holding firm to his opinions – if someone asked him what he thought of a piece of news that had been reported, he would ask himself what the person probably wanted to hear and then offer that as his opinion.

Three years into the therapeutic relationship, in what would turn out to be the concluding months of therapy, I asked his permission to record a session.

Here he talked of an emerging 'new me' in contrast to an 'old me'. The 'old me' was marked with 'a lack of self-respect', he said. 'I blame myself when things go wrong, I believe I'm not working hard enough.' His voiced droned on, body hardly moving.

This is what a four-second section of a pitch plot of his 'old me' voice looks like (Figure 4.1):

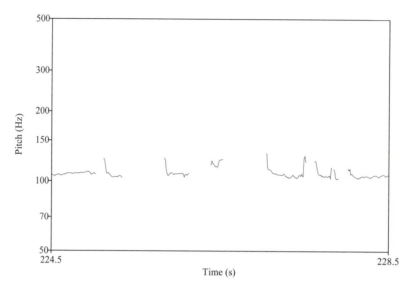

FIGURE 4.1 PITCH PLOT OF 'OLD ME'

After describing 'old me' he paused…his body relaxed, he looked up from the floor, his hands lifted from his lap, the volume of his voice increased, its pitch lifted, and he began talking of 'new me'. 'New me is more rational about life. This part says, "Well, I was uncommunicative this morning – that's all right, that's OK. That's just the way I was. Doesn't make me a bad person. Other times I communicate really well!"'

Below is a four-second pitch plot of 'new me' (Figure 4.2):

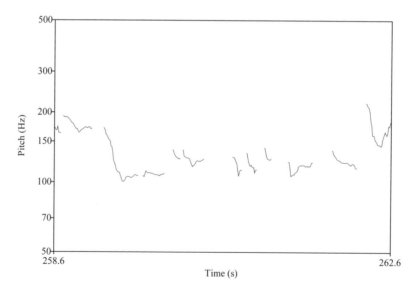

FIGURE 4.2 PITCH PLOT OF 'NEW ME'

The shift in the vitality of the musicality is clear.

Over the course of a number of sessions, many parts of a client's Self will become apparent to both of us – for example, Mark's 'old me' and 'new me'. Communicative Musicality is a mind–body expression – inner motivations are both expressed and created through the moving body in relationship.

It was proposed earlier that the IMF, through the IMP, acts to integrate and 'musically' coordinate the living, moving, communicating body. A possible reason our musicality is so complex when expressed as music or dance, when compared with birdsong or the movements of a chimpanzee, is because of the multitude of relatively autonomous 'moving parts' that make up our upright bodies. These require meticulous coordination if we are to move through our environment, into the future, with efficiency, efficacy, and without harm (Blacking 1976; Goodrich 2010; Trevarthen 1999; Trevarthen and Fresquez 2015; Trevarthen and Malloch 2000; also see Merleau-Ponty 2012 [1945]). Our brains have needed to become adept at centrally organizing a multitude of semi-autonomous movements tied to a number of potentially conflicting motivations. I am walking to work, and unexpectedly I see a friend in my peripheral vision. I turn my head and upper torso, wave my hand and say hello, while still walking in the same direction and avoiding others walking in the opposite direction. This is a highly intricate feat of coordination! I propose that this multiplicity of semi-autonomous movements could contribute to the existence in all people of the various parts of the Self – like 'old me' and 'new me' – parts that relate to the world through different motivational lenses.

At this point I want to draw on the work of Roberto Assagioli, an important figure in the development of humanistic psychology in the mid-20th century, and founder of the therapeutic movement known as psychosynthesis. His work emphasizes the existence of 'sub-personalities' and the possibility for the synthesis of these different parts.

> Sub-personalities, in psychosynthesis theory, have been defined as 'structured constellations or agglomerates of attitudes, drives, habit patterns' (Crampton [1981], p.712) and 'learned responses to our legitimate needs: survival needs, needs for love and acceptance, and needs for self-actualization and transcendence' (Brown [2004], p.41). They are, most simply stated, the *parts* of every individual, that may or may not be in service of the whole. (Firman 2007)

Often, these different parts come more into conscious awareness when we are in the process of trying to decide whether to do 'this' or 'that'. Does Mark continue to blame himself, or start to see himself in a more optimistic light? Behind each 'this' and 'that' will be a set of beliefs and emotions that make up a particular orientation towards how we move through the world and our life.

If coordinating well, these parts enable us to navigate our way into the future with grace, vitality and learning. A depth of understanding emerges from integrating multiple perspectives. Mark could come to realize that at times it is appropriate to see one's faults and give oneself a talking to, and at other times it is appropriate to overlook something that doesn't go quite as you wanted, and just get on with things. If our sub-personalities fail to weave together, just as if the head and eyes turn too far to say hello to a friend and the body walks straight into a wall, then harm can come to the whole. Mark could continue with 'old me', blaming himself when anything in his relationships goes wrong, while 'new me' remains merely a hope – he would continue to be dejected and lonely.[4]

As we saw, these different parts of the Self have their own dynamics of musicality. The piece as a whole can consist of the movements of both – a life can consist both of seeing one's faults and getting on with things with a sense of one's strengths. It is in the balance and coordination of the flow of their expression – a flow that will be mutually influencing on both – that health is to be found. Just as the body can move with greater or lesser grace and adaptiveness through its environment, so the selves move with greater or lesser grace and creativity through the changing demands on the Self (see also Stone and Stone 1989).

Discovering we have options, when we have felt condemned to live in just one particular way, is the re-finding of creativity. It is also the discovery of a broader, more inclusive perspective where we become aware of the larger overarching phrases of our unfolding musicality. Just like musicians do as they gain in experience, we learn how the smaller phrases fit within the larger narrative, rather than continuing to believe the smaller phrases *are* the larger narrative.

Bringing awareness to different musical sections

For the therapist working in the model of Communicative Musicality, all themes, all sections, are part of an unfolding composition, and all parts are to be respected as parts of the whole. The client, however, may fail to see them this way. For the client a particular theme may just not belong, or a particular section is leading in a direction that appears completely incompatible with another section of the composition that is jostling for attention.

By engaging with the various parts of the composition, and bringing awareness to the imbalances, a path is navigated where the parts may begin

---

4   This way of thinking resonates with McGilchrist (2009, p.9), who argues, citing Sir Charles Sherrington, Roger Sperry and Marcel Kinsbourne, that the brain is a series of opponent processors, 'in other words, it contains mutually opposed elements whose contrary influence makes possible finely calibrated responses to complex situations'.

to cohere more successfully into a balanced composition. The overall structure successfully accommodates the diverse thematic offerings, which work together to create a healthily functioning Self.

In a final example we'll look at larger scale integration of musical sections. In this story, an underlying theme dating from the client's early childhood becomes the basis for unifying motivations and experiences into a larger-scale musical structure. This structure enables the client to more effectively 'conduct' her different musical sections, which had all been competing for attention.

Becoming the conductor

Helen came into my consulting room, confidently and with a warm smile. She looked and behaved older than her 16 years, sitting comfortably on the couch opposite me, engaging me in easy conversation. Born in England, her story was that she had lived in Indonesia with her parents for some years. They had come to Sydney three years before and Helen was now attending a private (non-government) school, living in the affluent Northern Beaches area of Sydney, and apart from some doubts about her abilities, she reported doing well in her school subjects.

She told her story in a way that suggested she had told this story before, and indeed later I learnt she had seen her school counsellor on a number of occasions because she was feeling down. She said it had been good to talk with the counsellor – it had helped to get things off her chest, she said.

With her father's encouragement she was seeing me because 'sometimes my head just gets so full!' She was also having strong doubts about the direction her studies were taking. She loved writing, and planned to study English Literature at university, so was opting for as many English subjects as she could. She was getting good marks, but she was starting to find the whole topic 'so boring!' It was far too theoretical. There was no exploration of its beauty.

She just felt so dissatisfied with everything! 'But,' she said, 'I have no reason to. There are people so much more worse off than me – what do I have to really complain about! But sometimes I just want to tell everyone to just fuck off! No one is really doing anything to make the world a better place – we all just keep talking about it!'

This was the first major section of the piece of music we were creating together in our first meeting. Then I asked a question.

'What do you enjoy?' Her body relaxed, her face softened, as she started to tell me about surfing. She feels connected with the wave when she surfs, she told me. She loses herself in the sound and movement as she moves with the board. She feels connected with the ocean, and she feels good to be alive. Her movements and the melody of her voice were flowing. The piece moved into a different mode

– lilting and warm. There was less effort involved in its production. The calm was all the more noticeable because of the previous tension.

In terms of musicality, prior to my question I had felt an imbalance in our conversation. After the initial pleasantries, it had grown staccato, jagged, very dramatic. Her voice had been covering a wide pitch range, her hand movements were abrupt, she had at times been red in the face. Her body was tense. After some time spent in that style of musical expression, it felt to me like her emotion peaked, and she, and the predominant music, was coming to a natural pause or shift. I wanted to give her space to explore other possibilities, for the piece to perhaps move on, and for her to have an opportunity to tell me something else about herself. Or, to put it another way, it felt like the piece was ready for another, balancing type of expressive movement.

In subsequent sessions I learnt that her mother had been ill with a heart condition for some time, and her father was often absent due to work. She found herself caring for both her mother and her younger brother. As she told her story, she would return to her theme of criticizing herself – 'There is so much suffering in the world, what right do I have to feel down?'

There seemed to me to be at least three major musical themes present. The most noticeable one for me (though not the one with the most energy) was characterized by a whole body movement of low-level contained tension. It felt like a melody that seemed at first to be aiming for a climax, but then it turned away and went down into itself. This melody sat beneath the words that said she did not have the right to be feeling down. Then there was the second principal melody – a variation on the first. This second melody would, at times, continue up towards its climax and reach its goal and then flow quickly towards its goal, again and again. This second melody was associated with words that expressed anger – towards her parents, towards her teachers, towards the world of people who didn't do anything to make the situation better!

Then there was a third, very different, melody – the contrasting theme that had a width and flow. It grew and swelled, would come to rest, and then move again – just like the sea, and her companionship with it which she described.

These three melodies were all integral to the piece that she and I were creating. My role was to notice if one of the themes felt over-represented or failed to flow – if the piece felt unbalanced – and then to encourage new themes, or the reappearance of existing ones, so that the piece could unfold in a way that felt to me, and to Helen, satisfying, whole and creative.

In a session fairly early in our therapeutic relationship, Helen's first two melodies were particularly strong, and the topics kept changing every few minutes – 'I can't take compliments', 'I'm terrified it will all fall apart', 'I feel panicked I will make the wrong decision about my studies', 'I've argued with my dad.' I started to feel lost in the constantly changing variations – probably how Helen was feeling as she moved from topic to topic. I then remembered her image of surfing and the sea, and so I brought that image to my mind, and allowed it to imbue my body with the feeling of graceful movement that I saw in her on our first meeting. The piece she was composing was tightly bound, and perhaps in search of a way to resolve its tension. So I encouraged her to sit with her emotions as she raised each topic. She would sit with the feeling for a moment before whirling onto her next subject. But those moments seemed to be enough. At the conclusion of our session she said she felt better for letting it all out. And I felt I had found an image that I could hang on to in the midst of her storm that helped to balance the music so that the piece could continue its progress.

As our meetings progressed, she talked less of her anger towards others and more of wanting to live more easily with all the different stresses in her life – all the different interlinking melodies. She was starting to take responsibility for her own music – to be the conductor, aware of the whole, shaping the music as it passes. Around the same time she recalled a moment, she thought she was about four years old, when she made a contract with the ocean. 'I agreed always to be with it – to trust it.'

Her surfing melody was gaining depth. There is an approach to understanding the structure of music called *Schenkerian Analysis*. Named after its founder, it posits that great examples of Western tonal music, that is 'masterworks' as Schenker called them, written around the period 1700–1900 can be understood as hierarchical structures. One of the ways these pieces gain their unity is through 'deep' structures (that often unfold over large stretches of a composition) influencing and at times repeating in miniature on the musical 'surface' (Schenker 1979 [1935]). This for me is a useful way of thinking about what was unfolding for Helen.

As therapy progressed, so her music of her love for surfing had begun to point to the deep structure that lay beneath it and deeply influenced it – her existential trust and connection with Nature that took birth at the age of four. Having connected with this broad deep-structural context, her 'inner conductor' could now hold a larger musical span in mind. Helen could now shape her music of anger and her music of not believing she had a right to be angry into a more balanced whole. She began talking of her thoughts on what happens when her own and others' wish to make the world a better place meets with the human limitations on that wish. She talked of her appreciation of the love she had for her mother and the love her mother had for her, despite her feeling her mother had never really mothered her. These insights calmed her. Her musicality of voice and body flowed with a depth of connection only hinted at in our first meetings; I let go of tension when I was with her that I hadn't even realized I had been holding in previous sessions; both of us spoke with more space between ideas. And all these themes worked their way through our companionship.

Helen's therapy continued for 12 months. Near the end of the school year she said she wanted to take a break, and would be in contact in a couple of months. I received an email:

> I finished school and got really good marks – so happy! I then jumped on a plane with a friend and went to a great surfing beach I know. It's great over here, and I'm staying here for a while, while I think.
>
> Thanks for all your help – really helped me to clear my head and put things into perspective.
>
> Helen

Coda

The unfolding musical narratives of our lives create ordinary masterpieces of stirring anthems, quiet lullabies, tentative explorations and deep hymns of interconnection. All of them are part of the whole, beautiful piece – if we can stand back far enough to see, hear, appreciate and conduct it.

I will end with a story from my own past.

I was raised by my maternal grandparents, my parents separating when I was three. Subsequently I had intermittent contact with my mother as I grew up, and no contact with my father until much later in life. I was cared for, educated and nurtured with love and unfailing commitment by my grandparents, Edith and Noel, but along the way I learned that it was not OK to say what was on my mind. I learned passive acceptance was the best strategy for things that mattered. After all, both my parents were virtual strangers to me for reasons that were never explained. Things of emotional significance were mostly not talked of.

At seven years old I began to learn the violin. I was reasonably good at it, and continued violin studies up to tertiary level. I still play. But at around the age of nine what I really wanted to play was the drums! I chose my moment carefully after school, when I judged the teacher would not be in the music room. My next memory is making wonderful sounds as I hit the drums louder and louder, and then had the courage to hit the cymbal – really hard! Some kids from my class walked by the window – 'Go Malloch!' they laughed. I couldn't work out if they were laughing at me, seeing me throwing myself into something so unusual, or laughing because of my own joy. I didn't care. I kept drumming!

I sometimes wonder what life would have been like if I had gone home that day and announced I was giving up the violin and taking up the drums. I didn't. I never played the drums at school again. I persevered with the task of getting my arms and fingers to obey the demands of the violin.

The drums and the violin cultivate such different physical musicalities. The drums for me are about taking up space with large, swinging movements of the arms, the sound radiating out and pushing into the world – it can't be ignored. The violin's movements feel thinner, more about precision of control, a fineness of sound that beguiles and at times amazes, rather than demands.

These are two very different ways of moving through the world – pushing into the world and demanding; precision and beguiling. Just as I chose to keep playing the violin, despite the yearnings of my mind and body for the larger more carnal movements of the drums, so for many years I have defaulted to an approach of precision and requesting, rather than pushing and demanding as I have travelled through my life.

This is changing. I am getting more skilled at incorporating both approaches, and flowing with them depending on what the circumstances require. There is a place for both.

Our outer and inner musicality – the gestural narrative expressions of the body and the Self – create the ways we approach our moment-by-moment experience, and our decisions of which paths to take. I will continue to practise listening to it, playing with it and conducting it, and encouraging others to do the same. It immerses me and others more deeply into the flow of life.

References

Berrol, C.F. (2006) 'Neuroscience meets dance/movement therapy: mirror neurons, the therapeutic process and empathy.' *The Arts in Psychotherapy 33*, 302–315.

Birdwhistell, R.L. (1970) *Kinesics and Context: Essays on Body Motion Communication*. Philadelphia, PA: University of Pennsylvania Press.

Bjørkvold, J-R. (1992) *The Muse Within: Creativity and Communication, Song and Play from Childhood through Maturity*. New York: Harper-Collins.

Blacking, J. (1976) *How Musical is Man?* London: Faber and Faber.

Brown, M.Y. (2004) *The Unfolding Self: The Practice of Psychosynthesis*. New York: Helios Press.

Buber, M. (1970 [1923]) *I and Thou* (W. Kaufmann, trans.). New York: Touchstone.

Bullowa, M. (ed.) (1979) *Before Speech: The Beginning of Human Communication*. London: Cambridge University Press.

Crampton, M. (1981) 'Psychosynthesis.' In R. Corsini (ed.) *Handbook of Innovative Psychotherapies*. New York: J. Wiley and Sons.

Cross, I. and Morley, I. (2009) 'The Evolution of Music: Theories, Definitions, and the Nature of the Evidence.' In S. Malloch and C. Trevarthen (eds) *Communicative Musicality: Exploring the Basis of Human Companionship*. Oxford: Oxford University Press.

Dissanayake, E (2000) *Art and Intimacy: How the Arts Began*. Seattle: University of Washington Press.

Firman, D. (2007) 'A Transpersonal Orientation: Psychosynthesis in the Counselor's Office.' In N. Young and C. Michael (eds) *Counseling in a Complex Society: Contemporary Challenges to Professional Practice*. Amherst, MA: Synthesis Center Press. Available at www.academia. edu/7389307/A_Transpersonal_Orientation_Psychosynthesis_in_the_Counselors_Office, accessed on 22 October 2016.

Goodrich, B.G. (2010) 'We do, therefore we think: time, motility, and consciousness.' *Reviews in the Neurosciences 21*, 331–361.

Jusczyk, P.W. and Krumhansl, C.L. (1993) 'Pitch and rhythmic patterns affecting infants' sensitivity to musical phrase structure.' *Journal of Experimental Psychology: Human Perception and Performance 9*, 627–640.

Malloch, S. (1999) 'Mother and infants and communicative musicality.' *Musicae Scientiae 3*, 1, suppl. 29–57.

Malloch, S. and Trevarthen, C. (2009a) 'Musicality: Communicating the Vitality and Interests of Life.' In S. Malloch and C. Trevarthen (eds) *Communicative Musicality: Exploring the Basis of Human Companionship*. Oxford: Oxford University Press.

Malloch, S. and Trevarthen, C. (eds) (2009b) *Communicative Musicality: Exploring the Basis of Human Companionship*. Oxford: Oxford University Press.

McGilchrist, I. (2009) *The Master and His Emissary: The Divided Brain and the Making of the Western World*. London, New Haven: Yale University Press.

Merleau-Ponty, M. (2012 [1945]) *Phenomenology of Perception* (Donald A. Landes, trans.). New York: Routledge.

Norcross, J. and Lambert, M. (2011) 'Psychotherapy relationships that work II.' *Psychotherapy 48*, 1, 4–8.

Osborne, N. (2009) 'Towards a chronobiology of musical rhythm.' In S. Malloch and C. Trevarthen (eds) *Communicative Musicality: Exploring the Basis of Human Companionship*. Oxford: Oxford University Press.

Papoušek, M. and Papoušek, H. (1981) 'Musical Elements in the Infant's Vocalization: Their Significance for Communication, Cognition, and Creativity.' In L.P. Lipsitt and C.K. Rovee-Collier (eds) *Advances in Infancy Research, Vol. 1*. Norwood, NJ: Ablex.

Ram Dass (1978 [1971]) *Be Here Now*. New York: The Crown Publishing Group.

Rogers, C.R. (1951) *Client-Centered Therapy: Its Current Practice, Implications and Theory*. Boston, MA: Houghton Mifflin.

Rogers, C.R. (1961) *On Becoming a Person: A Therapist's View of Psychotherapy*. Boston, MA: Houghton Mifflin.

Scharmer, O. (2007) *Theory U: Leading from the Future as It Emerges*. Cambridge, MA: Society for Organisational Learning.

Schenker, H. (1979 [1935]) *Free Composition* (E. Oster, trans.). New York: Longman.

Stern, D.N. (2000) *The Interpersonal World of the Infant: A View from Psychoanalysis and Developmental Psychology* (2nd edn). New York: Basic Books.

Stern, D.N. (2004) *The Present Moment in Psychotherapy and Everyday Life*. New York, NY: W.W. Norton.

Stern, D.N. (2010) *Forms of Vitality: Exploring Dynamic Experience in Psychology, the Arts, Psychotherapy, and Development*. Oxford: Oxford University Press.

Stern, D.N., Hofer, L., Haft, W. and Dore, J. (1985) 'Affect Attunement: The Sharing of Feeling States between Mother and Infant by Means of Inter-modal Fluency.' In T.M. Field and N.A. Fox (eds) *Social Perception in Infants*. Norwood, NJ: Ablex Publishing Corporation.

Stone, H. and Stone, S. (1989) *Embracing Our Selves: The Voice Dialogue Manual*. Novato, CA: New World Library.

Thich Nhat Hanh (1991 [1975]) *The Miracle of Mindfulness*. London: Rider.

Thich Nhat Hanh (1998) *The Heart of the Buddha's Teaching*. Berkeley, CA: Parallax Press.

Trevarthen, C. (1998) 'The Concept and Foundations of Infant Intersubjectivity.' In S. Bråten (ed.) *Intersubjective Communication and Emotion in Early Ontogeny*. Cambridge: Cambridge University Press.

Trevarthen, C. (1999) 'Musicality and the Intrinsic Motive Pulse: evidence from human psychobiology and infant communication.' *Musicae Scientiae 3*, 1, suppl.157–213.

Trevarthen, C. (2001) 'Intrinsic motives for companionship in understanding: their origin, development, and significance for infant mental health.' *Infant Mental Health Journal 22*, 1–2, 95–131.

Trevarthen, C. and Aitken, K. (1994) 'Brain development, infant communication, and empathy disorders: intrinsic factors in child mental health.' *Development and Psychopathology 6*, 4, 597–633.

Trevarthen, C. and Fresquez, C. (2015) 'Sharing human movement for well-being: research on communication in infancy and applications in dance movement psychotherapy.' *Body, Movement and Dance in Psychotherapy 10,* 4, 194–210.

Trevarthen, C. and Malloch, S. (2000) 'The dance of wellbeing: defining the musical therapeutic effect.' *Nordic Journal of Music Therapy 9,* 2, 3–17.

Trevarthen, C. and Malloch, S. (forthcoming) 'Grace in Moving and Joy in Sharing: The Intrinsic Beauty of Communicative Musicality from Birth.' In S. Bunn (ed.) *Anthropology and Beauty: From Aesthetics to Creativity.* Oxford: Routledge.

Watts, A. and Huang, A.C. (1975) *Tao: The Watercourse Way.* New York: Pantheon Books.

Wittman, M. and Pöppel, E. (1999) 'Temporal mechanisms of the brain as fundamentals of communication – with special reference to music perception and performance.' *Musicae Scientiae 3,* 1, suppl.13–28.

5

FINDING OUR WAY TO RECIPROCITY

Working with Children Who Find It Difficult to Trust

DANIEL HUGHES

Many, many years ago I reflected on my frequent inability to help children who had been abused and neglected to resolve their traumas and get on with their lives. My initial goals were to help them to be less terrified by the traumatic events of their past. When I found I wasn't successful with this I developed other goals, which focused on helping them to reduce the deep sense of shame they felt and which underpinned their conviction that they deserved the maltreatment that they had received. Still later, I hoped to help them – when they were living with foster carers or adoptive parents – to learn to trust their new carers who, I could say with confidence, would not hurt them as they had previously been hurt. Valuable and important goals yes, but I was starting too far ahead of their experiential reality and this was stopping me from being able to provide the help they so desperately needed. I needed to help them to trust me first. Still too far ahead. I needed first to help them to trust this here-and-now-moment-with-me. This one moment, and from there, if it proved to be safe, this next moment-with-me. And the next.

The children who I was attempting to 'treat' were children who were very isolated, very lonely. They were isolated from me as I attended to them, talked with them, noticed their new hair cut or shoes, asked about their day at school or their bedtime routine. After attending to them, they were still lonely. They were isolated when I watched them draw or construct a town out of toy houses and people. Moment to moment they were isolated because they did not seem to notice my initiatives or not to care about them if they did. They did not seem to notice my responses to what seemed to be their initiatives. Later I realized that their vocal expressions or movements were simply that – expressions made with no expectations of a response. Expressions, not communications.

Expressions made to the universe, long since having given up an expectation of a returning expression meant to recognize theirs.

These children did not trust me, nor did they trust any other adult in their lives – caregivers, teachers, or social workers. They did not trust me enough to share their past or their future goals with me. They certainly did not share with me their memories of traumatic events. They did not even share with me the routine events of their day. They did not trust me or truly engage with me for one moment, no matter the content of the moment, whether it be accepting our being together with a reciprocal 'Hi' or the shared mild enjoyment of listening together to a bird sing outside the window, or sharing an interest in the dinosaur bone on my desk. What they seemed to be saying with their whole body was, 'I'm not interested in spending one moment with you. And I know you're not interested in spending one moment with me.'

Providing 'treatment' for these children was also a goal too far. I needed first to find a way for them to invite me to be with them. To invite me to be with them not for a year, a month, a week, a day or an hour, but to be with them for this one moment. And from this moment there might be a series of moments. From this attuned reciprocal moment-to-moment state a conversation might begin to form, a conversation that would integrate the nonverbal with the verbal. And from the child's increased comfort and confidence in this conversation with me, a dialogue could emerge that would invite both me and the child to explore and share memories and themes. And from this, the the co-creation of a narrative could truly begin. A narrative that could lead to resolution and integration of the many events that led to the child's need for treatment. This beginning involves moments-of-meeting, then a connection, then a conversation. The beginning involves reciprocity, reciprocal influence, and companionship. Helping children to feel able to invite me into this experiential, intersubjective present, opens the door for them to the discovery of self and other, to the meaning of trauma and relationship, to caring for and being cared for, to integration and resolution. I discovered that my original 'treatment goals' only had the possibility of being attained if they had been revised many times along the way, each time involving this moment-to-moment process. Only from there could the journey be a shared one that could creatively guide us both as to where we needed to go.

Let me pause for a moment and give an example of what these words mean to me. About 30 years ago an eight-year-old foster boy, Jake, was in my office with me. He was alone, as back then I primarily was a play therapist who saw children without their carer or parent being present. He was playing with wooden people, houses, and trees. One of his characters was having a difficult time finding someone to play with. I commented on my experience of his play, not expecting any response as he habitually seemed to be totally absorbed in his play and did not seem aware of my presence. I said, 'That must be hard for him. He might be getting tired of being so alone.' Jake paused in his play, seemingly waiting for me to say something else. 'He might be feeling kind of lonely and wishing that he had a friend to play with.' I added. I waited for a moment, Jake glanced at me, and then he said, 'I feel sad when you talk that way.' I leaned forward slightly and asked, 'Is it OK that you feel sad now?' 'Yeah', Jake nodded, and he resumed his play with no further signs of acknowledging my presence.

That evening I wondered about that brief moment with Jake. I knew that while my words were probably accurate in reflecting his experience at that moment, he had responded more to how I said the words rather than the words themselves. I knew that my voice conveyed a gentleness, a lightness. My prosody – how the voice expresses the meaning of words nonverbally – had most likely enabled him to be receptive to the words. I thought then that the word 'hard' (because of the softness in my voice as I spoke it) may have been experienced by Jake as my really knowing how hard his life had been. Jake may have sensed in my voice that he was safe to experience his sadness, with me, in that moment. I did not know it at the time, but later have come to realize that this is often a key moment in the successful treatment of children who have been abused and neglected. Before they can truly move forward in life, they need to be 'safe to be sad'.

With Jake, I began to be more aware of my nonverbal expressions, not just over his hard times but also over his confusion, his enjoyment, his excitement, and his pride. I had been taught in my early years as a psychotherapist to pause and understate my experiences by being less expressive nonverbally. At the time I had young children at home and I was aware of how natural it was for me to give clear expression nonverbally to my experience of our time together. So, I allowed myself to be similarly expressive with Jake, and he seemed to be engaged with me more strongly and more often. He seemed to trust and naturally respond to my nonverbal communications much more readily than to the words themselves. But it did not stop there. It seemed that as we both were more expressive nonverbally, we became more at ease to find words to talk about our experiences. And gradually our conversations included Jake's hard times.

My time with Jake reflected my early days in exploring the role of nonverbal communication in the treatment of children. At some point during those years I began to wonder why such communications were important. Words are so important in taking us into our minds and sharing experiences of people, places, and events. They are excellent in taking us away from the present into the past and the future. But often the words never came, or when they did, they seemed to be lacking in energy or felt meaning. They were expressed alone, without the body's synchronized nonverbal communications.

This chapter describes how trust might develop within the child's relationship with their therapist. The first stage involves reciprocal, here-and-now, nonverbal communications. Second, as these are developing, there emerges the presence of ongoing conversations – described here as affective–reflective dialogues. Third, within these reciprocal conversations between child and therapist, there is space for poorly integrated events of shame and terror to enter the dialogue and be met with the co-regulation of associated affect and co-creation of new meanings. Fourth, and finally, after the resolution and integration of these past events, the child is able to more fully enter into all manner of reciprocal communications with family and friends. These communications include the deepening moments of comfort and joy within which the relationships between the child and therapist, and the child and caregiver, are able to flourish. I will now briefly describe each of these four phases of engagement and then present a therapeutic approach developed to enhance them.

Reciprocal nonverbal communications

Within the healthy parent–infant relationship both infant and parent discover that the source of development, relationship, and enjoyment involves becoming engaged in reciprocal, contingent, nonverbal communications with each other. Within these moment-to-moment communications, infant and parent are having a mutual influence on each other. Each baby's unique response is contingent upon their parent's unique initiative, and the parent's subsequent response is contingent upon the baby's unique response to the prior one. And the same applies to the parent's responses to their baby's unique initiatives. Within the baby, this reciprocal, contingent process develops a level of trust that the parent's initiatives (and influence) will not cause harm.

The baby is bodily aware (long before the emergence of reflexive language in the pre-frontal cortex) that they need to engage with their caregiver in this manner if they are to develop and thrive while they organize and discover who they are. The baby's vocal and facial expressions, along with their overall bodily gestures, combine with the parent's responses to guide the baby into an experience of reciprocity that is both comfortable and that fully engages their interest and attention. And the caregiver also 'knows' that they need to engage in this spontaneous, attuned way. The baby initiates the tune and the caregiver follows. The caregiver introduces a bit of novelty into the tune, and the baby says 'yes' and they dance to that tune a bit until the baby says 'enough' and they fall back into something less stimulating. Sometimes the baby says 'no' and the parent needs to modify her initiative and make another start at developing a tune to the baby's liking. This has been called interactive repair (Tronick 2007) and is crucial if the baby is to learn that her preferences matter to her parent. The baby's 'yes' may last a moment or a minute – only the baby knows – so the caregiver needs to continuously be alert to the baby's cue as to when it is time to move on, continue, or fall back. This whole process occurs in a relaxed, open and engaged, manner. This allows the parent's experience of the child to be communicated nonverbally and creates the building blocks from which the art of conversation can develop. Such nonverbal expressions are rhythmic and tend to quickly become synchronized: parent with baby and baby with parent. Vocal expressions are harmonious with, and match, those of the other. The baby's facial expressions become synchronized with the parent's bodily movements and vice-versa in a process of mutual influence and engagement. The synchronization of these expressions is called 'attunement' by Stern; he defines 'attunement' as 'the intersubjective sharing of affective states' (Stern 2004, pp.12–13). This is the mutual experience of sharing shifting states of affective energy – or 'vitality' (Stern 2010) – and is best envisioned by a 'vitality contour' defined by quality, rhythm, beat, duration, and shape (Stern 2010, pp. 47–48). Colwyn Trevarthen also speaks of this joint process, which he considers to be inherently a form of music; he describes this principle as 'musicality' (Malloch and Trevarthen 2010). When the parent and infant – or, I would add, the therapist and child – enter into this relational dance, Trevarthen describes it as 'synrhythmia'.

How to create this synchronized rhythm with the child who does not know how to sing or dance or who long ago discovered that such dancing – with an abusive or neglectful parent – would only lead to pain, loneliness, disappointment, or terror? It is not always easy even with a baby who loves such mutual rhythms, but with children who do not trust because they were abused or neglected it is a huge challenge. Abused children often dissociate in fear from any opportunity for attuned interactions while neglected children fail to respond to or even to recognize such opportunities. The therapist must anticipate this difficulty for the child and this then becomes the first therapeutic goal: to focus primarily on creating the beginnings of trust through establishing reciprocal, synchronized, nonverbal rhythms with children who are terrified of such interactions or, more basic still, who do not know how to join the rhythmic flow. This is the challenge that comes inherently with the opportunity and privilege of being with the children we seek to help; the challenge at the heart of creating this living moment together.

Reciprocal conversations

In my early years as a therapist I was often surprised how very hard it was for most of the children that I saw to have a conversation with me. I certainly anticipated that they would have difficulty talking about past traumatic events, and might well become avoidant, withdrawn, and/or oppositional and evasive when I brought up their past traumas or current challenges. But this was something more basic. They had difficulty just with the process of having a conversation itself. Taking turns, talking and listening, focusing on the same events or themes, reflecting on and developing a deeper, joint understanding of what was being discussed – all proved to be very difficult. These children often asked countless questions. Many times they changed the topic to something seemingly unrelated to what we had been exploring. I became aware that the reciprocal nature of having a conversation with someone, talking and listening, was hugely difficult for them.

This might not be surprising if we notice how parents and infants – long before the infant is able to use words – have ongoing 'conversations' about what is happening and what is present. The attuned moment extends to include sharing affective states, engaging in joint interests, and developing cooperative activities. There is something between the infant and parent that holds them together. Something that does not exist when they are apart. They are taking aspects from the perspectives of each and forming a joint narrative. The present event or object takes on more complex and richer meanings when explored together. This joint activity adds to the lives of each. Taking turns talking and listening, initiating, and responding, they are forming an intersubjective experience that could not be formed by either alone. Knowing and being known, cooperating in a joint endeavor, both are feeling safe and both are contributing to the meanings being created. In the absence of these early attuned rhythms of communication, it is not surprising that the abused or neglected child finds the basic structures of conversation so alien.

Reciprocal creation of safety and meaning regarding traumatic events

Therapists rightfully worry that it might be re-traumatizing to explore and attempt to resolve and integrate a trauma. The verbal recall of a trauma might create a level of anxiety and confusion that is similar to the traumatic event itself. In addressing this dilemma, many therapists have chosen a non-directive approach, though too often the traumatic event is then avoided by the child for months or years. In response to this avoidance other therapists have been more directive in addressing the trauma. But this directive stance can become troublesome when the child either seems to detach himself emotionally from the discussion, or becomes very emotional and has difficulty staying regulated or cooperative in the act of exploration.

This problem with the highly stressful nature of trauma exploration is more easily managed when the therapist has first established the rhythms of reciprocal communication – both nonverbal and verbal. Safety is better insured and maintained when the therapist is acutely responsive to the child's affective state. In this way, moment to moment, the therapist is able to co-regulate any emerging affect, while taking the lead in changing the focus and tempo of the dialogue so that it is easier to address the trauma. The child feels safe in the knowledge that the sensitive therapist will respond to any signs of distress that he is making and accompany him to a place of greater safety. The child is never trapped in the exploration of any theme. Safety is present before the traumatic theme is addressed and safety is continuously re-established whenever it weakens.

Within the safety of flowing, reciprocal communication the child will often accept a natural shift in the topic of exploration: a synchronous movement from the day-to-day, light and casual, to the more intense event that was experienced as trauma. Having first established the momentum of the conversation, when the therapist moves the focus onto the areas of shame or terror the child often follows and remains engaged with the traumatic content. This continues as long as the therapist maintains the reciprocal rhythm of the conversation whatever the content. When this happens the child is able to experience the therapist's experience of the traumatic event (and the therapist's experience of the child's experience of the traumatic event). The child's original experience of the event (embedded in terror and shame) is now joined with the therapist's experience and the child is able to create with the therapist a new, intersubjective meaning of that event. Doubt has been cast on the child's original meanings of the event (meaning given to the child by the perpetrator of the event). The child is now open to new meanings, influenced by the meanings experienced by, and through, the therapist.

The fullness of reciprocal communications

As the child comes to trust the process of engaging in attuned moments of reciprocal nonverbal interaction – becomes ready and able to enter into conversations – she uses these conversations to explore and integrate traumatic events. The child becomes more able to take full advantage of being with an adult who both knows and cares about them. The child is now able to enter into states of companionship with an adult who is both known and trusted.

Such companionship opens up a wide range of experiences, which are now experienced more deeply because they are shared. The caregiver or therapist, being older and wiser than the child, has much to offer the child that will enhance his safety, enjoyment, and ability to learn about self, other, and the world. When these experiences involve fear, sadness, shame, or other very stressful emotions, the child is now able to turn to the adult for comfort. With comfort, safety and understanding are able to follow quickly, often preventing the development of a traumatic experience. With comfort, if trauma does emerge it is often kept smaller and resolved more quickly. When these experiences involve enjoyment and the development of skills, the child is able to go more deeply into those experiences at the side of his caregiver. Enjoyment develops into opportunities for deep reciprocal joy and delight. The child's developing skills, as well as their ability to experience that they are loved, create a deep sense of pride and worth.

The therapeutic journey toward reciprocity

When we focus on this here-and-now rhythmic relating, we can see an opportunity to create safety within a therapy session. This safety can be fostered even with children who never usually feel safe with adults, and even when the child enters into conversation about traumatic events which violated every sense of safety that a child needs to feel with their parent. It is through such flowing, synchronized experience within verbal and nonverbal communication between child and therapist that the awareness, empathy, and intentions of the therapist begin to be known and trusted by the child. Words are embedded in the vitality of each reciprocal moment. And these moments are expanded into musical conversations in which all content is more likely to be rendered safe.

The therapeutic paradigm known as Dyadic Developmental Psychotherapy (DDP) was developed to utilize the developmental processes described above. Within this paradigm, 'musical' conversations became known as affective–reflective dialogues (a–r dialogues) and form the central activity of DDP. An a–r dialogue has narrative content; together the child and therapist explore events from the child's experience. As this is unfolding, the goal of each a–r dialogue is twofold: to create an intersubjective therapeutic relationship in which the child first experiences safety through the co-regulation of affective states, while at the same time co-creating new meanings – again intersubjectively – of the events being explored. These a–r dialogues are therapeutic conversations in which the child gradually develops the readiness and ability to create coherent stories that contain new meanings about the events of his life. The goal of these dialogues is to enable the child to develop, understand, and communicate her inner life. Many children who have experienced relational trauma do not have these skills.

DDP attempts to empower them to both discover and express words that help them to make sense of their life story. It is the act of developing this story, with an attuned therapist, that enables the child to revisit past traumas, re-experience them with less terror and shame, and reintegrate them into their life narrative.

How to begin this journey with a frightened, defensive, mistrustful child?

It is first necessary to remain committed to establishing a truly attuned rhythm. The therapist must maintain the intention to create and preserve this joint presence with the child. But it is hard! The therapist is human and all of us seek truly reciprocal interactions with others. Failing to receive a reciprocal response, the therapist – like the rest of us – is likely to become defensive. The therapist might begin focusing on reciprocity but when the child does not respond the therapist might think that it is better to take another approach. This could involve relying on reason to identify the problem, presenting behavioral solutions to resolve problem behaviors or trying to elicit a commitment (a contract) from the child to engage in the therapist's or carer's solutions. If none of these work, the therapist might modify the recommendations, and try again. Or they might give up hope. Reason justifies the therapist's retreat to words and the cortex when experiential, bodily-based communications are not successful in developing cooperative synchronized rhythm. If reason fails, the danger then is that the therapist will present home-based contingency plans to the child's caregivers in the hope that they will create cooperation and success. These are not likely to be successful if the child continues to mistrust the caregivers and their motives. What impact can structured solutions have when the child remains trapped in a bubble of isolation and shame that was constructed during the original abuse and neglect?

Given the child's lack of safety and trust in their experience with adults, they are likely to approach interactions in a very defensive manner. Protecting themselves at all times from psychological or physical acts of aggression is *the* top priority. The defensive strategy might either be to make the adult uncomfortable with the interaction and so withdraw from it, or to act in an overly compliant manner so as not to cause a conflict. These highly vulnerable children are attempting to control the interactions so that they cannot be hurt. One way to establish control is to control the emotional response of the adult. Many children who have been abused or neglected become experts at making the adults in their lives feel angry, anxious, inadequate, or like they want to give up. When the child elicits such a reaction from the adult, it is likely to cause the adult to become defensive or move into a position of blocked care that mirrors the child's blocked trust. With both child and adult now defensive it is very unlikely that they will enter into a reciprocal, attuned relationship. To prevent the development of ongoing defensiveness, it is imperative that therapists anticipate this likely defensive reaction in themselves, reflect on it, and crucially still maintain the intention to initiate and respond to co-create a reciprocal dialogue. This takes practice, perseverance, and a safe place in supervision where the therapist can reflect on the unique struggles each therapist–child relationship engenders, make sense of it and discover new ways forward to connect with the rhythm of each unique child.

Our responses to the child's nonverbal communications are often the strongest guide for that child when she is tentatively feeling for potential safety: the safety to share more about a traumatic event, the safety to feel and express sadness. Our eyes, our voice, our facial expressions, movements, gestures, and the timing of our response are all cues to the child as to whether or not we are listening, interested, accepting, understanding, and empathic. For mistrusting children, if our nonverbal expressions are ambiguous, understated, or 'professional', this may well represent to them that we are not interested, we do not care, and we are not personally engaged. They anticipate that we are either just doing our job or don't really believe the words we are saying. Mistrusting children fill in the blanks resulting from our ambiguity by assuming the worst. This is likely to mean that they assume we have an attitude toward them similar to that held by the adults who abused or neglected them.

The open and engaged state of mind I am talking about is described so well by Stephen Porges as representing the Social Engagement System: a system-wide neurophysiological state (Porges 2007, 2011). In a child, the Social Engagement System comes online when stress responses are dampened. It orchestrates holistic changes which facilitate reciprocity, attunement, and mutual influence. The Social Engagement System is the opposite of defensiveness. When a defensive, controlling child is met in interaction by an open and engaged therapist, the experience tends to activate the child's Social Engagement System. However briefly this occurs, over time and repetition the experience will gradually lead the child into an open and engaged state of mind which matches that of the therapist. The therapist must remain aware of what being open and engaged is like and return to that experience every time she becomes a bit defensive.

Within such a relationship, the therapist will engage in continuous modification of expression based on the responses and initiatives of the child. These frequent, often minute, alterations in the engagement are known as *acts of interactive repair*. The same processes were described by Ed Tronick (2007) when speaking about the continuous acts of repair that occur between an attuned parent and infant. In each of these acts, the therapist experiences the child's response to her initiative and then modifies that initiative so that it is more comfortable and interesting to the child. Such ongoing repairs are are the heart of attunement.

Interactive repairs also facilitate the child's sense of safety and confidence in the fact that she does influence the engagement, and her communications are understood and responded to. When the therapist initiates an interaction and the child communicates discomfort with it, the therapist then follows the child's response and modifies their initiative. The child quickly learns that the content of the a–r dialogue is a joint decision. She will not be trapped in any discussion. Here too, the therapist gains more confidence in her ability to initiate a discussion of difficult themes whilst enabling the child to remain safe in the process.

So, then, when engaging in this delicate process of interactive repair, where does the therapist direct his open, engaged, flexible awareness? It begins with focus on the child's nonverbal expressions. The therapist needs to be aware of:

- eyes that look away, look down, look around, searching, flit about, bore through us, distant, wandering

- facial expressions that are flat, exaggerated, rapidly changing, seemingly conveying one or more emotions, directed toward us or not

- movements of turning away or turning toward us, passivity or agitation, sudden, repetitive, frozen

- vocal expressions that are very intense, barely audible, monotone or rhythmic, with sighs, loud breathing.

All of the above may seem to occur in response to, or independent of, the therapist's expressions or both. Each one is a glimpse into the child's inner life, guiding the therapist as to how best to join with the child in this moment, leading or following depending on its likely meaning.

In DDP, this process of continuous interactive repair (or fine tuning) is known as follow-lead-follow. The DDP therapist gives priority to the child's initiatives, joins them, and may gently lead them into areas the child may have some difficulty thinking about. The therapist then immediately follows the child's response to that leading comment. There is no effort to pressure the child to focus on material that the child indicates, verbally or nonverbally, is too difficult for him. The therapist's goal is not to explore particular content on a given day. Rather, the goal of the therapist is to maintain an open and engaged relationship with the child while maintaining the rhythm of the dialogue, regardless of its content.

Here is an example of an early treatment session involving a 15-year-old girl, Betty. She had considerable mistrust of the therapist's motives and perceptions of her. As a result, she was definitely reluctant to enter into a reciprocal dialogue.

Therapist: I think that's a new coat. *(Matter of fact and inviting, after Betty entered the room for the second session and sat down)*

Betty: (Looks out window, strong sigh)

Therapist: You might not be interested in your coat or more likely, in my noticing your coat. *(Rhythmic voice, light awareness, not intrusive)*

Betty: (Even stronger sigh, stronger expression of reluctance to engage)

Therapist: Possibly not interested in being here as well. *(Recognizing that the increased intensity might reflect that there is a bigger desire not to engage)*

Betty: (Continues to look out the window, now without a sound)

Therapist: I don't know what you're thinking or feeling, which may be as you want it to be now. *(Accepting the quiet, seemingly inner focus of the teen; followed by a minute of silence)*

Betty: (Sitting quietly at first, then some fidgeting, restlessness – seemed to value the silence at first, now becoming uncomfortable with it)

Therapist: I'm not sure if you'd rather be quiet now or you'd like my help to find the words to say what's on your mind.

Betty: I don't want your help, asshole, you work for my parents and their help always comes with a demand attached. *(Intense, challenging, with good eye contact and appearing to be waiting for a response. This seems like an opening toward reciprocity, depending on whether or not the therapist is able to accept, be curious about, and maybe experience empathy for the child's experience)*

Therapist: Thanks for helping me to understand! *(Matching the intensity of Betty's voice – accepting her experience)* Of course you're not likely to tell me anything this week if you've lost the bit of trust that I think you had toward me last week. Is there something that makes you think that there are strings attached to my interest in you? *(Still intense, not challenging, but conveying a sense of urgency to understand)*

Betty: I saw her give you the check after the session, asshole. That's when I figured it out. You're working for them and what I think and feel doesn't really matter to you.

Therapist: Got it! You think that I'm taking your mom's money to fix you, rather than what I think, which is to help the family work well, without sacrificing what is special about each unique member of the family.

Betty: What's that supposed to mean?

Therapist: It means that I help families, not fix kids. I see my job as helping every member of the family to feel safe in expressing what is unique about each one. Without hurting or being hurt by each other. And right now, all I want is to understand you. What is special about you. What you bring to the family. What is hard for you about the family. What is good for you about the family.

Betty: Sounds nice but how do I know you mean it?

Therapist: You keep part of your brain focusing on any strings that might be attached to the way I am with you and what I say. If you find a string, push me about it. Start with calling me an asshole again.

Betty: OK, asshole.

Therapist: (Lightly, with a bit of playfulness) Hold on, you can only call me that if you see a string attached. What string do you see?

Betty: (Laughs) OK, you get a pass now. But the first time I see a string I really nail you.

Therapist: And if you don't see any strings at all? Do you trust me then?

Betty: We'll see. What's your first question?

In this session, Betty gradually became open and engaged in the reciprocal dialogue. She became open to being influenced by the therapist and interested in the possibility that she might be influencing the therapist as well. Both in a way that might be of value to her. Not that it lasted. Many times Betty pulled back to defensively reappraise the therapist's intentions. That defensive response then influenced the therapist to repair their relationship rather than to go forward in the dialogue. Repair proceeded with the therapist remaining open and engaged with every initiative and response that Betty made.

A–r dialogues are genuine conversations, and conversations are not lectures. For full engagement in any conversation, the dialogue itself needs to be rhythmic: with variations in intensity, tempo, latencies; with elements of suspense, surprise, and fascination. The dialogue does not proceed in a monotone voice. There is an emotional tone with implied meaning during the description of events and when raising questions. The conversation is inherently interesting through the act of its telling as much as through the content. This is similar to how a storyteller tells a story to an audience. Prosody, facial expression, and gesture all convey meanings that increase the child's interest in what is being discussed.

When the rhythm of the conversation demonstrates reciprocal engagement between the child and therapist, the therapist now has the opportunity to introduce elements of a particular theme for the child. This will relate to the shameful and/ or traumatic themes of the child's experience. The therapist maintains the flow and momentum of the dialogue, the rhythmic nature of the prosody expressed, whilst making this introduction. The therapist does not adopt a stern, serious monotone when focusing on this stressful event, but rather moves from one theme to the next in as seamless a manner as is possible. In doing so, the momentum of the conversation often leads the child to becoming engaged in the shame/trauma event for a minute or two before the child is likely to show any sign of distress. At that point, the therapist slows, pauses, and focuses on re-establishing the child's sense of safety before going forward. These conversations, which include the therapist's intersubjective experience of the event being explored, are very important for the child to be able to re-experience those events so that they are less terrifying or shameful. Without those dysregulating affective states, the child is then free to explore the event for new meanings, meanings which will facilitate the creation of a more coherent narrative.

The conversation prior to, and following, the exploration of the shame/trauma event is just as important to the course of the treatment as is the attention given to the trauma and/or problem. These light and routine aspects of the conversation are not simply techniques that enable the actual treatment to begin. Rather they enable the therapist to come to know many aspects of the child, not just the trauma or problems. The child is a unique individual to the therapist – not a case, diagnosis, or group of symptoms. When children sense that they are experienced as the unique person that they are, they will be more likely to trust the motives of the therapist. When the therapist senses what is unique about the whole child, the therapist will understand more fully the reasons why the child is in treatment.

The following example presents how the therapist successfully maintained the intention to establish a reciprocal interaction with a child. The therapist was able to bring the child into a difficult conversation through continuing with an open and engaged state of mind and responding to the child's challenges in a flexible, non-defensive manner.

A nine-year-old boy, Stan, (who was quite aggressive with his foster carer, Jane) got up and walked around the room when the therapist wondered about the hard time he had with his carer the day before.

Therapist: I think that your feet are saying that you'd like to get away from talking about you and Jane.

Stan: LA, LA, LA, LA. *(Loud and forceful, talking over words)*

Therapist: And now your voice is too. Well done! *(Equally loud, matching his energy, but with no vocal annoyance)*

Stan: Shut up! Shut up! *(Forcefully refusing to engage in conversation about his aggression)*

Therapist: (*Turning away from Stan, the therapist looks at the foster carer and speaks quietly to her. While speaking about Stan to his foster carer rather than directly to him, the therapist is able to convey empathy for him in a manner that he is more likely to accept)* I think that Stan really does not like talking about his anger toward you. It is so hard for him – and for most kids – to do. I think that he might rather forget it and hope that you do too. And I bring it up! No wonder he might be annoyed with me!

Stan: Why don't we just forget it! *(Intense and angry but engaged with some openness to therapist's experience)*

Therapist: Great question! *(Matching his intensity)* I worry that it might keep happening if we can't figure it out. I hope that I might help you two to figure it out!

Stan: I swore at her because she just doesn't care about what I want! She needs to know that what I want is important too! Not just what she wants! *(Anger remains, but intensity now includes his efforts to figure why she had said 'no' to him. He might also be testing to see if carer and therapist care what he thinks)*

Therapist: Thanks, Stan! That really helps me to begin to make sense of this! You think that Jane does not care about what you want! Of course, if she doesn't care about what's important to you, of course you'd be angry about that! *(A reciprocal dialogue is beginning, with both voices matched in intensity and faces showing the same heightened, joint focus on this important event)*

PACE: Playful, Accepting, Curious, Empathic

It begins with an attitude: one that will enable the therapist to remain open and engaged with the child; remain attuned to the child's nonverbal expressions; maintain a reciprocal conversation in which every aspect of the child's life is able to be explored with regulated affect and an openness to new meanings. This attitude is common in our relationships with healthy infants. It is also the attitude which tends to be effective in creating the treatment relationship being described. This attitude is characterized by being playful, accepting, curious, and empathic. Now briefly to consider each of them.

With an attitude of *playfulness* the therapist remains open to discovering features of the child that are a source of delight, hope, and mutual relaxation. These features are never forced upon a child, especially one who is frightened, sad, angry, or shameful. However, when there is space for these qualities in the present moment, the therapist is ready to assist the child in being aware that there are reasons for laughter and joy. The therapist helps the child to be aware of the positive events of life and when ready, the child might begin to actually experience them. Within the playful attitude, the child also discovers the ability to bring laughter and joy to others. There is room in the child's life for a sense of self that goes beyond being a victim or survivor.

Acceptance applies to every aspect of the child's inner life: every thought, feeling, wish, dream, memory, perception, value, and judgment. There is no intent to change anything, simply to understand. (Assaultive or dangerous behaviors of the child are not met with acceptance, though their motives are. The therapist is clear that there is no place for certain behaviors in the session and if such behaviors occur they are addressed. However the therapist remains openly curious about why the child wants to engage in a given behavior.) Acceptance requires that there is no evaluation of the child's expression, no judgment about its meaning. The therapist is open and responsive to the expression, acknowledging it openly, with full interest.

This degree of acceptance helps the child to feel safe. It also helps the therapist to remain fully present with the child since the therapist does not need to change the child's experience. If the child is challenging or dismissive, but the therapist is able to accept the child's expression and maintain openness to its deeper meaning, the therapist is much less likely to become defensive. From here, the therapist will be in a better position to simply understand the child.

Curiosity, embedded in acceptance, is entirely nonjudgmental. The therapist is wondering who this child is, what this event means, how the child makes sense of things. The act of wondering embodies an act of reflecting and facilitates the child's own interest in self-reflection.

Empathy is likely to be a core aspect of the therapist's natural experience of the child and the difficult realities of the child's life.[1] The child's mistrust of adults is very likely an adaptive response to the child's ongoing experience of her inner narrative – a narrative containing a great deal of betrayals, violations, shame, and terror. Giving expression to this sense of empathy for the child's experience, the therapist shows nonverbally that he is being impacted by those narrative events. Awareness of this new shared nature of narrative has an impact on the child (i.e. the therapist is touched by my sadness, feels my sadness with me, maybe he sees me as someone of worth, maybe I can trust the therapist?) As the child comes to feel that the therapist cares, accepts, and understands, this opens up the potential for the therapist and the child together to explore the traumatic narrative anew. Now the therapist's experience of the child's past enables the child to re-experience those traumatic events and discover new meanings. These meanings are likely to reduce the shame and terror associated with past traumas and enable the child to be open to a new manner of experiencing self and other. As the child is now likely to be more open to the therapist's experience of them,

---

1   As do many therapists, I use the term 'empathy' to refer to the relational quality of being with another, affectively joining and understanding their experience. Many scholars consider the word 'sympathy' to more accurately describe this process.

the child will be more ready to allow the therapist to influence his sense of self, other, and the world. The therapist's nonverbal, affective, empathic response to the child enables the child to begin to experience herself in new ways: as being lovable, courageous, good, and able to evoke compassion and joy when relating to others.

An 11-year-old girl, in anger, pushed her adoptive mother, who fell and broke her arm. The girl was now in a 30-day assessment program to determine what was needed for her and her family. An excellent program; she saw her therapist twice a week. During the fourth session, the following dialogue occurred.

Therapist: (In a slow, quiet, rhythmic voice, as if she were telling a story. Reflective, while conveying a sense of sadness over how hard Rayna's life must have been) Rayna, as I get to know you, and after talking with your adoptive parents, my sense is all your life…all your life…you've really never quite had the experience of feeling loved by a mom. Your first mom, we don't know much, but we do know that during the two years you were with her, we know that she was on drugs, moved a lot, and left you with many people. *(Rayna's nonverbal responses, as the story progresses, indicate that she is engaged with it, that she and her therapist are actually having a conversation)* Then you were in an orphanage for four years and you did not have a mom there. Then when you were six, you got a mom, and I think that you were not ready to trust her. I think she loved and loves you, but that you have not been able to feel it, and you think she is mean when she says 'no' to you. So I think that during your whole life, you've never known what it is like to be loved by a mom.

Rayna: (Sitting quietly, she continues to look out the window, seeming pensive, unlike her usual fidgeting and unfocused manner. She then looks at the therapist) I miss my mom. *(Her face now seems soft and vulnerable and she shows a touch of sadness)*

Therapist: (Seeing the softening of Rayna's face, she experiences Rayna's emerging sadness and the therapist's eyes now water, while focusing on Rayna) I can see that you do. I'm glad.

Rayna: (Notices the therapist's eyes and her face further softens and there is a bit of yearning in her voice) When will she be here?

Therapist: Tomorrow *(Gently, with even more empathy for Rayna who now looks much younger than her 11 years, with even greater vulnerability than before)* I think that you've been missing a mom all your life. *(Rayna now seeing a hint of a tear in the therapist's eye, begins to cry)*

The story about Rayna's history with her two mothers and the lack of a mother in the orphanage was, in fact, a conversation, even though Rayna did not say a word. As the story developed, Rayna responded to it nonverbally: Rayna became quieter and her face became more pensive and then softer. In reciprocation, as the therapist spoke, Rayna's nonverbal responses had an influence on the therapist too. In real time, the therapist altered the nature of how the story developed – both nonverbally and verbally.

In summary

DDP encourages the child and therapist to enter and maintain states of attuned rhythmic reciprocity. These sustained experiences will include the nonverbal, as well as rhythmic conversations (a–r dialogues). These therapeutically contained conversations enable safe exploration of events characterized by shame and terror. All traumatic experiences are welcomed by PACE. In this context, trauma narratives become safe and malleable – together the child, carer, and therapist re-write these narratives giving them new meaning. And then, when comfort and joy emerge within the reciprocal communications, there remains little reason to continue therapy. At that point, the child and caregiver are likely to move forward within the fullness of their relationship. Certainly there will be messy moments in the days ahead when the lingering impact of trauma is evident. Yet there are messy moments in all intimate relationships. But with a commitment to evoking reciprocal engagement in the present moment, the healing power of the relationship is likely to bring the child home.

References

Malloch, S. and Trevarthen, C. (2010) 'Musicality: Communicating the Vitality and Interests of Life.' In S. Malloch and C. Trevarthen (eds) *Communicative Musicality: Exploring the Basis of Human Companionship.* Oxford: Oxford University Press.

Porges, S.W. (2007) 'The polyvagal perspective.' *Biological Psychology 74,* 116–143.

Porges, S.W. (2011) *The Polyvagal Theory: Neurophysiological Foundations of Emotions, Attachment, Communication, and Self-regulation.* New York: W.W. Norton.

Stern, D.N. (2004) *The First Relationship: Infant and Mother.* Cambridge, MA: Harvard University Press.

Stern, D.N. (2010) *Forms of Vitality: Exploring Dynamic Experience in Psychology, the Arts, Psychotherapy, and Development.* Oxford: Oxford University Press.

Tronick, E. (2007) *The Neurobehavioral and Social–Emotional Development of Infants and Children.* New York: W.W. Norton.

6

FROM COCOON TO BUTTERFLY

Music Therapy with an Adopted Girl

COCHAVIT ELEFANT

Noa was two and a half years old when I first met her: a beautiful, lively girl with long dark hair and wide open brown eyes. She was brought to music therapy by her adopted mother with the complaint that Noa was hitting, biting and pushing children at her nursery school. Noa had lived in several foster homes from the time she was two weeks old until she was nine months, when she was finally adopted. Her biological mother and Noa stayed together in a foster family but, after a few weeks, her mother ran away with Noa. Soon after, they were assigned to a new foster family to assist the mother in raising Noa. However, when it was evident that she couldn't care for her baby, it was decided to take Noa away from her biological mother and Noa continued to stay in foster care. At age six months the father in the foster family became ill and Noa was moved to yet another foster family that adopted her at age nine months. The hardship in her short life could have ended at that point. However, two months after the adoption, her adopted parents divorced and the father left the home.

From this brief history we can assume that attachment and detachment were themes in young Noa's life. Noa's security in her basic attachment bond to her mother will have been severely shaken and compromised. Her impulse and ability to attach to new carers (the various foster carers along the way) will have been worn down over time and through challenging experience. Her innate impulse to reach out to connect through healthy interpersonal rhythms – to feel connected, to fulfil her need for emotional learning – may have faded. She may have learnt to defend herself from emotional uncertainty, probably becoming more guarded and less open to others. She will have become less naturally social, interacting with others as objects of suspicion *just* as she was treated as an object, being moved from one place to the next.

This chapter will describe two and a half years of music therapy process with Noa. It will be illuminated by examples from our 45-minute-long weekly sessions. These examples illustrate stages along the way, as our relationship was slowly woven through musical and verbal interplay and communication. We will explore intricate movements in physical, emotional and musical space and regulation; from total distance (both physical and musical), to closeness; from chaos and turmoil, to self-control and responsibility. I will attempt to connect psychological process and musical nurturing, by carefully utilizing various musical elements and nuances (tempo, rhythm, dynamic, melody, harmony, timbre and form) within vocalization and playing. We will see how these changes took form in the therapeutic process.

Beginning

Noa, two and a half years old, enters the music therapy room with confidence. She says goodbye to her mother and begins to explore the room.

The first session was mostly chaotic and disorganized. Noa went from one instrument to the other, throwing everything that came to hand. She went to a bowl full of mandarins and began throwing them at me while laughing. I began picking up the fruits, putting them in the bowl while singing:

In the bowl, in the bowl,
in the bowl we put the mandarins.
All the mandarins are now in the bowl and
the bowl goes on the shelf.

Noa was surprised by my reaction and began singing:

Yes, all the mandarins are back in the bowl
and we put them on the shelf,
and we put them on the shelf!

This little scene of throwing mandarins came as quite a surprise to me. However, instead of reacting with, 'No, we don't throw mandarins' (thus emphasizing the 'bad behaviour'), I began organizing the event, provided a frame, which in turn gave internal and external borders. The singing provided a natural structure and organization, with clear repetitive phrases that contained binary words (in the *bowl*; on the *shelf*). For each rhythmic phrase, Noa seemed to make a small body movement on each accent. Noa, who was surprised by my response, went along with me, imitating the song. For the next session I made sure there were no objects around that Noa could destroy or break.

Drake (2011) describes her experiences in the early sessions with adopted children and discusses how their behaviour 'can appear unregulated and erratic and they may present with heightened anxiety. This may be evident through avoidant, controlling or withdrawn behaviours' (p.22).

This was quite true in Noa's case. During the first sessions she was busy exploring the instruments, moving from one to the other while asking me, 'What is this? What is this? How do you use it?' She wanted me to name each instrument and show her what it does and how to play it. She did not, however, want me to play the piano or the guitar. She only 'allowed' me to improvise singing when I was describing what she was doing. Reflecting each of her movements every time she picked up an instrument, I described her actions and facial expressions through my song. If I stopped, she asked me to continue my descriptions.

Physical and musical space

Noa ordered me to sit as far away as possible from her (the farthest end of the room), while she was exploring the instruments. There was no eye contact between us. I began reflecting, through my singing, a simple description of what she was doing.

> Reflecting the person's words or feeling state [or actions] allows the client
> to stay in the moment and explore it more fully. In many respects this is
> a unique aspect of therapy – we allow clients the time to uncover feelings
> at a pace that is comfortable for them. (Grocke and Wigram 2007, p.31)

However, whilst reflecting, my singing during this period was quite emotionally detached, without much expression or emotionality. My physical and emotional distance felt appropriate. It felt as though this was the level of interaction Noa could currently handle. And so, I attempted to meet Noa's needs and abilities in her self-exploration process as *she* expressed them to me, telling me exactly what she could contain at that period in our relationship.

In a later session Noa found a box full of pictures representing children's songs. She tossed all the cards on the floor. My singing reaction was to the tune of 'London bridge':

> *Oh, oh, all the cards are on the floor*
> *on the floor, on the floor*
> *All the cards are on the floor,*
> *out of the box.*

She asked me to pick up the cards and put them in the box as she began singing to the same tune:

We are putting all the cards in the box, in the box
We are putting all the cards in the box.
They are no longer on the floor, on the floor
Now they're in the box.

She then asked me to sit far away, as she once more tossed all the cards, and I sang:

Oh, oh, all the cards are on the floor, on the floor, on the floor
All the cards are on the floor, out of the box.

The tossing and picking the cards was repeated about five times. Then Noa began picking one card at a time, putting them back into the box. I began singing the song represented by each card, as she picked it up, but as soon as she put the card in the box, I stopped singing. She looked surprised and smiled when she realized what had occurred. Noa felt the potential for control. She continued picking up one card at a time, now with control over how short or how long I was supposed to sing the song. She waited with anticipation for my singing to stop as each card entered the box. We were totally synchronized, our cycles of shared rhythm coming to a natural crescendo as Noa put the card in the box.

Noa was at the beginning of her self-exploration. She was experiencing the sense of her emergent self, 'experiencing being alive while encountering the world' (Stern 2000, p.22). As I synchronized myself to her movement and mirrored her actions in my singing, she was able to see herself in my performance. This synchronous mirroring, over time and many iterations, will help Noa to learn about herself and others (Bruscia 1987; Wigram 2004).

She then lifted the card representing the 'Bee song'[1] and I began singing it. She held the card with the picture of the bee while I sang the whole song. At the end of the song, Noa said, 'Again'. I sang the whole song one more time and she said, 'Again'.

I would like to explain what happened during this song. The first time I sang Noa the song, I sang it in a steady, quite fast tempo with moderate dynamic. I did not employ any emotional or musical attunement. It was sung with restrained musicality and emotional distance, just like our physical distance. Then Noa began to reduce that emotional distance. Her intrigued energy – communicated in her body positioning, tone and expression – led me to respond by singing the song again, but this time singing it a bit slower and extending

---

1   The 'Bee song' is a famous children's song: 'I'm bringing home a baby bumble bee, won't my mummy be so proud of me. I'm bringing home a baby bumble bee, oops the bee stung me.' The song can be extended by adding 'bzzzz, oops, the bee stung me, bzzz, bzzz, oops the bee stung you'.

the ending by adding the 'bzzz' part to the song. Now I was using 'attunement' to simultaneously communicate and connect with Noa's emotional state. Stern (2010b, p.42) defined 'attunement' as, 'matching and sharing dynamic forms of vitality, but across different modalities'. Then Noa asked for the song again, and I extended the song even further by adding two 'bzzzz' parts. I sang the song with attunement and greater emotionality and she began to anticipate the 'bzzz' and the 'oops' in the song, asking me to sing it again and again.

Our synchronized interaction took another step forward as Noa allowed me to 'play' with the song by expanding the ending sequence. She was able to contain the fine changes and the associated emotional tension, as she now had safety and enough predictability in her experience of the song's basic structure. Daniel Stern used the term vitality affects (Stern 2000) to describe the temporal contour of energetic experience as it arises. Vitality affects comprise narrative structured patterns that involve heightening excitement with an ending in resolution. The experience of sharing vitality in a synchronous temporal structure, over a moment of time, gives mothers and infants a sense of meeting. Stern (2000, 2010a) describes an example in which a mother is playing with her infant, suspending each time the end moment in which she will 'get him' and tickle him. They interact through a play of temporal variations that regulates the infant's state, and as the mom tickles him the game resolves and the dyad shares a unique moment. Similarly, we can see vitality affect in our improvisation which occurred within the clear structure of musical phrases – Noa allowed and enjoyed the anticipation of climax, acquiring meaningful and safe experiences of, and for, constructing her self-with-others (Stern 2000). This made for a potential growth of intimacy as a result of these encounters.

At one stage I tried singing a new song, but Noa shouted, 'NO, the Bee song'. I responded accordingly and continued with the Bee. However, after about ten times of singing the Bee song, she showed me a new song card. Slowly, Noa began requesting different songs and I sang them now, with greater degrees of emotional and musical attunement. Noa could tolerate this (and enjoy the connection) if, at the same time, I continued to maintain my physical distance. Her self-regulatory capacity progressed as she was able to receive and react more and more to my actions (Trevarthen 1980). It was evident in the change of the dynamic forms of our music that an intersubjective relationship was forming (Pavlicevic 1997).

In one of the sessions Noa held all the mallets she could find in the room (about ten of them). She held them tightly and began walking around the room. I picked up the tempo and quality of her walking, which sounded to me like a march, and began playing and singing it on the piano, accentuating each word:

Noa is marching with the mallets, with the mallets with the mallets
Look at her while she's marching with the mallets, with the mallets.

Noa began shouting, 'No, no!' I continued to play and sing, 'No, no! No, no! You don't want me to sing while you are marching!'

All of a sudden, Noa approached the piano and bit me. I asked her, 'Did you bite me?' Noa: 'Yes, it's your fault!' She then continued marching around the room with the mallets telling me to continue to play.

Young children are music listeners, and can be sensitive to musical changes even between octaves, harmony or simple frequency ratio (Trehub, Schellenberg and Hill 1997). Accordingly, in mother–infant interactions, each change in the form and/or pattern of the temporal shifts of sound intensity can have its own emotional reaction (Stern 1996). In our interaction, my music elucidated with intensity Noa's acts, words and movements. Noa was faced with a multisensory mirror – one that could illicit strong self-regulatory reactions.

The biting was the first close physical contact that occurred between us. Although I was quite surprised and puzzled, I did not react with a strong emotional reaction. I contemplated whether my playing was too dominant and was too much for her to handle, although after she had bit me she *did* want me to continue to play.

It could be that Noa wanted something else from me, something unknown to me when she said 'NO, no!' – something she was not able to explain in words. And possibly when I in return imitated the 'No, no!' I triggered her frustration. The reason I continued playing throughout was that I believed our communication could continue and be supported through the playing and singing. I amplified Noa by singing: 'No, no! No, no! You don't want me to sing while you are marching!' This amplification would help her in her self-awareness and show Noa that I was always alongside her. I did not set a specific boundary around hurting/biting, etc. at this stage in Noa's therapy. I felt quite safe and felt that our delicate and intricate work of building borders should grow from within rather than from external limit setting. I did, however, ask Noa if she had bitten me, as I thought it was important to acknowledge that the biting came from her.

When Noa was done marching, she came to the piano and began playing on it with a rubber-head mallet. Previously, Noa had needed to keep a physical and musical distance between us. In the marching section she seemed to be exploring that distance, testing out my reactions and feeling for where her trust lay. As she approached the piano with her rubber-head mallet she seemed to be expressing a new level of trust in my ability to keep her safe. She stayed beside me at the piano.

I held the mallet (together with her), leading her on the piano while forming a melody. It seemed that the mallet represented an extension of her fingers, or a kind of an 'intentional object' (Stern 2000). The mallet was more than an extension; it enabled a safe distance from any potentially overwhelming direct experience on her skin. Through it, Noa safely continued to experience her emerging self – receiving body inputs, symbolizing, touching and creating.

I began improvising on the piano, a quiet melody, and she asked me to stop playing. It seemed that any move to generate my own input was still unwelcome. It had to be exactly as she wished. As long as I was synchronized with her, moving the mallet with her, she felt comfortable. But as soon as I initiated my own melody, this level of separation was felt by Noa as uncomfortable.

Towards separation (and so into relationship)

With her family history, Noa may have experienced disrupted, confusing interactions with the adults in her life. The usual consistent experiences which lead to strong, safe attachment bonds with caregivers may not have been available for Noa. She may never have felt consistently in sync with a caring adult. She may not have felt connected or 'held' rhythmically, emotionally – not enough anyway. Within the music therapy room Noa was beginning to experience that connectedness. And once Noa was safe enough to open to elements of the attachment experience, to allow herself to feel in sync and connected to me, she needed to experience this over and over again.

Next, I will move on to describe the beginnings of Noa's explorations into psychological separation (the development of her sense of autonomous self). It is important to note two things about this progress. First, Noa's separation needed to be proceeded and underpinned by many experiences of connectedness. An infant has to feel contained in the rhythm of her caregiver before developing the confidence to reach out to explore the world as a separate being. Second, this progress towards separation is never linear. Noa's forays into separation developed alongside a deepening of her connectedness. She would always need the base of attachment experience from which to explore.

In a later session Noa was again playing with the rubber-head mallets. Noa picked up all the mallets and one fell down. I reacted by saying, 'Oh, oh!' Noa laughed and threw another mallet on the floor and waited for my 'Oh, oh' reaction. This was repeated several times. Each time, when I added the 'Oh, oh', I would make it more dramatic with a wider melodic and dynamic range. The more I accentuated the second note, the more Noa laughed. I asked her if the mallets were falling by themselves or if she was throwing them? She replied, 'I am throwing them.' This was the first time Noa took real responsibility for her action. She was beginning to view herself separately from me.

This first incident in which Noa took responsibility for her action (identifying her role and control over it) can be seen to have occurred within a universal game structure, the game of 'Fort-Da'.[2] The term Fort-Da describes any game

---

2   Freud (1955) coined this word 'Fort-Da', meaning 'Here-There', when he noticed the joy his baby grandson showed watching the movement of a yoyo in front of his face.

in which the baby throws an object back and forth, noting when it is gone and is returned. Freud (1955) used this game to explain the notion of pleasure, suggesting that pleasure was derived from a sense of empowerment related to the mastery of task, other people and reality. In our game Noa explored the mastery of her 'gone' act, and received a musical reaction 'back' as she saw the mallets on the floor. This interaction was a progression from our base of synchronization as she took responsibility and identified herself.

For Noa, her emerging sense of psychological separation was occurring within a safe environment. When this is the case, a child's flourishing sense of autonomy will naturally lead her to play more confidently with psychological distance, to test and develop trust, to explore and take risks in relationship. In other words, we need to be individual before we can truly be in relationship.

A little later on in our sessions, Noa began to hide in the room, asking me to find her. The first time she hid, I sang, 'Where is Noa, where is Noa?' She came out from hiding and laughed. This game was repeated several times and became longer as I expanded on the singing, 'Where is Noa, where is Noa? Maybe she is in the piano? Maybe in the closet? Maybe she left the room? Oh, what will I do, I can't find her.' Not only did it become more tolerable for Noa to disappear for a longer time, it also became evident that she was becoming able to give me more control through a musical structure. When I found Noa, I sang out loud, 'Here you are. I finally found you.' She asked me to sit far away while she was hiding and was especially happy when I called out her name in a worried intonation, 'Noa, Noa.' She replied immediately, 'But I am here, don't worry, I didn't go away.' In a safe, exciting context (defined by the shared musicality of our relationship) Noa was testing my consistency and reliability – would I always find her, would I always care enough to try? She was internalizing a sense of safety and consistency in relationship through experiencing the care in my musical, emotional and practical response.

Noa's story unfolding

In a development of the Fort-Da game with the rubber-head mallets, Noa spontaneously began to organize the mallets in a row saying, 'One for Noa, one for Cookie, one for Ron [her brother] and one for my mother.' Noa did not mention her older brother, who had special needs, nor her father. When I asked about them, she said that they are 'gone far away'. At this point, I decided not to ask any leading questions to explore this further. Noa's disclosure felt fragile, tentative and premature. Instead I marked this moment as a 'sign' and decided to see if this topic would reappear later. I trusted the slow process in therapy and believed that Noa would come back to her family later, and throughout her sessions – she did. This was the beginning. Noa went on to explore herself in relation to me and the meaningful others in her life. Themes of safety and confidence would arise, together with acts of construction and destruction.

Developing subtleties of relationship: A balance of structure and spontaneity

A year into our music therapy, together Noa and I had found a new level of shared musical structure which enabled Noa to develop her confidence in exploration and improvisation. This more sophisticated improvisational process became a vehicle for Noa to develop her social skills and engage in subtleties of relationship.

In one session I showed Noa how to play the kazoo. The kazoo can be an extension of our voice. It is a fun, emotive extension that can be likened to the babbling and playful sounds a baby will often explore in her pre-verbal developmental stage. Spontaneously, a dialogue began between us. At first the sounds were disorganized with no clear regulation, but slowly, as I began imitating her playing, her phrases became longer and more expressive. A basic musical structure – with an underlying beat, tempo and pulse of turn-taking – can hold a vulnerable child as she explores relationship and emotion in improvisation. Here, a balance between structure and measured unpredictability is so often essential. Together, Noa and I explored the subtleties of joint attention, turn-taking, collaborative intentionality and shared meaning making. We felt connected, in sync and happy. There was a lot of eye contact between us, and laughter and more freedom than ever. And all with a kazoo!

Intimacy

Noa had found safety and spontaneity in the structure of our musical play. The temporal framing, and the predictable emotional narrative (the vitality affect) of each iteration of play enabled Noa to improvise and explore with confidence. Noa now brought this sophisticated balance between structure and spontaneity into her physical play, enabling exploration of intimacy for the first time.

Noa took out all the kazoos from the instrument box (ten in all) and put them on her fingers. She began singing a well-known children's song about ten fingers. She asked me to put the kazoo on my fingers and I sang the song about the fingers. At the end of the song I walked my fingers towards her and tickled her. She seemed to like it. The following time, as I got close to her, she patted my glasses. I asked if she wanted me to take off my glasses and she replied, 'Yes'. I continued walking my fingers toward her slowly, while singing the finger song, and towards the end of each phrase of the song, I tickled her. We played through this pattern many times. Noa was able to tolerate the closeness when she could anticipate the tickling at the end of the phrase. Here Noa had the repetitious structure of each phrase of the game – the temporal patterning along with an energetic and emotional narrative – to hold her anxiety and help her anticipate what was to come.

Noa then asked me to tickle her even more. I now used my hands, instead of the kazoo, to very gently tickle her. I tickled her legs, her stomach, her back and her arms. Out loud, I named the body parts while doing so. She came very close to me and lay on my lap, took my glasses off my face and looked straight into my eyes. She began playing with my face, trying to put her small hands in my mouth and nostrils. She played with my hair. I sang softly as she played in this way, singing about the things she was doing. Then I tried a playful development of this interaction. I began pointing at different parts of Noa, while singing, 'Here is Noa's nose, your beautiful little nose. Here is Noa's mouth, your beautiful little mouth. Here are Noa's eyes, your beautiful brown big eyes, etc.' Noa asked me to repeat the song over and over again. She was engaged, connected and secure enough to hand over control of the game. Her body became totally relaxed as her breathing became deeper and slower. The reflexive, embodied nature of the joint attention integral to this experience helped Noa build her boundaries between self and other; helped her to begin to shape her body scheme and structure.

In the following session, Noa told me that her leg was hurting and asked me to take care of her. I said that of course I would take care of her. She lay on my lap and asked me to tell her that I would take care of 'all of her'. I began singing that I would take care of her legs, of her arms, of her tummy, of her nose, etc. But then she began to pinch me. I explained that she was hurting me, which led onto the following interaction.

Me: Would you like me to watch over you so you don't hurt me?

Noa: Yes, I want you to take care of me. You, Cookie bite me and hit me.

Me: Did I bite you?

Noa: Yes!

Me: And I hurt you?

Noa: Yes!

Me: And I hit you and scratched you? All this I did to you? So what do you need to tell me?

Noa: That it hurts me.

For the first time (possibly ever) Noa felt safe enough to make a clear statement about the pain that had marked her young life. This was hugely significant.

Noa then lay on the floor and covered her face with her arms and asked, 'Where am I? Where am I?' She laughed and hid her face again. Then she covered my face with a scarf and I asked, 'Where am I? Where am I?' Noa suggested that we hide together and gave me a big hug. Her invitation to hide together was an important step in our relationship.

Midway

During our second year of music therapy Noa began playing the instruments, rather than only exploring them. She began putting the bells around her arms and legs, dancing freely around the room with the music while singing the songs. She also let me play the piano whilst she moved back and forth from watching herself in a mirror, to coming close up to me with a big smile, to back to the mirror again.

The sessions were rich with music making. Noa now had a clear sense of her self in relationship with other – there was Noa and there was me. We had separate voices that at times could merge, and in that merge, Noa no longer worried that she would disappear. There was a lot of freedom, vitality, and it seemed that Noa had emerged into an independent person.

Noa's growing capacity as an independent, confident child was evident in her wider life. Noa was much calmer in the nursery school and had stopped hitting and biting. She was playing with the other children and had become quite popular. She was now able to accept and live positively with the separation of her parents within her adopted family. During her first year of therapy, Noa lived with her adopted mother – never staying overnight with her adopted father. Noa's adopted parents separated only a few months after she was adopted. The divorce was a mutual agreement and the father moved within a walking distance from the family. The adopted parents had shared responsibility for the children although the older brother stayed more often with the father.[3] In that first year, Noa liked being with her father as long as they stayed in her mother's home. This may have been due to her difficulty in accepting changes, difficulty leaving her secure surrounding. Now, into her second year of therapy, Noa was happy to stay overnight with her adopted father – in fact, she couldn't wait to spend more time with him.

Increasingly, Noa included all these meaningful characters from her life in her therapeutic process, a process in which she now took the lead.

---

3   Here, we get a little more insight into Noa's earlier statement about her brother and father having 'gone far away' (see 'Noa's story unfolding' above).

Symbolism and ending

Noa began to play with some of the dolls and other toys in the room. She organized all the dolls in rows and said that she was making a show and everyone needed to watch her while she was singing and dancing. For several sessions she performed her dancing and singing in front of me and the audience of dolls.

Noa's play with the dolls and toys then began to take on more of a symbolic quality. She began to tell stories. She dictated each story and asked me to put music to it.

In one example Noa used five dolls along with clear rhythmical patterns and melodic lines to create a story:

Noa: Here is a man, ah, ah, ah and here is a woman, ah, ah, ah. *(I repeated the exact line. I then continued)*

Me: Here is a man and a woman, ah, ah, ah. Here is their boy, ah, ah, ah.

Noa: Here is their girl, ah, ah, ah.

Me: Yes, the woman and the man have a very sweet girl and a boy, ah, ah, ah.

Noa: But they also have one more boy, la, la, la, la.

Me: The mother and the father, the girl and two boys.

Noa: They are one big family. They are all together. The mother plays with the girl and the boys and then the father plays with them.

After this session Noa's mother told me excitedly that Noa had said the following to her, 'My brother Ron came out of your tummy, my brother Ben came also out of your tummy. I came out from another mummy's tummy, but you are my *real* mother.' Needless to say how surprised and happy the mother was and no one could have worded it in a better way than Noa. The mother felt that from a cocoon Noa had become a beautiful butterfly.

Epilogue

A few weeks after our sessions had ended, and I had left for another country, I received an email from Noa's mother suggesting that Noa would like to meet me in a café when I next came to visit. We met in a café two months after I had left. Noa was five and a half. She told me about her new kindergarten and about her friends. She asked if she could meet me in the clinic to play and sing next time I came. I agreed to that and we set a date for almost two months later. We met in the clinic, played and sang. At the end of the session Noa said, 'Next time you come, I won't need to meet you, only talk to you on the phone.' And so it was. We had a long phone conversation almost two months later in which she said, 'I don't need to talk to you again, but I will send you pictures.'

References

Bruscia, K.E. (1987) *Improvisational Models of Music Therapy.* Springfield, IL: Charles C. Thomas Publications.

Drake, T. (2011) 'Becoming In Tune: The Use of Music Therapy to Assist the Developing Bond between Traumatized Children and Their New Adoptive Parents.' In J. Edwards (ed.) *Music Therapy and Parent–Infant Bonding.* Oxford: Oxford University Press.

Freud, S. (1955) 'Beyond the Pleasure Principle.' In J. Strachey (ed.) *The Standard Edition of the Complete Psychological Works of Sigmund Freud.* London: Hogarth Press.

Grocke, D. and Wigram, T. (2007) *Receptive Methods in Music Therapy: Techniques and Clinical Applications for Music Therapy Clinicians, Educators and Students.* London: Jessica Kingsley Publishers.

Pavlicevic, M. (1997) *Music Therapy in Context: Music, Meaning and Relationship.* London: Jessica Kingsley Publishers.

Stern, D.N. (1996) 'Temporal Aspects of an Infant's Daily Experience: Some Reflections Concerning Music.' Paper presented at the 2nd International Congress of the World Federation of Music Therapy, Hamburg, Germany, July 18, 1996.

Stern, D.N. (2000) *The Interpersonal World of the Infant.* New York: Basic Books.

Stern, D.N. (2010a) 'The issue of vitality.' *Nordic Journal of Music Therapy 19*, 2, 88–102.

Stern, D.N. (2010b) *Forms of Vitality: Exploring Dynamic Experience in Psychology, the Arts, Psychotherapy, and Development.* Oxford: Oxford University Press.

Trehub, S.E., Schellenberg, E.G. and Hill, D.S. (1997) 'The Origins of Music Perception and Cognition: A Developmental Perspective.' In I. Deliège and J. Sloboda (eds) *Perception and Cognition of Music.* Hove, East Sussex: Psychology Press.

Trevarthen, C. (1980) 'The Foundation of Intersubjectivity: Development of Interpersonal and Co-operative Understanding in Infants.' In D. Olson (ed.) *The Social Foundations of Language and Thought: Essays in Honor of J.S. Bruner.* New York: W.W. Norton.

Wigram, T. (2004) *Improvisation: Methods and Techniques for Music Therapy Clinicians, Educators and Students.* London: Jessica Kingsley Publishers.

7

PLAY AND THE DYNAMICS OF TREATING PEDIATRIC MEDICAL TRAUMA

Insights from Polyvagal Theory

STEPHEN PORGES AND STUART DANIEL

Kal and his polar bear

Kal was curled in the far corner of his hospital bed. His body was emaciated. He was six years old and suffering from every aspect of an especially nasty cancer. A few days earlier Kal had received an injection as part of a particular treatment procedure. Crying and fighting, Kal had been physically restrained by his mother and two nurses. Since that procedure Kal had refused to talk, make eye contact with anyone, or eat. His blood count was dangerously low.

Clare, the oncology psychologist, sat near Kal as he lay in bed. She introduced herself in a gentle voice and then sat quietly with Kal for a while. Clare tried a few playful initiations and, when Kal displayed a lack of interest, she used her melodic storyteller's voice to acknowledge this and lightheartedly 'tell herself off'. Kal smiled a tiny smile. Clare then told a little story out loud of what Kal might be feeling. She used large emotional gestures, sighs, and her rhythmical voice to accompany the words of this story. Kal was actively listening now.

'Hey Kal, I've brought something with me today, have a look at these...'

Clare took out a box containing a range of play figures and set it down on the hospital-bed tray.

'I wonder if you could choose one?'

Kal said nothing. But he looked at Clare for the first time, his eyes a little interested, a little hopeful.

'How's about I start…' Clare said, 'maybe this one, and maybe right here in the middle…'

Clare placed a tiny knight in the center of the tray. She looked at Kal. Kal was now shaking his head vigorously. He had half sat up from his prone position.

Clare admonished herself mockingly, 'Oh, I've got it wrong (*big sigh*)… You know I think I left my brain at home today… Kal, can you knock on my head to see if my brain is in there?'

Kal did.

They both laughed and Clare continued, 'Yep, no brain… I am really going to need you to help me.'

Kal swapped the tiny knight for huge polar bear. From this point on Kal started to talk. He talked about what he was doing as he developed a complex play configuration with many characters. From these moments of shared emotional state, Kal moved into a powerful therapy process. Kal continued to speak, and eat, from that day on.

Systems of safety: Introducing the Polyvagal Theory

This chapter introduces the Polyvagal Theory (Porges 1995, 2001, 2007, 2009, 2011), an innovative model that explores how human evolution has linked social behavior and health to the mechanisms which mediate our feelings of safety or danger. The Polyvagal Theory will be outlined and then used in an exploration of human connection, safety, trauma, and the potential healing power of play. Polyvagal Theory helps us understand how cues of risk and safety, which are continuously monitored by our nervous system, influence our physiological and behavioral states. The theory emphasizes that humans are on a quest to calm neural defense systems by detecting features of safety. This quest is initiated at birth when an infant's need to be soothed is dependent on the caregiver. This quest forms the motivation to develop social relationships that enable individuals to effectively co-regulate each other. The quest continues throughout the lifespan with emerging needs for trusting friendships and loving partnerships.

Polyvagal Theory describes a three-tiered hierarchy of survival-oriented adaptive strategies: the Social Engagement System, the Mobilization System, and the Immobilization System.

We look first at the Social Engagement System. Without cognitive awareness, our nervous system continuously scans the environment for features of danger or safety. This 'reflexive' process we refer to as *neuroception*. The term neuroception is used to contrast with classical notions of perception which, due to requiring cognitive awareness, result in a slower appraisal of risk. When there is a neuroception of safety, two important features are expressed. First, bodily state is regulated in an efficient manner to promote health, growth, and restoration (visceral homeostasis). This occurs when the influence of mammalian myelinated vagal motor pathways on the cardiac pacemaker increases. Increasing the influence of these vagal pathways slows heart rate, inhibits the fight–flight mechanisms of the sympathetic nervous system, dampens the stress response system of the hypothalamic–pituitary–adrenal (HPA) axis (e.g. cortisol) and reduces inflammatory reaction (e.g. cytokines). Second, through evolutionary processes, the brainstem nuclei that regulate the myelinated vagus were integrated with the nuclei that regulate the striated muscles of the face and head. This link enables a bidirectional coupling between spontaneous social engagement behaviors and bodily states. Thus, as mammals evolved, an integrated Social Engagement System emerged that not only expressed physiological state in facial expression and vocalizations, but also enabled social behavior to regulate physiological state. These concepts will be developed below (see 'The face-heart connection').

The human nervous system, similar to that of other mammals, evolved not solely for life in a safe environment but also to survive in dangerous and life-threatening contexts. On neuroception of risk, or when the Social Engagement System is compromised, the two more primitive neural circuits regulating physiological state may be recruited to support defensive strategies. The first of these is the Mobilization System, which orchestrates fight–flight behaviors, and the second is the evolutionary ancient Immobilization System (involving death feigning behaviors).

Central to the Polyvagal Theory is the conceptualization that these three survival-oriented strategies are dependent on a *parallel hierarchy* in the function of the three neural circuits in the autonomic nervous system. This hierarchical perspective is a defining feature of the Polyvagal Theory and is in contrast with the traditional perspective of the autonomic nervous system as a paired-antagonistic system: a model in which two subsystems, the sympathetic and parasympathetic nervous systems, have antagonistic functions (i.e. either activating or calming) on the same organ. In the Polyvagal hierarchy of adaptive responses, the newest circuit (the circuit which supports the Social Engagement System) is recruited first; if that circuit fails to provide safety, the older circuits are recruited sequentially to orchestrate defense responses (Mobilization then Immobilization). It is important to note that when these defense systems are recruited, the autonomic nervous system supports these survival related behaviors at the expense of health, growth, and restoration; social behavior, social communication, and visceral homeostasis are all incompatible with the neurophysiological states and behaviors promoted by the two defense systems.

The face–heart connection

In vertebrates, which are the phylogenetic ancestors of mammals, the vagus originates in a brainstem area known as the dorsal nucleus of the vagus. During the evolutionary transition from primitive ancient reptiles to mammals, a second vagal motor pathway emerged that originated in the nucleus ambiguus, a brainstem area ventral to the dorsal nucleus of the vagus. Although the vagal pathways originating in the nucleus ambiguus are the primary motor pathways regulating the heart, the nucleus ambiguus is also part of a brainstem column that regulates the striated muscles of the face and head. This evolutionary bootstrapping process allowed for integration between the myelinated vagus and the nuclei that regulate muscular control of the face and head: specifically the muscles controling facial expression, listening, and prosodic vocalizations. These emergent changes in neuroanatomy gave rise to a phylogenetically novel face–heart connection. The face–heart connection provided mammals with an ability to convey physiological state via facial expression and prosody (intonation of voice). This gave mammals, and subsequently humans, the potential to use social interactions to calm physiological state in others, through the facial expressions and vocalizations that form the core of social interactions. The face–heart connection enables humans to detect whether someone is in a calm physiological state and 'safe' to approach, or is in a highly mobilized and reactive physiological state during which engagement would be dangerous. The connection concurrently enables an individual to signal 'safety' through patterns of facial expression and vocal intonation, and potentially calm an agitated other to form a social relationship.

The face–heart connection is the crucial element of our Social Engagement System. The system detects and communicates bodily states and the intentions of behaviors. Social engagement behaviors by an adult are potentially capable of calming, eliciting spontaneous social behaviors, and down-regulating the stress responses (immediate and/or chronic) inherent in the two defense systems for a child.

The Social Engagement System is first expressed at birth when it is used to signal states of comfort and distress and to detect features of safety. For example, a mother's voice has the capacity to soothe her infant. As the infant listens to the mother's melodic vocalizations, 'feature' detectors in the infant's brain interpret the voice as reflecting the mother's state as calm and her presence as safe and supportive. This sequence is not learned, but an evolved adaptive process that enables social signals to regulate biobehavioral state. The sounds of the mother's vocalization signal safety, which is detected by higher brain structures. The higher brain structures dampen defense systems and facilitate the calming effect on the heart by ventral vagal influences. In parallel to this calming effect, the regulation of the muscles of the face and head are enhanced to enable reciprocal interactions between mother and infant. The reciprocal interactions function as a neural exercise between their Social Engagement Systems. The result is an infant–mother dyad that efficiently uses social communication to co-regulate, with both participants feeling calm and bonded. This neural exercise builds capacity for the infant to develop relations with others and to deal with state regulation challenges and disruptions through the lifespan. In all cultures, the presentation of prosodic acoustic stimulation, whether vocal or instrumental, is an effective strategy for signaling safety and calming infants. In our example above, Clare's use of melodic intonation was crucial for Kal to feel safe in relationship; her voice functioned to 'contain' Kal's emotional state.

The type of mutually modulated co-regulation of emotion described in the 'mother's voice' example occurs throughout all examples of healthy play; it is a defining feature of a healthy, playful relationship (Porges 2015; Stern 2004; Trevarthen 2001). Early play, within the infant–adult dyad, is a functional dialog of co-regulation experienced over time. It is a story of shared rhythm (the 'pulse' of play) and of the experience of traveling through energetic and emotional contours together (Malloch and Trevarthen 2009; Stern 2010). The rhythms of reciprocity of play are defined primarily by synchronous changes in facial expression, quality of eye contact, touch (changing patterns of position, intention, and intensity of the body) and vocalization (changing patterns of rhythm, timbre, pitch, and volume in voice) (Malloch and Trevarthen 2009). Play is a flowing series of face–heart connections defined by essentially musical parameters.

Medical trauma and patterns of immobilization

The dynamics of childhood medical trauma may be described by two qualities: overwhelming fear and inescapability (either physical or perceived). Posttraumatic Stress Disorder (PTSD) is an increasingly recognized childhood response to the experience of cancer and cancer treatment (Phipps *et al.* 2005; Taïeb *et al.* 2003). Recent research by Graf, Bergstraesser, and Landolt (2013) on the prevalence of childhood PTSD (onset preschool) in cancer survivors showed that 18.8 per cent of subjects met the age-appropriate criteria for full PTSD proposed by Scheeringa and Zeanah (2005) and 41.7 per cent met the criteria for partial PTSD.

What are the experiences, unfortunately common within the story of cancer and cancer treatment, which disrupt a child's ability to regulate physiological state? Primarily, these include any frightening procedure which involves being physically restrained, and/or intense and immobilizing toxic/physical shock, but also potentially MRI scans with anaesthetic restraint (not including a general anaesthetic). Sadly, despite many intelligent child-friendly hospital protocols, physical restraint continues to be used on a daily basis in most paediatric oncology wards. Studies by Diseth (2005) illustrate that children forced to undergo medical procedures, particularly in the context of their families holding them down, presented with significantly more dissociation than children treated less invasively. In our example above, Kal was repeatedly physically restrained for frightening procedures. It was one such experience that pushed him into what could have easily become a chronic trauma pattern. The following quote is from a mother I worked with, Angie, describing her son's early experiences on an oncology ward:

> Initially Kieran appeared unaware of hospital visits, other than the effect my own stress would undoubtedly have had on him. He first started to show recognition around 5–6 months old, he was very scared of strangers and would openly react to a 'blue' nurses' uniform, becoming very distressed and anxious. Kieran was 8 months old when I first witnessed his complete 'shutting down'. At the time he was a happy, chatty, lively little boy who was cruising round the furniture and didn't stay still for more than a few moments. We arrived at clinic at 10am and the instant we walked through the doors Kieran stopped moving, he kept his head dropped, making no eye contact or sounds at all. He stayed this way for about 5 hours until he went in for his examination under anesthetic, literally not moving or reacting to myself or his Grandma in any way. It was completely heart-breaking to see my son so broken.

The behavioral 'shut-down' that Angie describes above, the psychological and social 'dissociation' described by Diseth (2005), and Kal's almost total withdrawal from interaction in our initial example can be explained by the triggering of the Immobilization System. The Immobilization Defense System is our body's phylogenetically ancient response to the detection of an inevitable and significant threat to physical integrity and/or imminent death. It is triggered by the co-occurrence of two factors: fear and inescapability, both registered pre-consciously via neuroception. The Immobilization Defense System recruits the unmyelinated vagal motor pathways to the heart to produce an immediate and massive slowing of heart rate (i.e. bradycardia) and often the cessation of breathing (i.e. apnea), and is often associated with vasovagal syncope (i.e. fainting). This massive shift in metabolic resources results in the organism appearing to be inanimate. This defense pattern is a primary defense strategy for many reptiles. Not moving and appearing inanimate is an adaptive response of reptiles to avoid detection by a predator. This reaction is metabolically conservative, rapidly withdrawing resources from the highly oxygen-dependent central nervous system. Once activated the Immobilization Defense System may involve feigning death, behavioral shutdown, and dissociation. As mentioned above, once the Immobilization Defense System is triggered, it produces a physiological state that is incompatible with a functioning Social Engagement System. Once the Immobilization System is reflexively employed, the Social Engagement System is temporarily disabled, which immediately shuts down all coordinated regulation of prosocial behavior. A child being bombarded with shutdown cues will not perceive the environment as safe and will not have the ability to produce or accurately detect features of social communication.

For some children the initial immobilization experience becomes a chronic pattern. The process through which this occurs is not fully understood. Many of these unfortunate children develop partial or full childhood PTSD. Drell and colleagues (Drell *et al.* 1993) provide a clinical outline of the developmental progression of early PTSD signatures (summarized in Table 7.1).

Table 7.1 Symptoms of PTSD in children 0 to 36 months, based on Drell, Siegel and Gaensbauer (1993)

	0–6 months	6–12 months	12–18 months	18–24 months	24–36 months
Withdrawal and/or hypervigilance, exaggerated startle response, irritability, physiologic deregulation	★	★	★	★	★
Increased anxiety in strange situations, angry reactions, sleep disorders, active avoidance of specific situations		★	★	★	★
Clinginess to caretaker, over/under use of words related to the trauma			★	★	★
Nightmares, verbal preoccupation with symbols of trauma				★	★
PTSD symptoms seen in older children, as defined in the DSM-IVr					★

Play and co-regulation: Insights from Polyvagal Theory

From the perspective of the Polyvagal Theory, play can be seen functionally as a neural exercise in which social cues of safety and danger are alternately expressed and explored (Porges 2015). The ability to safely transition 'dangerous' states of disconnection – breaks in flowing emotional containment – is crucial to the development and internalization of a child's robust sense of self (Hughes 2004; Porges 2015; Schore 1994). During play, risks are taken, dangers are survived, and connections are repaired through co-regulation. As an example, we can think of the simple game 'peek-a-boo' that a mother may play with her infant. By hiding her face and removing the cues of safety normally generated by the Social Engagement System (prosodic voice, facial expressions), the mother is creating a state of uncertainty in the infant. This state of uncertainty is followed by the mother startling the infant by showing her face and saying 'peek-a-boo!' The sequence of the peek-a-boo game is ended when the mother uses a prosodic voice with warm facial expressions to calm the startled infant.

Deconstructing the behavioral sequence involved in peek-a-boo we see the neural exercise embedded in this play behavior. First, the initial hiding of the mother's face elicits a state of uncertainty and vigilance. This state is associated with a depression of the infant's Social Engagement System including a withdrawal of the myelinated vagal pathways to the heart. This puts the infant in a vulnerable state in which a 'startle' stimulus could easily recruit sympathetic activity to support mobilization (i.e. fight/flight behaviors). The mother provides the startle stimulus by showing her face and stating 'boo' in a relatively loud and monotonic voice. The acoustic features of the mother's vocalizations support the unpredictable presentation of the mother's face, since the vocalizations of 'boo' have acoustic features that are associated with danger and lack the prosodic features that would be calming. The cues of this sequence trigger a detection of danger, which recruits increased sympathetic activation. The next step in the sequence of this game provides the opportunity for a neural exercise that will promote resilience and enhance the infant's ability to calm.

After the infant is motorically and autonomically activated by the 'boo', the mother needs to calm the infant with her Social Engagement System using a prosodic voice with warm facial expressions. Her prosodic voice and warm facial expressions trigger a detection of safety. The infant calms as the Social Engagement System comes back online and the myelinated vagal pathways down-regulate the sympathetic activity. When effectively implemented, peek-a-boo provides opportunities for the infant to 'neurally navigate' through a sequence of states (i.e. from calm, to vigilant, to startle, and back to calm). Repeating this game provides opportunities for the Social Engagement System to efficiently down-regulate, via social interactions, sympathetic activation. The child will need this 'neural' skill to adapt throughout every aspect of life.

Building connections with traumatized children:
Polyvagal Theory informs therapeutic play

Tyler, who was nine years old at the time, was referred for play therapy with the following profile: social withdrawal punctuated by episodes of extreme anger and violence, hypervigilance, difficulty sleeping, difficulty making friends, problems at school and home. When Tyler was four he had been through an eighteen-month treatment for leukaemia. Like Kal, Tyler had been regularly physically restrained for certain medical procedures.

In his first session, Tyler *did* make it into the playroom. He sat on a little wooden chair near the window, doing tricks with his finger-board (a mini-skateboard he brought with him) on the window sill. He did this for an hour. The Polyvagal Theory provides a lens to understand Tyler's withdrawal behavior. At this point Tyler is likely to be experiencing one of two defensive states – immobilization or mobilization – or fluctuating between periods of both. Tyler could have a sense of generalized anxiety whilst also feeling disconnected from his emotional surrounding, experiencing dissociation. In this immobilized state his senses will be numbed, his thoughts ambiguous, his ability to detect and engage in a flowing interaction highly limited, and his motivation to socially interact would be non-existent. Or Tyler could be feeling highly mobilized with the necessary energy to flee or fight. Behaviorally, he might be easily triggered into anger and possibly violence. Although seemingly turned inwards, Tyler might be scanning every aspect and moment of his environment for cues of risk and danger. Internally, his heart rate might be elevated, his breathing shallow and rapid, his viscera, blood vessels, and muscle tone constricted, ready for action. In this hypervigilant and mobilized state Tyler is likely to perceive almost everything as a threat. The Polyvagal Theory explores why this might be the case. In the process of risk detection, external cues are not the only source of information. Afferent feedback from the viscera provides a major mediator of the accessibility of prosocial circuits associated with social engagement behaviors. Polyvagal Theory predicts that states of mobilization compromise the ability to detect positive social cues. Functionally, visceral states distort or color our perception of other people. Thus, the features of a person engaging another may result in a range of outcomes, depending on the physiological state of the target individual. If the person being engaged is in a state in which the Social Engagement System is easily accessible, a reciprocal prosocial interaction is likely to occur with the calming benefits of co-regulation. However, if the individual is in a state of mobilization, the same engaging response might be responded to with asocial features of withdrawal or aggression.

Sean, Tyler's play therapist, worked with the basic principles of non-directive play therapy as a foundation: acceptance, non-judgement, empathy, and emotional honesty (Landreth 2012). In that first session, Sean sometimes used whole-body gestures and empathic 'sighs' to accompany reflections like, 'Just not sure what it's all about in here' and 'Feeling kind of weird, what am I doing in here…?' After a while Tyler seemed to relax a little, his muscle tone dropped slightly, his play with the mini-board became a little less intense. Sean intuitively understood that the musicality – the rhythmic pulse, the contours of volume, and in particular the quality of intonation – in his voice was a crucial factor in helping Tyler feel safe and to stimulate Tyler's Social Engagement System. If in a state of partial immobilization, Tyler would probably respond to very little, but he would need the background tone to be playful, peaceful, and musical (never a monotone) to give him the best chance in engagement. If Tyler was in a mobilized state, hypervigilant to risk factors and prone to interpreting any stimulus as a threat, Sean would need to keep his voice melodic and avoid projecting low vocal frequencies; according to the Polyvagal Theory deep-sounding voices are signals of a predator and might trigger defense. If successful, Tyler's sympathetic nervous system would be down-regulated. In this 'safe' state, Tyler's innate prosocial ability would have an opportunity to be expressed in reciprocal and synchronous interactions promoting mutual feelings of connectedness between Tyler and Sean.

The ability to detect contour shifts in sound, especially in prosodic vocalization, is *usually* central to human connectedness through the healthy engagement of our Social Engagement Systems. But there are children for whom hearing is not accessible (profoundly deaf children) and children who have inherent difficulties with the particular emotional quality of human voice (e.g. children with autism and related disorders). Likewise, the visual exchange of information involving eye contact, facial expression, and hand gestures is *usually* central to play. These features functionally provide the pathways for co-regulation of physiological state, which optimize prosocial behavior and child development. Understanding the face–heart connection allows us to appreciate just how significant the human face is for co-regulation of emotion and biobehavioral states in support of psychological health. But there are many children for whom visual–facial information is not readily accessible; for instance, blind children and children with tendencies to avert their gaze, such as those with autism or related disorders. Somehow, we need to find ways to enable these children with experiences of safety, of flowing human connection, of healthy co-regulation within exploratory play. We need to do this without recourse to the regular sensory pathways of sight and sound that evolution efficiently selected to trigger our social engagement system (see Chapter 9 for a development of these ideas).

Conclusion

By deconstructing the play of mammals, whether we are observing kittens, dogs, or children in the playground, we see a common dynamic in social behavior – features of fight/flight are continually stimulated *and* actively inhibited by social engagement behaviors (e.g. facial expressions, gestures, prosodic vocalizations). Play is a natural and powerful therapeutic tool. From the Polyvagal perspective, play can be conceptualized as an efficient 'neural exercise' that uses social engagement to actively inhibit fight/flight behaviors. A sensitive adult can attune herself to a way of communicating which recruits a child's social engagement system and down-regulates defense. Therapists, who work actively through playful modes, consciously leverage this process. As illustrated in the clinical descriptions above, it is crucial that the therapist engenders a feeling of safety for the child via sensitive attunement. The experience of safety increases, in the child, the frequency of spontaneous reciprocal interactions. It is through these interactions that there is a resetting of the neuroceptive threshold from a defensive baseline to a robust sense of safety.

Frequently, children referred for therapy are in neurophysiological states that support mobilization, withdrawal, and shutdown. In these states, cognitive processes are greatly compromised and there is a loss in the awareness of the emotional states of others. Polyvagal Theory informs clinical practice that there is a neural circuit that can rapidly down-regulate mobilization behaviors to foster the calm states that optimize social behavior. Although play is frequently characterized by movement and often recruits many of the neural circuits involved in fight/flight behaviors, it may be operationally distinguished from defense, since during play mobilization is easily down-regulated by the social engagement system. However, the effectiveness and efficiency of the social engagement system to down-regulate fight/flight behaviors requires practice. Although this practice usually starts early in a child's development through play, trauma may disrupt the child's ability to feel safe and to exhibit spontaneous social engagement behaviors. Given this situation, similar to the clinical examples provided above, clinicians need to provide the child with unambiguous biological signals of safety through intonation of voice, facial expressions, and gestures. Moreover, once these signals effectively trigger a spontaneous engagement by the child, the intuitive therapist must be ready to respond with reciprocity. Reciprocal exchange of cues of safety, between therapist and child, function as playful neural exercise of the Social Engagement System: the mechanism that shifts mobilization from defense to play and trust. From a Polyvagal perspective this is the central objective of therapy.

References

Craig, A.D. (2002) 'How do you feel? Interoception: the sense of the physiological condition of the body.' *Nature Reviews Neuroscience 3*, 8, 655–666.

Diseth, T.H. (2005) 'Dissociation in children and adolescents as reaction to trauma – an overview of conceptual issues and neurobiological factors.' *Nordic Journal of Psychiatry 59*, 79–91.

Drell, M.J., Siegel, C. and Gaensbauer, T.J. (1993) 'Posttraumatic Stress Disorder.' In C.H. Zeanah (ed.) *Handbook of Infant Mental Health*. New York: Guilford Press.

Graf, A., Bergstraesser, E. and Landolt, M.A. (2013) 'Posttraumatic stress in infants and preschoolers with cancer.' *Psycho-Oncology 22*, 7, 1543–1548.

Hughes, D. (2004) 'An attachment-based treatment of maltreated children and young people.' *Attachment and Human Development 3*, 6, 263–278.

Landreth, G.L. (2012) *Play Therapy: The Art of the Relationship*. New York: Routledge.

Malloch, S. and Trevarthen, C. (2009) 'Musicality: Communicating the Vitality and Interests of Life.' In S. Malloch and C. Trevarthen (eds) *Communicative Musicality: Exploring the Basis of Human Companionship*. Oxford: Oxford University Press.

Phipps, S., Long, A., Hudson, M. and Rai, S.N. (2005) 'Symptoms of post-traumatic stress in children with cancer and their parents: effects of informant and time from diagnosis.' *Pediatric Blood and Cancer 45*, 952–959.

Porges, S.W. (1993) 'The infant's sixth sense: awareness and regulation of bodily processes.' *Zero to Three: Bulletin of the National Center for Clinical Infant Programs 14*, 12–16.

Porges, S.W. (1995) 'Orienting in a defensive world: mammalian modifications of our evolutionary heritage. A Polyvagal Theory.' *Psychophysiology 32*, 301–318.

Porges, S.W. (2001) 'The polyvagal theory: phylogenetic substrates of a social nervous system.' *International Journal of Psychophysiology 42*, 123–146.

Porges, S.W. (2007) 'The polyvagal perspective.' *Biological Psychology 74*, 116–143.

Porges, S.W. (2009) 'The polyvagal theory: new insights into adaptive reactions of the autonomic nervous system.' *Cleveland Clinic Journal of Medicine 76*, 86–90.

Porges, S.W. (2011) *The Polyvagal Theory: Neurophysiological Foundations of Emotions, Attachment, Communication, and Self-regulation*. New York: W.W. Norton.

Porges, S.W. (2015) 'Play as a Neural Exercise: Insights from the Polyvagal Theory.' In D. Pearce-McCall (ed.) *The Power of Play for Mind Brain Health*. Available from: http://mindgains.org

Scheeringa, M.S. and Zeanah, C.H. (2005) PTSD Semi-Structured Interview and Observational Record for Infants and Young Children. Department of Psychiatry and Neurology, Tulane University Health Sciences Center: New Orleans. (Note: Contains diagnostic algorithms since incorporated in the DSM-V).

Schore, A.N. (1994) *Affect Regulation and the Origin of the Self*. Hillsdale, NJ: Lawrence Erlbaum.

Stern, D.N. (2004) *The First Relationship: Infant and Mother*. Cambridge, MA: Harvard University Press.

Stern, D.N. (2010) *Forms of Vitality: Exploring Dynamic Experience in Psychology, the Arts, Psychotherapy, and Development*. Oxford: Oxford University Press.

Taïeb, O., Moro, M.R., Baubet, T., Revah-Lévy, A. and Flament, M.F. (2003) 'Posttraumatic stress symptoms after childhood cancer.' *European Child & Adolescent Psychiatry 12*, 255–264.

Trevarthen, C. (2001) 'Intrinsic motives for companionship in understanding: their origin, development and significance for infant mental health.' *Journal of Infant Mental Health 22*, 95–131.

8

SOMATIC EXPERIENCING®

A Body Oriented Approach to the Treatment of
Traumatized Infants and Children

PETER A. LEVINE

Consciousness has no more influence on our actions than a steam whistle has on
the locomotion of a train.

Thomas Huxley

Roger Sperry[1] (1952) made the distinct point that the fundamental basis of perception derives from motoric potentiality. It is through engaged movement that each infant generates a pre-verbal sense of 'body-self' – a sense of bounded self with agency and power (Bentzen, Jarlnaes and Levine 2004).

In experiments prompted by the 'Sperry Principle', Held and Hein (1963) asked their subjects to wear special prism goggles that made everything appear to be upside down. After some time (usually a week or two) the brain adapted such that the environment appeared to be normal (right side up) again. This occurred. however, *only* if the subjects were free to move about actively, touching and manipulating their environments. The subjects who were not allowed to move around and explore did not experience visual normalization. Similarly, infants or children who engage in successful motoric actions are able to 'renegotiate' experiences of terror, helplessness, and inescapability (Levine 2010; Payne, Levine and Crane-Godreau 2015).

The basis of an 'unconscious' readiness to act was demonstrated in a later landmark series of well replicated experiments conducted by Benjamin Libet[2] (1985, 1992, 1996). In a deceptively 'simple' experiment, Libet instructed his experimental subjects to move a finger 'at will'. However, based upon brain wave measurements he recorded electrical activity (in the pre-motor region) a full

---

1 Pioneering neurophysiologist and winner of the 1981 Nobel Prize for Physiology and Medicine.
2 Neurologist and neurosurgeon.

30 seconds before they were aware of deciding to move it. This research clearly demonstrated that motor action itself, and the sense of agency that comes along with it, depends on neurological events that 'we' (as in our conscious selves) do not control and that happen significantly *before* our conscious decision to act (i.e. before the awareness of our impulse to protect, defend, pursue, etc.).

The primacy of movement is essential in working with early and pre-verbal trauma. Motor patterns that have been thwarted, overwhelmed, or incomplete will color the entire perceptual field of the child and later the adult (Levine 2010, 2015). Hence, transmuting these thwarted motor actions can greatly alter the child's pre-reflective sense of self.

The essence of our core, pre-conscious 'body-self' is explored from an analytic and psychodynamic perspective by Krueger (1989). Krueger exemplifies an emerging view in developmental theory: that the core (pre-conscious) 'body-self' comprises an aggregate experience encompassing a wide range of (embodied) sensory, kinaesthetic, and proprioceptive input. Craig (2002, 2009, 2010) has shown how critical body sensations (interoception) are central to core regulation and, as such, to our sense of wellbeing.

Let us see how these principles can be put into action in the 'renegotiation' of a traumatic experience, from helplessness and overwhelm, to empowerment and agency. This physically sensed transformation is illustrated in the case of Jon, a 14-month-old, who suffered severe birth trauma and an abrupt separation from his mother along with invasive medical procedures. For Jon, this led to a subsequent failure to mold and attach to his mother. The second example is of Sammy, a two-and-a-half-year-old toddler, who had a terrifying emergency room visit after a bloody fall.

Baby Jon: A mother and child reunion

Jon is a bright and energetic toddler, yet at the same time painfully shy and reserved. He had been referred to me by a colleague because Jon had struggled through a very difficult birth and was presently contending with the sequelae to that ordeal. At 14 months old, Jon was now being evaluated for yet another invasive procedure: this time, to investigate a condition of intermittent gastric reflux. His mother, Erika, was dutifully following through with the pediatrician's recommendations and had scheduled an endoscopy for two weeks from the day of our first session. While she appreciated the pediatrician's thoroughness, Erika was hoping that there might be another solution, one that was not invasive and potentially traumatizing.

Jon had been in a breach position leading up to labor, with the umbilical cord wrapped three times around his neck while his head was caught high up in the apex of the uterus. Each push he directed with his tiny feet and legs drove his head into a tighter wedge, while further constricting the cinch around his throat. This was a 'no exit' ordeal evoking a primal strangulation terror, something that is difficult for most adults to comprehend (Macknik 2013). The doctors noted Jon's serious distress; his heart rate had dropped precipitously, indicating a potentially life-threatening situation and an emergency Cesarean section was performed. In addition to this, a forceful suctioning was required to dislodge Jon's head from the uterine apex. He was then whisked away from his mother. Jon's arrival into this world was accompanied by multiple clinicians poking and prodding him, plying their trade with the necessary needle sticks, IV insertions, aggressive examinations, and rushed interventions.

I saw Jon sitting astride his mother's hip as I opened the door and interrupted her second knock. She looked somewhat abashed as the follow-through on her rapping propelled her across the threshold and into my office. Regaining her composure and adjusting her son's position, she introduced Jon and herself. I countered by introducing myself to each of them as Peter and inviting them inside. As they moved through the entryway, I noticed a slight awkwardness in the shared balance of mother and son. I could have dismissed this as a general unease with a new environment, an unfamiliar stranger, and an unknown form of therapy. However, it seemed to be more fundamental than that; there was a basic discordance in their dyadic rhythm.

It is often assumed that when there is a disconnection between baby and mother, there has been a failure on the part of the caregiver to provide the 'good enough' environment required for bonding. This is not always true, and was clearly not the case with Erika. She earnestly and lovingly provided comfort, support, and attention. It was, rather, the traumatic birth that caused a jolt, splitting them apart at birth. The subsequent 'shock wave' disturbed their mutual capacity to participate in each other's most intimate moments, to fully bond and attach.

Following his gaze, I could see that Jon was intrigued with the colorful array of toys, musical instruments, dolls, and sculptures that were crowded onto the shelves above my table. I picked out a turquoise Hopi gourd rattle and began slowly shaking its seeds. Using the rhythm to engage baby and mom, I made eye contact with Jon and called out his name. 'Hi, Jon,' I intoned in rhythm with the rattle as I gently leaned forward towards him and his mom.

Jon tentatively reached out for the rattle, and I slowly extended my arm to offer the handle to him. He quickly pulled back in response to my overture, but then tentatively reached for the rattle again, this time with an open palm. On contact, Jon pushed the rattle away and turned toward his mother with a faint whimper of distress.

Erika responded by securing her hold on her son and rotating away from our interaction with a quick spin. He was distracted, looked away, and became quiet.

Keeping a comfortable distance, I began speaking empathetically to Jon about his difficult birth, talking *as if* he could understand my words. While it is, of course, unlikely that Jon would understand the precise meaning of my words, I believe that communicating as if he would conveyed more than the words themselves, that it was a reflection of his distress and a recognition that I 'got him'. My prosody and tonal modulations seemed to give him some comfort and reassurance, conveying the feeling tone that I was an ally and somehow understood his plight.

Recovering his calm, Jon reached out again with curiosity and then pointed toward the table. 'Apple, apple,' he said, extending his left arm toward a plate holding three pomegranates. I lifted the plate and offered them to him. He reached for the pomegranates, touched one, and then pushed it away. This time his push was more assertive. 'You're into pushing, aren't you?' I asked, again communicating not only with words but with rhythm and tone. 'I sure can understand how you might want to push, after all those strange people were poking and hurting you.' Wanting to reinforce his pushing impulse and his power, I offered my finger to him; he reached out to push it away. 'Yeah, that's great,' I responded, conveying my feelings of encouragement, warmth, and support. 'You sure want to get that away from you, don't you?' Jon let go another whimper, as if he agreed.

Erika sat down on the couch and began removing Jon's shoes. He seemed fearful and turned away from the two of us as we talked about his gastric reflux and its possible penetration into his lungs. When Erika mentioned that the pediatric surgeon was proposing an endoscopy, Jon seemed to show a flash of distress: his face scrunched downward in a frown of worry and anxiety as he called out, 'Mama'. Jon seemed to have recognized the meaning of our words (or was perhaps picking up on his mother's unease), and in a millisecond, his mid-back stiffened and he turned toward his mother. I quietly asked his permission and then gently placed my hand on his mid-back, resting my palm over his stiffened and contracted muscles while extending my fingers upward between his shoulder blades. Jon whimpered again and then turned to look directly at me. Given that he maintained our eye contact, I assessed that it was safe to proceed with the physical touch. Jon continued to connect with me visually as his mother recounted the history of his symptoms, treatment, and medical assessment.

Then suddenly, Jon pushed mightily against his mother's thighs with his feet and legs, propelling him upward toward her left shoulder. This movement gave me a quick snapshot of his previously, incomplete propulsive birth movements. These were the instinctual movements (the procedural memories[3]) that had

---

3   Procedural memories are impulses, movement, or action patterns that are experienced as body sensations through interoceptive awareness. See: Levine 2015, p.25.

driven him into the apex of her uterus and strangled his throat with the cord – exacerbating his distress while further activating his drive to push, creating in turn even more distress. As if following a dramatic, choreographed script, Jon pushed hard against his mother's legs twice more, propelling him again up to her shoulders.

This completion of his birth push – without the previously associated strangulation, intense cranial pressure, and 'futility' brought on by his head wedging into the uterine apex – was an important sequence of movements for Jon to experience. It allowed him a successful 'renegotiation' of his birth process in the here and now. His procedural memories had begun to shift from maladaptive and traumatic to ones that were empowering and successful. Maintaining a low to moderate level of activation in this renegotiation was essential. I quietly removed my hand from his back and allowed him to settle.

His mother responded to his thrusts by standing him up in her lap. While I maintained a soft presence with an attentive, engaged gaze, Jon looked directly at me with a fierce intensity that seemed to express his furious determination. His spine elongated and he seemed both more erect and more alert.[4] I again reached for Jon's mid-back and spoke soothingly: 'I wish we had more time to play, but since they are planning this procedure in a few weeks, I want to see if we can do something to help you.' Jon stiffened again and strongly pushed my hand away with his. He grimaced and flashed me a look of snarling anger while simultaneously retracting his hand and priming for another major defensive push away.

Leaning slightly toward Jon, I offered him some resistance by bringing my thumb into the center of his small palm. By matching his force and allowing him to push me away with his strength, I observed that, as his arm extended, he was able to harness the full-throttle power of his mid-back and then follow through with a robust thrust. We maintained eye contact and I responded to his expression of concerted aggression by opening my eyes wider in surprise, encouragement, excitement, and invitation. Jon continued to hold my gaze, and as he pushed my hand away with significant determination his response transformed into one of seeming celebration. I reflected back to him his great triumph over an unwelcome intruder, an intruder who characterized his earliest experience of a threatening and hostile world.

Jon pulled his hand back and let go with a small whimper. But still he maintained eye contact, giving me an indication that he wanted to go on. Jon's cry strengthened into deep sobs as he gave one more strong push to my thumb. He howled with apparent anguish, confusion, and rage. Slowly his cry

---

4   In my clinical work, I have observed that children who were born via Cesarean section often have a lack of power when they first attempt standing as toddlers. Then, as mature adults, they often have difficulties initiating actions in the world.

deepened, becoming more spontaneous after I placed my hand again on his back. This invited the sound to come through his diaphragm in deep sobs. As he pushed my hand away once more, I spoke to him about all those people touching and poking him and how much he must have wanted to push them away too.

Jon broke away from our eye contact for the first time in this series of pushes and turned toward his mom. She reciprocated by gently connecting with his need for ventral support. With that brief interlude of respite, Jon turned back to re-initiate our eye contact even as his cry deepened. I responded to his cry with a supportive, 'Yeah…yeah,' matching his anguish with a soothing, rhythmic prosody. Jon took a deep and spontaneous breath for the first time. He turned his chest fully toward his mom while looking over his shoulder to once again return my eye contact.

Jon continued to cry, but remained relatively relaxed. We paused for a moment, since I could see that Erika was consumed by many thoughts and feelings of her own. She took a deep breath and then looked down in amazement at her son. 'He never cries,' she said. 'Or rather, he cries with a little whimper, but never fully like this!' I reassured her that it seemed to be a cry of deep, emotional release. Erika paused and then added, 'I mean, I can't remember the last time I actually saw tears running down his face.' A grateful astonishment seemed to light up her face, while opening an energetic connection to her son.

When offered the opportunity, Jon reached out from his nested position and assertively pushed my finger out of the vicinity of his territory. I reinforced to Erika how profoundly disturbing it must have been for him to have strangers probing him with all those tubes and needles, how very small and helpless he must have felt. Erika repositioned herself as he burrowed deeper into her lap and chest.

Jon nestled into his mother's lap with a new molding impulse, hitherto unseen by her. Molding is the close physical nestling of the infant's body into the shoulder, chest, and face of the mother. When reciprocated it is a basic component of bonding – the intimate dance that lets the infant know that he is safe, loved, and protected. I believe that it also replicates the close, contained, physical positioning of the fetus in the womb and conveys similar primal physical sensations of security and goodness.

'I'm not sure what to do with this,' Erika commented, pointing with her chin to his nuzzling and snuggling shape. We paused together for a moment to appreciate this delicate contact between the two of them. 'Whoa!' she said, breaking the silence. 'He is really hot.' I commented that heat was part of an autonomic discharge that accompanied his crying and emotional release.

Jon settled down as Erika rocked him gently, maintaining full, yielding, chest-to-chest contact. He took in an easy, full inhalation and released it with a deep, spontaneous exhale that sounded both ecstatic and profoundly stress relieving. Indeed, Erika also let down her guard as well, shedding her doubt and beginning to trust that this new connection was 'for real'. She looked down at her son as he continued to mold deeply into her chest and shoulder. She bent forward to meet his molding with her head and face. The two could be said to be 'renegotiating their bonding'. Erika continued to gently rock her son while maintaining their connection. He continued to regulate himself with a gentle trembling and then took several deep, spontaneous breaths with full and audible exhalations. Erika quietly released her head backward and momentarily closed her eyes in an ecstasy of contact and connection.

After a few minutes, Jon peered out from his burrow and made eye contact with me. I recognized that he had had enough for one day, so I began to wind down the session. Erika acknowledged the closing, but needed to again share her own process of astonishment and hope. With a perplexed and startled expression, she noted, 'I've just never seen him be this still.' Then she asked Jon, 'Are you asleep?' And then on her next breath, 'So sweet, oh so sweet,' she intoned as if getting to know her baby for the first time.

Before the end of the session, Jon and I played Peekaboo with a warm and playful engagement for a few moments; however, at no time did he leave the cradle of his mother's lap. She nuzzled his head and mused: 'This really seems different. Usually he gives a quick hug and then is off on his way.' Almost as if smelling her newborn and drawing him in to her chest, she too let out an audible exhale and broke into a broad smile. 'This is so very strange,' she murmured quietly. 'He is affectionate, but never still…he never stays with me… he's always off to something new.' As they continued to snuggle, they smiled in tandem. Their absolute delight was visible and palpable. Her baby had come home and they celebrated, together, that reunion.

At our next session, one week later, Erika had a number of anecdotes she wanted to share. Her upbeat excitement and Jon's comfortable curiosity were contagious. They sat down together on the couch, Jon resting his head against his mother's chest. I leaned forward in my chair, eager to hear her report. She began by recounting an episode that had occurred the night after our first session. 'He woke up in the middle of the night and called out, "Mama", she reported, adding that she went to pick him up as usual. Jon sat quietly on her lap and pulled his head down deeper into her chest. 'When I picked him up, he was doing this,' she added, pointing with her chin to his comfortable snuggling. I watched with an appreciative smile. 'Looks to me like he's making up for lost time,' I suggested.

Erika resumed her story: 'Well…and then he said, "Apple, apple." I thought he wanted something to eat, but normally this would include him wiggling out of my arms and running to the kitchen. So I realized he must have been talking about the "apples", the pomegranates on your table.' She explained that after their last session with me, later in the week, they had an appointment with the pediatrician, which had upset Jon. While they drove home in the car he kept calling out to Erika from his car seat, 'Pita, pita, apple, pita.' 'Again I thought he was hungry,' Erika continued, 'and responded by asking him if he wanted pizza. "No," [he answered] "pita, pita, apple!" I realized he was talking about you, trying to say "Peter". Pretty amazing, isn't it, how much he recognized and wanted to talk about the change he felt?' she queried, looking up at me for validation.[5]

I smiled with shared enjoyment and appreciation, and then asked about his energy. Erika replied, 'He has been so much more talkative, much more interactive. He wants to show us lots of things and then wants our feedback. He seems much more engaged and interested in having us play with him.' She bent down and kissed his head as he curled up in her lap. 'But really, this is the biggest change,' she said. 'I can't tell you – for him to sit and just be cuddled, it's a complete change, completely different. It's not him…or…it's…it's the new him.' 'Or maybe it's the new us,' I responded. Erika tipped her head shyly and spoke, ever so softly. 'It's wonderful for me.'

Jon and I played for much of the rest of this session. I recognized that much of the birth trauma and interrupted bonding was resolved and that his social engagement systems were awakening and coming online with gusto. As previously noted, lack of attachment is far too often attributed to the mother's perceived lack of availability and attunement. It was Erika's and Jon's shared trauma that disrupted their natural rhythm and mutual drive to bond, trauma that displaced the chance of a mother–child reunion. Now that reunion had happened. And the invasive procedures regarding gastric reflux were never needed.

Sammy: Child's play

You can discover more about a person in an hour of play than in a year of conversation.

Plato

Often, children's symptoms or behavioral changes can present puzzling questions that baffle parents and pediatric professionals alike. This is especially true when the child has 'good enough' parents who provide a stable and nurturing home environment. Sometimes the child's new actions, although anything but subtle,

---

5   I believe that Erika's report demonstrates the formation of pre-logical associational networks (procedural memory engrams), which remained in place when they returned for a two-year 'checkup' at age four and a half.

are a mystery. The bewildered family might not connect the child's conduct or other symptoms with the source of his terror. Rather than expressing themselves in easy to comprehend ways, kids frequently show us that they are suffering inside in terribly frustrating ways. They do this through their bodies. They may act 'bratty', clinging to parents or throwing tantrums. Or, they might struggle with agitation, hyperactivity, nightmares, or sleeplessness. Even more troubling, they may act out their worries and hurts by 'steam-rolling' over a pet or younger, weaker child. For other children, their distress may show up as head and tummy aches or bed-wetting. Or they may avoid people and things they used to enjoy in order to manage unbearable anxiety. Parents ask, where in the world can these childhood symptoms possibly come from? There are often hidden culprits in the day-to-day physicality of childhood. When unresolved, fairly regular childhood events – such as falls, accidents, and invasive and emergency medical procedures – become suspects in the case to uncover what underlies a child's distress.

Children, by their nature, enjoy play. Therapists and parents can use the vehicle of guided play to help them to rebound and move beyond their fears to gain mastery over their scariest moments. As children express their inner world through play, their bodies are directly communicating with us.

What follows is an example of showing parents (in this case, also a grandparent) how to work with a child who may be traumatized. I believe that this is an invaluable function that therapists can provide to parents and other caregivers so that *they* can prevent traumatic symptoms from occurring in the wake of potentially overwhelming events (Levine and Kline 2006, 2008).

The story of Sammy's strange behaviors

Here is the case of a two-and-a-half-year-old boy in which a 'play session', set up by me and defined by a series of five principles, led to a reparative experience with a victorious outcome. The principles offered after this case history provide simple suggestions for therapists, medical professionals, and parents. This case is an example of what can happen when an ordinary fall, requiring a visit to the emergency room for stitches, goes awry. It also shows how several months later, Sammy's terrifying experience was transformed through play into a renewed sense of confidence and joy.

Sammy had been spending the weekend with his grandparents, where I was their guest. He was being an impossible tyrant, aggressively and relentlessly trying to control his new environment. Nothing pleased him; he displayed a foul temper every waking moment. When he was asleep, he tossed and turned as if wrestling with his bedclothes. This behavior was not entirely unexpected from a two-and-a-half-year-old whose parents have gone away for the weekend.

Children with separation anxiety often act it out. Sammy, however, had always enjoyed visiting his grandparents and this behavior seemed extreme to them. They confided to me that six months earlier, Sammy fell off his high chair and split his chin open. Bleeding heavily, he was taken to the local emergency room. When the nurse came to take his temperature and blood pressure, he was so frightened that she was unable to record his vital signs. This vulnerable little boy was then strapped down in a 'pediatric papoose' (a board with flaps and Velcro straps). With his torso and legs immobilized, the only part of his body he could move was his head and neck – which, naturally, he did, as energetically as he could. The doctors responded by tightening the restraint and immobilizing his head with their hands in order to suture his chin. This imprinted him with an overwhelming sense of powerlessness and helplessness.

After this upsetting experience, mom and dad took Sammy out for a hamburger and then to the playground. His mother was very attentive and carefully validated his experience of being scared and hurt. Soon, all seemed forgotten. However, the boy's overbearing attitude began shortly after this event. Could Sammy's tantrums and controlling behavior be related to his perceived helplessness from this trauma?

When his parents returned, we agreed to explore whether there might be a traumatic charge still associated with this recent experience. We all gathered in the cabin where I was staying. With parents, grandparents, and Sammy watching, I placed his stuffed Pooh Bear on the edge of a chair in such a way that it fell to the floor. Sammy shrieked, bolted for the door and ran across a footbridge and down a narrow path to the creek. Our suspicions were confirmed. His most recent visit to the hospital was neither harmless nor forgotten. Sammy's behavior told us that this game was potentially overwhelming for him.

Sammy's parents brought him back from the creek. He clung dearly to his mother as we prepared for another game. We reassured him that we would all be there to help protect Pooh Bear. Again he ran – but this time only into the next room. We followed him in there and waited to see what would happen next. Sammy ran to the bed and hit it with both arms while looking at me expectantly.

'Mad, huh?' I said. He gave me a look that confirmed my question. Interpreting his expression as a go-ahead sign, I put Pooh Bear under a blanket and placed Sammy on the bed next to him.

'Sammy, let's all help Pooh Bear.'

I held Pooh Bear under the blanket and asked everyone to help free Pooh. Sammy watched with interest but soon got up and ran to his mother. With his arms held tightly around her legs, he said, 'Mommy, I'm scared.'[6] Without

---

6   This trust of safety would not happen without a solid attachment. Where healthy bonding is not the case, or where there is abuse, therapy is of course much more complex and also generally involves therapy for the parents or caregivers.

pressuring him, we waited until Sammy was ready and willing to play the game again. The next time grandma and Pooh Bear were restrained with the blanket together. And this time Sammy actively participated in their rescue. When Pooh Bear was freed, Sammy ran to his mother, clinging even more tightly than before. He began to tremble and shake in fear, and then, dramatically, his chest expanded in a growing sense of excitement and pride.

Here we see the transition between traumatic re-enactment and healing play:

The next time Sammy held on to mommy, there was less clinging and more excited jumping. We waited until Sammy was ready to play again. Everyone except Sammy took a turn being rescued with Pooh. Each time, Sammy became more vigorous as he pulled off the blanket and escaped into the safety of his mother's arms.

When it was Sammy's turn to be held under the blanket with Pooh Bear, he became quite agitated and fearful. He ran back to his mother's arms several times before he was able to accept the ultimate challenge. Bravely, he climbed under the blankets with Pooh while I held the blanket gently down. I watched his eyes grow wide with fear, but only for a moment. Then he grabbed Pooh Bear, shoved the blanket away, and flung himself into his mother's arms. Sobbing and trembling, he screamed, 'Mommy, get me out of here! Mommy, get this off of me!' His startled father told me that these were the same words Sammy screamed while imprisoned in the papoose at the hospital. He remembered this clearly because he had been quite surprised by his son's ability to make such a direct, well-spoken demand at two-and-a-half years old.

We went through the escape several more times. Each time, Sammy exhibited more power and more triumph. Instead of running fearfully to his mother, he jumped excitedly up and down. With every successful escape, we all clapped and danced together, cheering, 'Yeah for Sammy, yeah! yeah! Sammy saved Pooh Bear!' Sammy had achieved mastery over the experience that had shattered him a few months earlier. The trauma-driven, aggressive, foul-tempered behavior used in an attempt to control his environment disappeared. And his 'hyperactive' and avoidant behavior during the reworking of his medical trauma was transformed into triumphant play.

Five principles to guide children's play towards resolution

The following section includes an analysis of Sammy's play experience. This will help clarify the outlined principles and support therapists and caregivers in their application.

1 Let the child control the pace of the game

Healing takes place in a moment-by-moment slowing down of time. In order to help a child feel safe, follow her pace and rhythm. If you 'put yourself in the child's shoes' through careful observation of her behavior, you will learn quickly how to resonate with her. Let's revisit the story to see exactly how we did that with Sammy.

By running out of the room when Pooh Bear fell off the chair, Sammy 'told' me loud and clear that he was not ready to engage in this new activating 'game'. Sammy had to be 'rescued' by his parents, comforted, and brought back to the scene before continuing. In order to make him feel safe we all assured him that we would be there to help protect Pooh Bear. By offering this support and reassurance, we helped Sammy move closer to engaging with the game – *in his own time at his own pace.*

After this reassurance, Sammy ran into the bedroom instead of out the door. This was a clear signal that he felt less threatened and more confident of our support. Children might not state verbally whether they want to continue, so take cues from their behavior and responses. Respect their wishes in whatever way they choose to communicate. Children should never be rushed to move through an episode faster or forced to do more than they are willing and able to do. Just like with Sammy, it is important to slow down the process if you notice signs of fear, including: constricted breathing, stiffening, or a dazed (dissociated) demeanor. These reactions will dissipate if you simply wait quietly and patiently while reassuring the child that you are still by their side and on their side. Usually, the youngster's eyes and breathing pattern will indicate when it's time to continue.

2 Distinguish between fear, terror, and excitement

Experiencing fear or terror for more than a brief moment during traumatic play will not help the child move through the trauma. Most children will take action to avoid it. Let them! At the same time, try to discern whether it is avoidance or escape. The following is a clear-cut example to help in developing the skill of 'reading' when a break is needed and when it's time to guide the momentum forward.

When Sammy ran down to the creek, he was demonstrating avoidance behavior. In order to resolve his traumatic reaction, Sammy had to feel that he was in control of his actions rather than driven to act by his emotions. Avoidance behavior occurs when fear and terror threaten to overwhelm. With kids, this behavior is usually accompanied by sign(s) of emotional distress (crying, frightened eyes, screaming). Active escape, on the other hand, is exhilarating. Children become excited by their small triumphs and often show pleasure by glowing with smiles, clapping their hands, or laughing heartily. Overall, the response is considerably different from avoidance behavior. Excitement is evidence of the child's successful discharge of emotions that accompanied the original experience. This is positive, desirable, and necessary.

Trauma is transformed by changing intolerable feelings and sensations into desirable ones. This can only happen at a level of activation that is similar to the level of activation that led to the traumatic reaction in the first place. If the child appears excited, it is OK to offer encouragement and continue as we did when we clapped and danced with Sammy. However, if the child appears frightened or cowed, give reassurance but don't encourage any further movement. Instead, be present with your full attention and support, waiting patiently until a substantial amount of the fear subsides. If the child shows signs of fatigue, take a rest break.

3 Take one small step at a time

You can never move too slowly in renegotiating a traumatic event with anyone; this is especially true with a young child. Traumatic play is repetitious almost by definition. Make use of this cyclical characteristic. The key difference between 'renegotiation' and traumatic play (re-enactment) is that in renegotiation there are incremental differences in the child's responses and behaviors in moving towards mastery and resolution. The following illustrates how I noticed these small changes with Sammy.

When Sammy ran into the bedroom instead of out the door, he was responding with a different behavior indicating that progress had been made. No matter how many repetitions it takes, if the child you are helping is responding differently – such as with a slight increase in excitement, with more speech or with more spontaneous movements – he is moving through the trauma. If the child's responses appear to be moving in the direction of constriction or compulsive repetition, instead of expansion and variety, you may be attempting to renegotiate the event with scenarios which involve too much arousal for the child to make progress. If you notice that your attempts at playful renegotiation are backfiring, ground yourself and pay attention to your sensations until your breathing brings a sense of calm, confidence, and spontaneity. Then, slow down the rate of change by breaking the play into smaller increments. This may seem contradictory to what was stated earlier about following the child's pace. However, attuning to children's needs sometimes means setting limits to prevent them from getting wound up and collapsing in overwhelm. If the child appears tense or frightened, it's OK to invite some healing steps. For example, when re-negotiating a medical trauma, you might say, 'Let's see, I wonder what we can do so Pooh Bear (Dolly, GI Joe, etc.) doesn't get so scared before you (the pretend doctor/nurse) give him the shot?' Often children will come up with creative solutions showing you exactly what *they needed – the missing ingredient* that would have helped them settle more during their experience.

Don't be concerned about how many times you have to go through what seems to be the 'same old thing'. We engaged Sammy in playing the game with Pooh Bear at least ten times. Sammy was able to renegotiate his traumatic responses quickly. Another child in your care might require considerably more time. You don't need to do it all in one day! Resting and time are needed to help the child internally reorganize her experience at subtle levels. Be assured that if the resolution is not complete, the child will return to a similar phase when given the opportunity to play during the next session.

4 Become a safe container

Remember that biology is on your side. Perhaps the most difficult and important aspect of renegotiating a traumatic event with a child is maintaining your own belief that things will turn out OK. Once held, this feeling of positivity and confidence comes from inside you and is projected out to the child. It becomes a container that surrounds the child with a feeling of confidence. This may be particularly difficult to maintain if the child resists your attempts to renegotiate the trauma.

If the child resists, be patient and reassuring. A deeply instinctive part of the child wants to re-work this experience and become free of it. All you have to do is wait for that part to feel confident and safe enough to assert itself. If you are excessively worried about whether the child's traumatic reaction can be transformed, you may inadvertently send a conflicting message. Adults with their own unresolved childhood trauma may be particularly susceptible to falling into this trap. Please be kind to yourself.

5 Stop if you feel that your child is genuinely not benefiting from the play

In *Too Scared to Cry* (1992), Lenore Terr, the esteemed child psychologist, warns clinicians about allowing children to engage in repetitive traumatic play that re-enacts the original horror. She describes the case of three-and-a-half-year-old Lauren who was the victim of sexualized abuse. Here, Lauren is playing with toy cars: 'The cars are going on the people,' Lauren says as she zooms two racing cars towards some finger puppets. 'They're pointing their pointy parts into the people. The people are scared. A pointy part will come on their tummies, and in their mouths, and on their…[she points to her skirt]. My tummy hurts. I don't want to play anymore.' Lauren stops herself as her bodily sensation of fear abruptly surfaces. This is a typical reaction. She may return over and over to the same play, each time stopping when the fearful sensations in her tummy become uncomfortable. Some therapists would say that Lauren is using her play as an attempt to gain some control over the situation that traumatized her.

Her play does resemble 'exposure' treatments used routinely to help adults overcome phobias. But Terr cautions that such play ordinarily doesn't yield much success. Even if it does serve to reduce a child's distress, this process is quite slow in producing results. Most often, the play is compulsively repeated without resolution. Unresolved, repetitious, traumatic play can reinforce the traumatic impact in the same way that re-enactment and cathartic reliving of traumatic experiences can reinforce trauma in adults.

The re-working or renegotiation of a traumatic experience, as we saw with Sammy, represents a process that is fundamentally different from traumatic play or re-enactment. Left to their own devices, most children, not unlike Lauren in the above example, will attempt to avoid the traumatic feelings that their play evokes. But with guided play, *Sammy was able to 'live his feelings through' by gradually and sequentially mastering his fear.* Using this stepwise re-negotiation of the traumatic event and Pooh Bear's companionship, Sammy was able to emerge as the victor and hero. A sense of triumph and heroism almost always signals the successful conclusion of a re-negotiated traumatic event. By following Sammy's lead (after setting up a potentially activating scene), joining in his play, and making the game up as we went along, Sammy got to let go of his fear. In this example, it took minimal direction (30–45 minutes) and support to achieve the *unspoken* goal of aiding Sammy to experience a corrective outcome. In this way, as Sammy's motoric potentiality changed, so did his embodied perception of the world, from dangerous to safe,[7] exciting and inviting.

References

Bentzen, M., Jarlnaes, E. and Levine, P. (2004) 'The Body Self in Psychotherapy: A Psychomotoric Approach to Developmental Psychology.' In I. Macnaughton (ed.) Body, Breath and Consciousness. Berkeley, CA: North Atlantic Books.

Craig, A.D. (2002) 'How do you feel? Interoception: the sense of the physiological condition of the body.' *Nature Reviews Neuroscience 3*, 655–666. DOI: 10.1038/nrn894

Craig, A.D. (2009) 'How do you feel – now? The anterior insula and human awareness.' *Nature Reviews Neuroscience 10*, 59–70. DOI: 10.1038/nrn2555

Craig, A.D. (2010) 'The sentient self.' *Brain Structure and Function 214*, 563–577. DOI: 10.1007/s00429-010-0248-y

Held, R. and Hein, A. (1963) 'Movement-produced stimulation in the development of visually guided behaviours.' *Journal of Comparative and Physiological Psychology 56*, 872–876.

Krueger, D.W. (1989) *Body Self and Psychological Self: A Developmental and Clinical Integration of Disorders of the Self.* New York: Brunner Mazel.

Levine, P.A. (2010) *In an Unspoken Voice, How the Body Releases Trauma and Restores Goodness.* Berkeley, CA: North Atlantic Books.

Levine, P.A. (2015) *Trauma and Memory, Brain and Body and a Search for the Living Past: A Practical Guide for Understanding and Working with Traumatic Memory.* Berkeley, CA: North Atlantic Books.

---

7   See Chapter 7.

Levine, P.A. and Kline, M. (2006) *Trauma Through a Child's Eyes: Awakening the Ordinary Miracle of Healing.* Berkeley, CA: North Atlantic Books.

Levine, P.A. and Kline, M. (2008) *Trauma-Proofing Your Kids: A Parent's Guide for Instilling Confidence, Joy and Resilience.* Berkeley, CA: North Atlantic Books.

Libet, B. (1985) 'Unconscious cerebral initiative and the role of conscious will in voluntary action.' *Behavioral and Brain Sciences 8*, 529–566.

Libet, B. (1992) 'The neural time-factor in perception, volition, and free will.' *Revue de Metaphysique et de Morale 2*, 255–272.

Libet, B. (1996) 'Neural Time Factors in Conscious and Unconscious Mental Functions.' In S.R. Hammeroff, A.W. Kaszniak and A.C. Scott (eds) *Toward a Science of Consciousness: The First Tucson Discussions and Debates.* Cambridge, MA: MIT Press.

Macknik, S.L. (2013) 'Neuroscience in Fiction: Fear and panic in Jaden and Will Smith's After Earth.' *Scientific American.* Available at http://blogs.scientificamerican.com/illusion-chasers/2013/06/08/after-earth, accessed on 22 October 2016.

Payne, P., Levine, P.A. and Crane-Godreau, M.A. (2015) 'Somatic experiencing: using interoception and proprioception as core elements of trauma therapy.' *Frontiers in Psychology*, February 4. DOI: 10.3389/fpsyg.2015.00093

Sperry, R.W. (1952) 'Neurology and the mind–brain problem.' *American Scientist 40*, 291–312.

Terr, L. (1992) *Too Scared to Cry: Psychic Trauma In Childhood.* New York: Basic Books.

9

FINDING TOGETHERNESS

Musicality in Play Therapy with Children with
Severe Communication Difficulties

STUART DANIEL

With thanks and love to Lea

Mark and Jonathon

It was just a regular classroom. I was there, by the window, with Mark and Jonathon and a collection of musical instruments. I was a special needs assistant 'doing music'. Using a drum, I was trying out a rhythmic pattern full of deliberate pregnant pauses – silences held just longer than the natural on-beat demanded – jazz pauses. This kind of pause (which I will talk more about later in this chapter) plays with the natural human capacity for musical time-keeping – a beat is expected, the attention is tied with anticipation over the pulse where that beat should be. A jazz pause has the energy of needing to be filled. And thrown into that pause, I was pointing at different bits of Jonathon's body: his knee, his chin, etc. It was working pretty well. Jonathon had the impetus and was learning (and shouting out) the names for the parts of his body. With Jonathon, though, it was easy. He was keen to engage.

In my enthusiasm I turned around to Mark, thinking he might have been swept up in the fun. No. Mark was a silent 12-year-old with a severe and fairly classical matrix of autism symptoms. In seven months in his class I had only seen him initiate interaction to get food or to scratch another child. Mark was rocking side to side. He always did. Educational psychologists told me he was self-calming or self-stimulating. Most people, including me, usually ignored Mark and his rocking. On that day I decided to do something different. Why not? I rocked with him. This bit was not too impressive for Mark. But then I noticed that we were rocking precisely in time with the almost inaudible ticking of the second-hand of a clock above Mark's head. Rocking together, I pointed at the clock. Mark gaze-tracked. A first for us. Mark smiled. A first for us.

141

I smiled back and held my arms up. Mark rested his hands on my forearms and we spent a few minutes in a slow kind of waltz. Turning circles. For those circles Mark and I were in sync, totally together. And in those moments, I know that something in both of us knew, without hesitation, just how important that was.

Introduction

Togetherness and musicality

This chapter is mostly about *togetherness*. By this I mean the *quality* of connectedness, of natural rhythmic flow, which permeates and defines the interaction of two (or more) people when they are in sync. It is also about the *feeling of togetherness*: a deep sense of relaxed 'okayness' felt by those experiencing togetherness.

Togetherness is the essence of healthy infant–mother play (Trevarthen 2001). From birth, most infants are naturally equipped with impulses to engage in reciprocal, playful interaction with their equally in-tune parents (Stern 2004; Trevarthen 2001). But for some children this impulse is absent or disorganized. This chapter contains stories about spending time with children who find the usual routes into togetherness elusive. These stories describe a deliberate attempt to emulate the essential patterns of togetherness through alternative routes. We will need some tools. And we will need to get some understanding of the mechanics of early interaction – the mechanics of 'musicality'.

So what enables two or more people to have the experience of being in sync? Malloch and Trevarthen (2009) have given us helpful refinements in the study of 'communicative musicality' – the study of the essentially musical nature of human interaction. The two fundamental tools we will explore here are the concepts of 'pulse' and 'quality' (Malloch and Trevarthen 2009).

Pulse

To help us connect, Mark and I had the pulse beat of the clock on the wall. We also had our *internal* biological clocks: 'clusters of rhythmically pulsing neurons that keep time for living organisms, regulate metabolism, procreation, movement, communication and even the temporal nature of human thought' (Osborne 2009, p.545). Our bodies equip us with biological imperatives to feel patterns of time. We perceive our worlds and engage with other people all within parameters of rhythm. So, on one hand, 'pulse' refers to the time-keeping and pattern generation of our biological clocks (Malloch and Trevarthen 2009). And, on the other hand, 'pulse' simultaneously refers to the related (temporally patterned) behaviour we produce: 'Pulse is the regular succession of discrete behavioural steps through time, representing the "future-creating" process by which a person may anticipate what might happen and when' (Malloch, p.65 in this book).

Healthy infants are born with organized impulses to reach out and engage with other people in temporally regulated playful interaction (Malloch and Trevarthen 2009). A mother's social pulse is met and complemented by her infant's. Part of Mark's biology meant that usually he did not display these types of organized impulses. But somehow the external pulse of the clock became something Mark and I could share, something that brought our biological clocks in phase together. And our sharing did not stop at simple phasic synchronization. Once engaged, Mark's biological clock motivated a natural flow of pattern-generation; Mark initiated a level of creative change in our rhythmic play.

Quality

When Stern (2010) reflected on his early observations of healthy infant–mother play he evoked the term 'vitality contour' to describe the shared energetic experiences he saw. Here, 'vitality' refers to the energetic impetus of human experience, including interaction (Stern 2010). Stern (1985) had noticed how healthy infant–mother play was characterized by the experience of 'moving' through patterns of energy and emotion together. These patterns were often defined by an energetic contour involving a shared heightening of excitement with a clear ending in resolution (Stern 1985). The dynamic, mutually modulated experience of sharing this basic vitality contour is at the essence of togetherness (Stern 2010). For us, the 'quality' of human interaction, 'consists of the contours of expressive vocal and body gesture, shaping time in movement' (Malloch, p.65 in this book). These contours are defined by temporally organized changes in facial expression, quality of eye contact, touch (changing patterns of position, intention, and intensity of the body) and vocalization (changing patterns of rhythm, timbre, pitch, and volume in voice) (Malloch and Trevarthen 2009).

Musical shapes of play

As an infant develops in relationship with her parents, the nature of the play they share develops too. We see different structured patterns of play at different developmental stages. In this chapter we will be exploring therapeutic work with children who, for various reasons, have not experienced or integrated certain play patterns. We will be exploring how to emulate these patterns in therapy for children who cannot access such experiences through developmentally 'normal' perceptual modes. Using the terms of pulse and quality, these different play patterns can be described as musical shapes.

In this chapter we will look at the earliest developmental pattern – the 'metronomic'. The quality of its shape is a curved sway; its pulse is regular, simple, on-beat: two bodies rocking, swaying, in sync.

We will also look at the quintessential pattern of infant–mother play, the next developmental step up from the metronomic – the 'basic contour'. Both its pulse and quality change over time; its shape is a skewed contour (see Figure 9.1). We gave a broad-brush stroke of this pattern above, when discussing the vitality contour described by Stern (1985, 2010). As we will require more detail here, we will be using a map of the basic contour by Trevarthen and Daniel (2005), adapted from Brazelton, Koslowski and Main (1974) (see Figure 9.1).

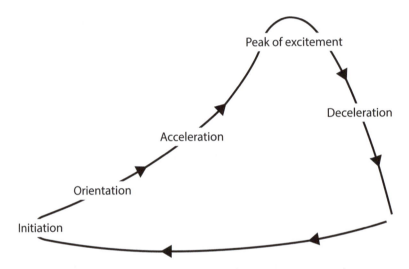

FIGURE 9.1 THE BASIC CONTOUR (ADAPTED FROM BRAZELTON *ET AL.* 1974)

Here, we will use Brazelton *et al.*'s temporal map as our guide and standard when attempting to emulate the basic contour in therapy. The flow through from Initiation, to Orientation, to Acceleration, to Peak of excitement, to Deceleration and back round to Initiation once again, represents one iteration of play – one 'play-phrase'.

To illustrate this map in healthy play and, conversely, to illustrate how this map differs in asynchronous play with a child with severe communication difficulties (here, autism) we can summarize the findings of a study reported in more detail elsewhere (Trevarthen and Daniel 2005).[1] In this study home video recordings of two 11-month-old monozygotic twin sisters were subjected to micro-analysis. Sarah was later diagnosed with infantile autism at 18 months

---

1   Both authors have given permission for the reproduction of graphical elements (Figures 9.1 and 9.2) and details of the study featured.

according to the ICD-10, while Rachel developed normally. Time-coded videos of two face-to-face interactions, in which the father attempts to engage each sister separately in a Monster-on-My-Belly game, were analysed. In the game the father uses humour and a ritualized build-up of excitement through looming in and growl noises towards a climax of nuzzling and 'biting' each infant's stomach. Categories of interactive behaviours were logged and charted to produce graphical representations of the interactions. These behaviours were defined to identify the occurrence in time of functional states of alertness, orientation between partners, communicative expression, emotion, body contact, and postural tension. By scoring combinations of behaviour, periods of *attention on and off partner, anticipation,* and *emotional build-up* could be charted for each subject (see Figures 9.2 and 9.3). Given that the twins were viewed at the time as identical (i.e. pre-diagnosis, with no signifiers detected consciously by either parent), any differences in behaviour would most likely be attributable to differences in prenatal brain development for Sarah, but the intuitive responses of the father would also be important.

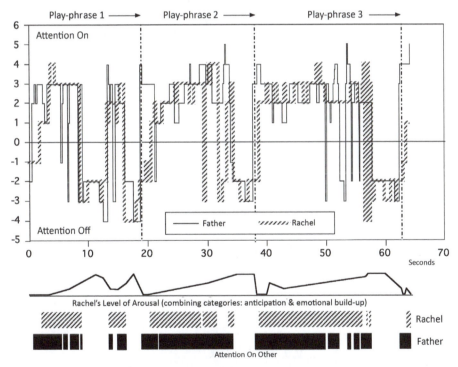

FIGURE 9.2 THE FATHER'S MONSTER-ON-MY-BELLY GAME
WITH RACHEL (DEVELOPMENTALLY NORMAL)

Figure 9.2 describes the clear rhythmic patterns of mutual-modulation within the Rachel-father game. The game follows a cyclical pattern of almost identical play-phrases, with each play-phrase being almost identical to the map of our basic contour (Brazelton *et al.* 1974). Each play-phrase begins with an Initiation on the part of the father – he brings his attention clearly to Rachel's eye-line, makes minimal physical contact and a preliminary anticipatory noise. This is met with a quick re-Orientation by Rachel who immediately locks eye contact. What follows is the Acceleration stage, where the father (in constant dynamical response to Rachel's expressed build-up of anticipation) adds interactive, teasing behaviours in an energetic progression towards the monster-belly-blow. The Peak of excitement is the belly blow, accompanied by loud, playful 'monster growls'. Here Rachel's whole body releases anticipatory tension and she laughs loudly. A natural period of Deceleration, self-regulated by Rachel, follows in which Rachel withdraws all interactive behaviours whilst maintaining a functional level of attention on her father. Even in Deceleration, Rachel is anticipating the social cues which mark the Initiation of the next play-phrase. The *Attention on Other* patterns clearly demonstrate how eye contact, social cueing, and gaze-tracking are normally in sync and essential in mutually modulated rhythmic play. The flowing trajectories of Rachel's *Level of Arousal*, as she moves through the stages of our map – from Initiation, flowing steadily up to a crescendo in the Peak and immediately down in the Deceleration – are clear examples of vitality contours.

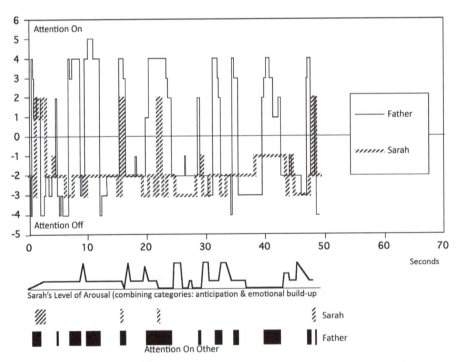

FIGURE 9.3 THE FATHER'S MONSTER-ON-MY-BELLY GAME WITH SARAH (AUTISTIC)

Figure 9.3 illustrates how the Sarah–father interaction lacks all of the cyclical elements of healthy game play. Replacing the interactive stages of our map of the basic contour are static periods (with no interactive emotional build-up) punctuated by frequent bursts of purely physical stimulation by the father. In these bursts the father does the monster-blow, 'growls', and tickles Sarah. Over time, it seems the father has adapted his 'style' – without knowing it – to a non-social pattern of engagement with Sarah. This was a natural response to repeatedly receiving no synchronous eye contact or social cueing whatsoever. The Sarah–father interaction is not really a game at all. It includes no shared experience, no mutual vitality contours, no togetherness.

Narratives, gaps, and co-regulation of emotion in play

Contained within every single interactive play-phrase is a rich and flowing emotional story. In healthy play the story is a happy one, one which involves two people meeting and valuing each other. We shall call these momentary emotional stories 'micro-narratives'. For us, these micro-narratives will take place within our two basic musical shapes: the metronomic and the basic contour. In every healthy micro-narrative there is the potential for *co-regulation* of the infant's arousal states. Togetherness gives an infant well-timed, felt experiences of her mother's emotional response to potentially stressful experiences. Piggy-backing on her mother's feelings, the infant learns to self-modulate her emotions in the face of these potential stressors (Schore 1994). Over time, affect co-regulation allows the infant to develop and maintain a relatively robust sense of emotional self. We can think about this emerging continuity of inner experience as the development of a child's 'big story of self'. And this big story takes a million writes, rewrites, and edits. The process is endless. And it all happens in play.

Healthy play and healthy co-regulation involve navigation of naturally occurring gaps within the flow of emotional narrative. In any relationship – infant–mother, therapeutic, person to person – these moments of disconnection punctuate our shared emotional flow; the experience is possibly uncomfortable, disruptive, disturbing, or even shocking. We will call these gaps 'micro-narrative gaps'. The nature of a child's experience in exploring, transitioning, and repairing these micro-narrative gaps is crucial to the child's developing sense of trust and her internalized sense of self (Hughes 2004; Schore 1994). 'The core of the (*healthy*) self lies in patterns of affect-regulation that integrate a sense of self across state transitions, thereby allowing for a continuity of inner experience' (Schore 1994, p.33). It is a crucial part of the development of every child to go through these gaps and survive. And it is crucial that their adult partner-in-play is accessible to co-regulate the emotional experience –

this enables that survival. Both mother and infant naturally initiate games that play in and around micro-narrative gaps. In peek-a-boo and hide-and-seek for instance, moments of vulnerability are sought, created, extended, survived, and repaired all in synchronous play.

Within a sensitive, playful, therapeutic relationship there is the opportunity for a child to rewrite a previously painful experience in a new way. There are many factors involved here, one of which will be the way the therapist reacts to, and supports, the child to explore micro-narrative gaps. In a therapy context, Hughes (2004) describes these gaps as 'disruption': 'the attachment sequence of attunement, disruption, and repair occurs frequently in an attachment-based model of therapy, just as it does in the parent–child relationship' (p.269). In therapy, as in life, there is something essential in the experience of safely transitioning these gaps. Hughes (2004) explains that 'the therapist does not avoid these…disruption(s), but rather provides a safe setting in which they can occur and then the therapist repairs the relationship before proceeding' (p.269). Sensitive co-regulation repairs emotional continuity in the immediate aftermath of micro-narrative gaps, allowing the child to survive and grow from the experience. The feeling of being 'held' by a sensitive therapist, throughout transitioning and repair, is central to a safe therapeutic relationship. The feeling of being 'held' by an attachment figure, throughout transitioning and repair, is central to the secure attachment experience for any child (Hughes 2000).

A core idea for us, which will be explored in detail as this chapter unfolds, is that it is the *musical nature* of play which holds the impetus for micro-narrative gaps to be safely transitioned. What is crucial here is that an energetic flow of shared connection is somehow maintained between infant and play-partner, even throughout the gap in directly modulated emotional connection. This energetic impetus contains the possibility of immediate reconnection and repair through co-regulation. It is the groove of the underlying pulse-beat of play which 'holds' a child safely and carries her through the unknown and out again.

Case stories

I work as a play therapist, but you will quickly notice that the type of play discussed in the following case stories is often physical and body to body. Sometimes the described play looks more like classical play therapy, flowing in and around symbolic play with toys. But more often it looks elemental and pre-symbolic and could have equally emerged in a session of movement, dance, music, or drama therapy. The case stories presented here explore the possibility of emulating healthy developmental patterns of play (our two musical shapes: the metronomic and basic contour), of fostering the feeling of togetherness, of facilitating affect co-regulation (including expression of otherwise 'hidden' emotions), and of engaging in the exceptionally sensitive process of playing with, extending, and transitioning micro-narrative gaps within our two musical shapes – all with children who do not easily access organized impulses for interactive play.

Tony: Emulating the basic contour – co-regulation and expression of emotions

I spent a year with Tony, twice a week, in a colourful soft-play room. The padded room supported the highly physical nature of Tony's play therapy and was considered a good precaution; sometimes Tony was dangerous. He was 15 and had the unusual diagnostic combination of Down's syndrome and autism spectrum disorder. Tony had lived in a residential unit for some time. His painful childhood was epitomized by neglect and rejection from his parents. When I met him, Tony spoke only single words or very short phrases. He displayed many disturbances in organized prosocial behaviour including an aversion to eye contact in general, specific difficulties with synchronous eye contact and gaze-tracking, flat affect, awkward prosody, and problems turn-taking and initiating proto-conversational turns. Tony lacked any real sophistication in emotional intelligence or expression. His strongest manifest emotion, anger, appeared as purely physical violence.

Tony had never reached out with organized impulses for rhythmical interaction and, as such, he had an extremely limited experience of play. His games had never progressed beyond the directly physical: tickling, chasing, falling down, passing a ball, etc. He did *love* this type of play though. And he had lots of energy. Here, in physical play-phrases, was where our therapeutic relationship would most likely begin. Our play would attempt to build on these physical interactions and move on to emulate the basic contour of early infant–mother play – a *social* play pattern which was painfully absent from Tony's infancy. But with only disorganized, painful impulses underpinning potential eye contact, tracking, and monitoring, the usual sensory pathways into rhythmic play would not be available. In any attempt to emulate our basic contour, I would have to rely on an alternative combination of sensory modalities, emphasizing physical contact whilst bypassing the visual exchange of emotional signals. But would this really be possible? Could togetherness be found through a different route? In describing the fundamentals of communicative musicality, Malloch and Trevarthen (2009) give us our answer: the *essence* of togetherness is 'musical' but amodal. Our two fundamentals of rhythmically modulated human interaction – 'pulse' and 'quality' – can be effectively communicated via various modality combinations (Malloch and Trevarthen 2009).[2] For Tony, *his* modalities would be *touch* (the direct experience of changing patterns of position, intention, and intensity of the body) and *hearing* (the experience of changing patterns of timbre, pitch, and volume in voice).

In our first session together, I sat quietly on the floor with Tony as he took in the room, the play stuff I had arranged, and me. Tony was sitting but in constant motion, flashing his fingers or tapping his feet, shifting his body posture. I felt like he was a box of fireworks, a lid of self-restriction barely containing the explosions within. I used whole-body 'sigh' gestures and big, wondering eyes to try to connect with Tony's sense of 'just-not-sureness'. I also took on his body shapes, shifting along with him. Tony showed the very beginnings of interest in my attuned, accepting behaviour: a sideways glance, · a mini-pause in his repetitions. To me, it felt as though Tony was looking for some sign of silent permission to accelerate. His whole body communicated the need to extend his minimal, contained movements into powerful expression.

Wanting to gently facilitate a playful physical interaction with Tony, I looked for inspiration from Sherborne Developmental Movement (SDM) (Sherborne 2001). I recommend exploring SDM to any therapist whose work takes them into physical interaction. The tools of SDM are a great foundation when playing with the experience of emotions in physical, embodied relationship. For children with severe communication difficulties, or with physical/motor disability, we can enable them with experiences of vitality and emotion through physical relationship which otherwise would never have been possible. For instance, how does a child who uses a wheelchair know how it feels to be a strong support for another person? Or how does that child know the sensation of free-flowing, spontaneous motion? Without those embodied experiences, what is that child's point of reference when internalizing and regulating related emotions? Can that child ever feel strong and supportive of others (and as such, feel supported or 'contained' herself)? Can that child ever feel the vibrancy of spontaneous action and risk-taking? The therapist's use of supportive contact and positioning to help a child into her *own* physically supportive role can help that child feel strong and compassionate. The use of a blanket to aid in being slid fluidly across a smooth floor can help that child feel the vitality of free-flow. Over time, the child accumulates these embodied experiences which can help anchor and regulate previously undefined emotions. The emotional landscape Tony would explore included his undisguised anger, the underlying sadness, and the more hidden compassion. My approach with Tony combined the ideas

---

2   Many modality combinations and personal preferences can be supported through music therapy (Trevarthen and Malloch 2000). For a great overview of a music therapy focus on communicative musicality with children with autism spectrum disorder and related communication difficulties see Wigram and Elefant 2009.

of SDM with an attempt to emulate our basic contour (Brazelton *et al.* 1974) and an openness to move into different levels and modes of play.

It was a particular SDM tool (the bum slide!) that helped Tony and me into our first mutual interaction. Feeling the inherent drive for movement *and* contradictory self-restriction in Tony's actions, I developed our sitting posture into something more free flowing. Propelling myself backwards with my legs, I slid around the floor on my bum. Tony smiled and joined in. With children with severe communication difficulties I find myself initiating direction in play more than I do with most other children. Working towards being open to the flow of vitality in the playroom can help us know when to gently encourage a child's play towards new patterns. There are some children who never actively reach out to play, and times when a child's vitality flow seems stagnant or habitually stuck. Direction *can* help. But the moment a child takes her own spontaneous initiative, it is crucial to follow that impetus. That initiative could be: reaching out for interaction (with even the most micro-gesture), by indicating that the direction was unwanted (either by active or passive communication), or by taking the play content, developmental play structure, modality, or quality in a new direction.

Tony and I slid around on our bums for quite some time! And then, with no eye contact or words spoken in the entire session, our bodies met back to back. Tony and I sat like that for a while, legs stretched out in front of us. Tony wriggled a bit, getting comfortable. He calmed down. A lot. I matched his postural release. Backs are big and strong – sensitive, supporting, and 'containing'. We had found our natural point of Initiation and Orientation in our basic contour map. Our back-to-back meeting would also become a natural anchor for calming co-regulation in the Deceleration stage. For children who cannot stand eye contact, I have often found that meeting back to back is extremely helpful. From a back-meeting you can even push against and slide down each other's backs, ending in a lying position with heads on each other's shoulders (Sherborne 2001)! From there I sometimes find the tiniest moments of eye contact from even severely autistic children. From there, so much becomes possible.

From our back-to-back position, Tony and I developed a play-phrase which would remain similar in structure for many months. It was Tony's container for exploring and expressing the anger which permeated his body. Each phrase would be Initiated by one of us, through a shift in posture, a change in the intensity of back wiggling, an anticipatory noise. The other would immediately Orientate to this gesture. The Acceleration started tentatively – wiggling, pressing, feeling our backs, starting to push against each other. Tony and I would then increase the force and rate of variability in quality of contact, building up anticipation and intensity in a shared vitality contour. Tony would add vocalizations in increasing pitch, frequency, and volume as the contour heightened. He would make quiet, disparate sounds that slowly grew in volume and intensity to form a period of staccato anger. The sounds then morphed into a continuous, fluid tone which flowed up to a roar just at the Peak. Close to the Peak, Tony would be pushing and shoving against my back with his full force. I would try to maintain enough stability to resist without ever overpowering Tony – a tricky balance!

Tony's anger was raw. I needed to communicate empathy through intensity without communicating anger itself. If I communicated anger, I would have been just another reactive, confrontational adult in Tony's life. Here Stern's concept of vitality (2010) is so helpful for us. 'Vitality' explores the nature and intensity of energetic expression underlying the more obvious communicative patterns we call 'emotions'. We can describe it through the musical elements of 'quality'; we can feel it in our bodies and hearts in the playroom. An understanding of vitality-matching, as opposed to emotion-matching, enables us to match the energetic tone and impetus beneath the more obvious manifestation of emotion. We can play with this idea in two ways. First, when Stern talks of 'attunement' he is describing, 'matching and sharing dynamic forms of vitality, but across different modalities' (Stern 2010, p.42). For example, if Tony made a loud staccato shout, I could make a quick, double-footed stomping jump on the ground. If he punched out at the air with a closed fist, I could make a loud but blunt 'huuugh' sound full of energy. Second, I would explore vitality-matching *within* the same modality – usually here within the modality of vocal sound. For instance, if Tony was shouting and swearing angrily, I would try to make loud sounds alongside him which matched the increasing energy contours of his vocalization but which held none of the verbal content or angry vibe. Through these two approaches I would focus on mirroring the energy rising in Tony's vitality contour – through postural, behavioural, and vocal shifts in intensity – whilst never displaying the facial, bodily, or verbal expressions of anger itself. With sadness we can match a pattern of subdued, folding energy – posturally, behaviourally, vocally becoming small and internal – so avoiding feeding the other's sadness, whilst staying present in empathy. The vitality of sadness is very tender. Vitality-matching is a conscious process to connect on a level more fundamental than emotion.

Initially, Tony's angry vitality contour would move through the Acceleration stage and would reach its height in a very simple Peak of Excitement. Basically, we slipped out of physical contact and fell over. Usually, we burst out laughing. We would then scramble back into our back-to-back position and sit for a while in Deceleration. Here the contact of our backs helped Tony calm himself and learn to self-regulate. It was co-regulation without eye contact, facial expression, or words.

Then, after a few weeks, a different Peak emerged. We would control our back-to-back force enough to push us both upright into a standing position. The motion would sometimes carry us up into a jump and release of tension. On one occasion we found ourselves standing face to face. Tony was shocked; it caused a break in the contour flow. But something in Tony felt the significance of the change. Despite the self-regulatory challenge it posed, Tony started to repeat this Peak in order to return again and again to face-to-face contact. We began spending time in Deceleration within this new face-to-face relationship. This was very different from our regular back-to-back co-regulation. It had a different quality. Through vitality-matching and a non-judgemental presence on my part, and a deal of courage on Tony's, he now stood in eye contact – surviving, self-regulating, calming down. Now we were co-regulating the extremes of Tony's anger, particularly his anger at other people and what they had done to him. This Deceleration evolved naturally into new expressive elements including grounded feet-stomping, body shaking, foam-sword fighting, punching cushions, and kicking the air. And all of these followed vitality contours that led to face-to-face, calming co-regulation. Together, Tony and I had evolved a series of play-phrases which each adequately emulated the basic contour. Within the phrase structure, Tony and I were in sync. Tony felt togetherness. Within co-regulation, he was able to express his painful emotional extremes and learn to self-calm and let go.

After a few months, play-phrases of support and compassion began to appear within Tony's play. The back-to-back vitality-build would, at times, simply lose its angry impetus. Following this lead, I could initiate new types of physical relating. We played with being an immovable rock whilst the other tried to dislodge us. We played with balances, holding each other stable at arm's length. And slowly, on Tony's initiative, we moved into a series of quiet play-phrases which included resting our heads on each other – one supporting, one resting. To begin with Tony was always the supporter. But slowly he came to feel safe enough to be supported. It was in a Deceleration stage, Tony's head supported on my chest, that Tony first cried. And it was in such a Deceleration stage, a little later on, that Tony spent some time in a place of deep relaxation. He returned from that place with a whole bunch of new, creative energy.

This new energy led Tony into playing with toys (a long series of mother and baby-doll play) and the creation of symbols using paint, textures, and water. Now, only occasionally Tony would return to our back-to-back or rest-support Deceleration positions. The rhythmic structure of his play had evolved.

As Tony's play therapy progressed, the violent episodes in his life became less frequent until one day, they stopped completely.

Bryn: The metronomic – playing with micro-narrative gaps

Bryn was seven when we met. It was a unique introduction. We spent the first ten minutes chasing each other around the waiting room, pretending to be mice after I scratched my nose! A single index-finger twist to the side of the nose can mean 'mouse' in British Sign Language (BSL). I did not know this back then. I thought I was just alleviating an itch! It was a very happy accident.

Bryn was born profoundly deaf. And, at age five, he underwent two years of intensive treatment for a particularly nasty form of cancer involving multiple traumatic experiences. There are often early developmental implications to being raised profoundly deaf by hearing parents, as was the case for Bryn. Bryn's family are wonderfully loving. Yet even in this close to ideal family environment, deafness takes time to acknowledge and diagnose, and sign skills take time to learn. As such, early development often lacks, to some degree, the experience of synchronous play. It was likely Bryn had missed out on much of the togetherness within healthy infant–mother play before heading straight into two years marked by medical trauma. Bryn's deaf-specific education was sadly lost as a priority during this period, and so, when I first met him, neither of us had developed our BSL skills beyond the basic.

Bryn was referred for play therapy due to a behavioural presentation remarkably similar to that of a child with Reactive Attachment Disorder (RAD). Bryn was hyper-vigilant, violent, quick to anger, had difficulty self-regulating to a calm state, and was constantly pushing the adults around him to elicit reactive responses. Children with RAD ironically, given the label, do not often display disturbances in *primary* attachment. Their developmental profile seems to stem from disrupted early inter-subjectivity (Minnis *et al.* 2006), from a lack of consistency in early togetherness. Without togetherness in interaction, these children have rarely experienced shared, co-regulatory play. Children with RAD come to experience themselves as isolated and insubstantial, essentially asocial (Hughes 2000). For children with a classical matrix of autism symptoms, the roots of disconnectedness are different from RAD (innate, as opposed to parental) – but the pattern of inter-subjective disturbance, lack of togetherness, and resulting asocial self-narrative is remarkably similar (Maestro *et al.* 2005). Despite his family being consistently loving and sensitively able, Bryn's early disconnectedness (rooted in deafness and trauma response) resulted in a similar trajectory. Like a child with RAD, Bryn controlled his social environment relentlessly. He could accept and enjoy emotional connectedness at the level of intact primary attachment; he often sought hugs and close proximity. But beyond this, like a child with RAD, Bryn was incapable of incorporating affection and love into his sense of self.

In the playroom Bryn's work began with an energetic expression of his sense of internal chaos. This expression was free flowing but in no way social. I was accepted as a necessary observer, but one that was held at a rigid psychological distance. Bryn used hundreds of play figures, all of the different spaces of the room, and an imposing mixture of elements (sand, water, red paint) to create a dark whirl of movement. At this stage the energy of Bryn's trauma patterning was tangible and raw. There was nothing to do but accept, keep Bryn safe, and connect empathically with Bryn's vitality through whole-body gesture. This lasted a long time. Many weeks.

It was acceptance, empathy, patience, and a mermaid that led Bryn and I into interactive play. At some stage, in the middle of all that chaos, I noticed an unusually personal level of care Bryn displayed for a mermaid figure. There seemed a vibrant tie between Bryn and that mermaid – perhaps a symbol of self? I pointed to the mermaid. Bryn gaze-tracked for the first time. Then I pointed at Bryn. He splashed himself with water, fell down theatrically on the floor, and flapped his two legs up and down like a mermaid's tail! I joined in.

The mermaid was a doorway into interactive play and a feeling of togetherness for Bryn. It was, however, a narrow doorway. Initially it opened onto our basic contour map at the Peak of excitement stage. Being mermaids was a high-energy routine: we flapped our legs, laughed out loud, and then collapsed the rest of our body tension in a heap. This play flowed out as a release of emotional tension from Bryn's chaotic solo adventures – a self-regulatory valve. And to begin with, this is where the doorway shut. Like Tony in his early stages, and Sarah in the Monster-On-My-Belly, Bryn's habitual patterns of control welcomed the physical, but shut down quickly at the approach of social stimulation. Like a child with RAD, Bryn's patterns of social control were firmly established. Being mermaids together had the glimpse of something alive and special, but it also represented a vulnerability that was difficult for him to let in.

For the next few weeks Bryn's play oscillated between periods of asocial self-expression and doorway moments of tentative social contact. Bryn was walking a knife-edge between control and relationship. On his part, this took an amazing level of courageous, intelligent self-regulation. For me, this meant engaging in a fragile balance of Follow-Lead-Follow (Hughes 2011). I would follow Bryn's vitality up to each tentative social doorway. There I would try a sensitive lead into interactive play. Then I would follow again, as our play developed only slightly and the door was shut. But no matter how slightly, our play *was* evolving. Slowly, in this tentative way, Bryn and I led each other into a series of play-phrases that unfolded from the Peak mermaid routine to include the rest of our basic contour. Bryn was deaf, and so the normal use of timbre, pitch, and volume when modulating the shared experience of vitality contours was impossible. Like Tony, Bryn was open to physical play. Unlike Tony, when engaging socially, Bryn was relatively comfortable with eye contact and had a sensitive understanding of basic emotional expression. It seemed the foundations of our interactive relationship would likely be built from physical contact and theatrical physical–emotional gesture.

The first complete play-phrase structure Bryn and I developed went something like this: one of us would Initiate the phrase with tentative eye contact and a gestural reference to the sink and the water in it. The other would immediately Orientate – locking onto, and maintaining, eye contact. Then I would begin the Acceleration. I would creep up to Bryn, my features and posture drawn in with the anticipation of a playful 'hunt'. I would try to build vitality through theatrical expression, whilst Bryn responded with alternating playful shyness and retaliation in synchronous reciprocation. Bryn would hide behind his hands, peek-a-boo style, and giggle. I added to the increasing vitality by making little darts forward, splashing Bryn (the mermaid) with tiny amounts of water. At the Peak of our contour, Bryn would break the tension and we would fall down into the mermaid routine. We would then spend some time calming and co-regulating in Deceleration. Here, to begin with, eye contact was too intense. We maintained our thread of contact through connected arms and legs. For any deaf child, contact without eyes is contact without language. So, just like Tony, Bryn's initial experiences of co-regulation happened without language, eye contact, or shared facial expression. Through physical contact Bryn could remain in relationship. Experiencing my physical stability and calm state helped his system self-regulate.

Once established, Bryn and I repeated this particular phrase over and over. We had found a play-phrase which emulated the basic contour of play in early infancy. The developmental level was appropriate in addressing the lack of synchronous play in Bryn's early years. The experience was of togetherness.

Our mermaid phrase continued as a theme throughout much of Bryn's play therapy, a powerful anchor in togetherness and co-regulation. Alongside this, Bryn also led us into developmentally earlier rhythms of play. He intuitively began to seek calming, metronomic social rhythms as a support for Deceleration. Our simplest socially oriented biological clocks are metronomic oscillators; they keep a simple on-beat and tend towards phasic sync with another person (Osborne 2009). These are the simplest developmental rhythms of togetherness. In Bryn's case his impulse pulled us into rocking and swaying in time together. Just like with Mark and our 'waltz'.

Bryn and I now shared two different developmental patterns of play: two different musical shapes – the early metronomic and the basic contour – within which we could go on to explore micro-narrative gaps. To recap, the 'micro-narrative' is our term for the shared emotional story of each play-phrase; it is the flowing pattern of mutually modulated emotional connection. The gaps which occur in emotional connectedness, through playful exploration or shocking 'disruption', we are calling 'micro-narrative gaps'. In therapy with children with RAD, micro-narrative gaps often appear within the themes of shame and terror (Hughes 2004). The child with RAD is used to controlling, manipulating, and provoking reactive responses from the adults around her. As the therapist remains stable and accepting, she naturally disrupts the tide of those reactive patterns. The therapist's shift to a non-reactive response can lead the child into gaps of confusion, confrontation, and discomfort. The therapist welcomes these gaps, providing a safe place for exploration, and then repairs the relationship before moving on (Hughes 2004).

Both Bryn and Tony experienced such periods of vulnerability as the therapy relationship got close to shaking their patterns of control. In the early stages, these gaps could lead to more protracted periods of social withdrawal for both of them. Without a thread of spoken narrative, and before we had established the rhythmic structures of interactive play, it was difficult to maintain a sense of vitality-connection throughout periods of natural emotional disruption. This is what my experience suggests is made possible through the shared rhythmic pulse and flowing vitality contours of interactive play: at a level more basic then expressed emotion, a pulse-beat of connection is maintained between partners in play, a pulse that maintains a feeling of togetherness in the temporary absence of emotional connection, a pulse that has the energy of requiring completion, and as such, inspires reconnection and repair.

Bryn and I played with micro-narrative gaps in our simplest metronomic rhythms. Rocking together to a basic on-beat, we would pause and close our eyes. Then we would wait to see who would start the motion again, who was impelled by the silent expectant pulse. This was a playful exploration of the jazz-pause discussed earlier with Jonathon. The pulse needed to be filled, the action completed. And the longer the potential remained on pause, the more the anticipation built within our shared vitality. On Bryn's initiation we then began to extend the gap in time. When the gap reached a certain felt duration, we began to share a sense of creeping vulnerability. We were starting to explore the potential for real disruption in emotional connection: riding the knife-edge of rhythmic vital connection where emotions are unclear, on the boundaries of trust and doubt. Feeling how this exploration was benefiting Bryn, I introduced a further element to our disruption. I carefully stepped away from physical contact with Bryn. Now Bryn was deaf, eyes closed, and disconnected physically. He was exploring his emotional vulnerability all on his own with only the impetus of our on-pause beat keeping us connected. Bryn took this even further, moving back from me a little. And then, each time, the expectation of the beat would bring us back into emotional contact in a moment of happy relief. The repair of our emotional connection came as we opened our eyes, laughed, and hugged. I had a palpable sense of how these repeated experiences – of held vulnerability, skirting the unknown, culminating in delightful repair – really did help Bryn to regulate his emotions and build a stronger sense of self.

In working with Nigel Osborne on his chapter in this book, I was drawn to reflect on my memories of the duration of each experience that Bryn and I shared. Sometimes those moments of vulnerability would feel like forever. So, on a few occasions, I remember deliberately clocking them. The maximum duration of rhythmically contained vulnerability, before Bryn would seek a repair of emotional contact, seemed to be around six or seven seconds. Interestingly, 'the current consensus in music psychology and cognitive neuroscience is that the ability to associate beats or perform them meaningfully as a pulse stops at around six seconds or 0.16Hz' (Osborne, pp.18–19 in this book). 'It is at this point that the mind and body can no longer "lock on" – either actively through playing, or passively through listening – to the rhythm as a pulse' (p.18).

Within the 'basic contour', playing with micro-narrative gaps seems to come most naturally within the Acceleration stage. With Bryn, this would be in the social build-up to the mermaid routine. Mid-vitality build-up, I would sometimes stop cheekily and pretend to be doing something else or walk away. This is clearly a bit of a risk and I would only recommend trying it within the sensitive practice of Follow-Lead-Follow (Hughes 2011). If I got my timing wrong, and the disruption was inappropriate, Bryn's gestures would let me know immediately and I would follow his vitality into something different. But most of the time Bryn loved it. The anticipation would build as the pulse of the rising vitality-contour was put on pause. And again, we intuitively extended the duration of the gaps to approach a real sense of emotional disruption. But always, the underling pulse-beat of the rhythmical play-phrase structure kept us connected in anticipation, and drew us back to the expected Peak of excitement (the mermaid routine) and Deceleration. I introduced similarly playful micro-narrative gaps into the Acceleration stages of play-phrases with Tony. He loved this exploration too.

Held safely by the rhythmic structures of our play, both Bryn and Tony were able to remain in connection and co-regulation whilst directly experiencing their pain. For Tony, this enabled a safe level of exploratory self-regulation and a playful remoulding of his early trauma – a rewriting of the emotional narrative from his past. For Bryn, his play therapy unfolded like this: He also developed the confidence to remain in direct eye contact within our Deceleration stages and rocking-rhythms. Bryn began to learn to self-regulate his extreme emotions within the safety of face-to-face co-regulation. Then one day our mermaid play-phrase changed. During a Deceleration stage, Bryn spent a while in deep relaxation. It was not long. But whilst there, something significant changed for Bryn. He stood up and brought me the doctor's kit. I took on the role of doctor, administering symbolic surgery and emotional/physical soothing to the intense trauma patterning in Bryn's system. The spring-coiled energy which had been leaking out in Bryn's mermaid movements became apparent in his stomach area. Bryn directed me in 'surgery' to the area of his original tumour. We played in this way for many sessions. Then the surgery was over. The intensity and focus left that pattern. From here, Bryn returned to the chaotic themes of his initial solo play but this time with the intent to restructure. He added safety, categories, and delineation to the previously chaotic elements, bringing these qualities to his internal world. And this time, his process was interactive. Through BSL, Bryn regularly let me know what he was up to. Within this restructuring Bryn returned to the mermaid figure. It was time for him to evolve his relationship to his symbol of self. Bryn built a shallow hollow of sand and water for the mermaid and covered her in red-paint blood. He then cleaned and healed her carefully. Bryn wrapped her like a new baby in sheets of pure white tissue and kept her safe. Bryn is still making progress in therapy today.

References

Brazelton, T.B., Koslowski, B. and Main, M. (1974) 'The Origins of Reciprocity: The Early Mother–Infant Interaction.' In M. Lewis and L.A. Rosenblum (eds) *The Effect of the Infant on its Caregiver.* New York: Wiley.

Hughes, D. (2000) *Facilitating Developmental Attachment: The Road to Emotional Recovery and Behavioural Change in Foster and Adopted Children.* London: Jason Aaronson.

Hughes, D. (2004) 'An attachment-based treatment of maltreated children and young people.' *Attachment and Human Development 3,* 6, 263–278.

Hughes, D. (2011) *Attachment-focused Family Therapy Workbook* (Pap/DVD Wk edition). New York: W.W. Norton.

Malloch, S. and Trevarthen, C. (2009) 'Musicality: Communicating the Vitality and Interests of life.' In S. Malloch and C. Trevarthen (eds) *Communicative Musicality: Exploring the Basis of Human Companionship.* Oxford: Oxford University Press.

Maestro, S., Muratori, F., Cavallaro, M.C., Pecini, C., *et al.* (2005) 'How young children treat objects and people: an empirical study of the first year of life in autism.' *Child Psychiatry and Human Development 35,* 4, 383–396.

Minnis, H., Marwick, H., Arthur, J. and McLaughlin, A. (2006) 'Reactive Attachment Disorder – a theoretical model beyond attachment.' *European Child and Adolescent Psychiatry15,* 336–342.

Osborne, N. (2009) 'Towards a Chronobiology of Musical Rhythm.' In S. Malloch and C. Trevarthen (eds) *Communicative Musicality: Exploring the Basis of Human Companionship.* Oxford: Oxford University Press.

Schore, A.N. (1994) *Affect Regulation and the Origin of the Self.* Hillsdale, NJ: Lawrence Erlbaum.

Sherborne, V. (2001) *Developmental Movement for Children.* London: Worth Publishing.

Stern, D.N. (1985) *The Interpersonal World of the Infant.* New York: Basic Books.

Stern, D.N. (2004) *The First Relationship: Infant and Mother.* Cambridge, MA: Harvard University Press.

Stern, D.N. (2010) *Forms of Vitality: Exploring Dynamic Experience in Psychology, the Arts, Psychotherapy, and Development.* Oxford: Oxford University Press.

Trevarthen, C. (2001) 'Intrinsic motives for companionship in understanding: their origin, development and significance for infant mental health.' *Journal of Infant Mental Health 22,* 95–131.

Trevarthen, C. and Daniel, S. (2005) 'Disorganised rhythm and synchrony: early signs of autism and Rett syndrome.' *Brain and Development 27,* 25–34.

Trevarthen, C. and Malloch, S. (2000) 'The dance of wellbeing: defining the musical therapeutic effect.' *The Nordic Journal of Music Therapy 9*, 2, 3–17.

Wigram, T. and Elefant, C. (2009) 'Therapeutic Dialogues in Music: Nurturing Musicality of Communication in Children with Autistic Spectrum Disorder and Rett Syndrome.' In S. Malloch and C. Trevarthen (eds) *Communicative Musicality: Exploring the Basis of Human Companionship*. Oxford: Oxford University Press.

10

HARNESSING THE DRAGON

Using an Image of Unbridled Life Force in Play Therapy[1]

DENNIS MCCARTHY

With wise and playful insight Tolkien wrote, 'It does not do to leave a live dragon out of your calculations, if you live near him' (Tolkien 2007). Every day in my play therapy practice, in a setting that is filled with a variety of materials and options for playful expression, children use the dragon image in their play configurations with the greatest frequency. It may be used in the making and unmaking of worlds in the deep sandbox. It may be used as inspiration in the various types of aggressive discharge that children engage in, or in the spontaneous narratives children tell me. But it is the single most used figure, and the penultimate catalyst of change and healing in a child's play process. This alone should command our attention and interest. It also informs us about how the child experiences life, something we really should know about if we are going to help them.

This past week alone there have been a dozen play sessions in which the dragon played a pivotal role, although these roles varied greatly from child to child. The dragon image is used by very young children and by adolescents as well. It is used by both girls and boys, and seems to span many developmental stages as well as the variety of childhood problems and life situations that children bring with them into the play space. This is not so surprising, as the dragon image has been a central figure, exalted and/or maligned, in folklore, mythology, and literature throughout the world for at least 6000 years. It shows up in every culture and the various roles it has played in folklore are similar to the roles it plays in treatment with children. Dragons are monsters and gods, royalty and the destroyers of royalty, hero makers, and hero un-makers. They create problems and resolve them and the fluidity of their roles is central to their potency.

---

1   Some of the material in this chapter was explored briefly in *Deep Play – Exploring the Use of Depth in Psychotherapy with Children* (McCarthy 2015), as well as in the *Healing Power of the Imagination Journal*, December 2015.

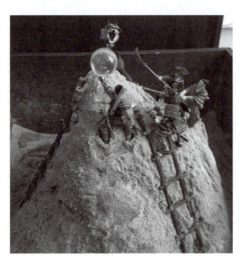

FIGURE 10.1 FOUR SAMURAIS WAKE UP A DRAGON AS THEY ARE TRYING TO STEAL 'THE ORB OF LIFE' (CREATED BY A FIVE-YEAR-OLD BOY DIAGNOSED WITH ADHD)

The great child psychology theorist and play therapy champion D.W. Winnicott focused on the intensity of aliveness in his writings about children. This seems to me to be the underpinning of his work and it is the underlying issue in all the children I work with, no matter what the presenting symptoms are. Paradoxically, life force contains the potential resolution of the very problems that may be caused when it is dysregulated, suppressed, or imploded. All children are waiting to be related to on this level. They are all waiting to have us help them with the expression and regulation of life force. Dragon and all that it implies can help us help them.

The idea of the dragon is rooted in part in a deep and universal apprehension about our own nature and the threats presented by the universe in which we live (Niles 2013) The dragon is a manifestation of an actual energy and form that exist in the human psyche. We won't find its bones buried in bogs or deep in the ground. But we will find them in the bogs and underworld of the human psyche, and the imagination of the playing child. The dragon is the nature of spirit and the spirit of nature. It is an external form of an internal process (Huxley 1979). It is life personified, in all its manifestations, and therein lies its power and appeal to the child. In children, especially the playing child, the dragon lives very close to the surface, making its potency readily accessible.

Dragon as catalyst

The most frequent use of dragons by children in the play therapy process is as a catalyst for change. This is a basic aspect of dragon power and the underpinning of its function in all the various roles dragons play. The simplest manifestation of this is as a figure that forces two opposing armies or sides to unite. An embattled child may depict two armies at loggerheads in the world they have made in the sand, stuck in a seemingly unresolvable state of stasis. Then out of the sky swoops a fire-breathing dragon and the armies immediately unite, their initial quarrel forgotten. Or a dragon emerges up out of the depths of the earth and the same immediate unifying response is triggered. Often it may be three armies or many more, and there may be great chaos in their battling, and it is unclear who is on whose side. Then a dragon enters and the chaos organizes; the myriad forces unite. This simple act of joining forces can, at the right time in the child's process, reflect and facilitate a shift in their inner and outer conflict.

An oppositional child may become more able to be a part of his or her family system or peer group. A child whose own neurophysiology has rendered them in a state of defensive opposition may soften as the two sides align. The process of change may have been fostered in weeks of preparatory play. This play probably involved the same child battling me in various ways or using materials that express and discharge negative aggression safely. I am sure that I initially joined them in their dysregulated play, mirroring them with the unspoken goal of fostering a sense of regulation. They may have fought me unfairly to secure victory and I may have both allowed and challenged this. But at last the child's defense system is ready to find a new, more functional form. The dragon makes this happen, arising in this case out of the very dysregulated aggression that was part of the problem. Its destructive power makes it a potentially creative presence. And there are other impasses that the dragon as catalyst helps to resolve.

Seven-year-old Michael had been attacked by two large dogs and came for treatment to address what was becoming an escalating phobia. He wasn't badly hurt by the dogs but was very shaken emotionally. He had become phobic, not only of dogs but also of going outside in case he might see one, or they might see him. He was contracting into himself.

In meeting with his parents, initially I asked them what might have concerned them about their son prior to the dog attack. I usually do this when a child has experienced situational trauma such as a dog attack to have a sense of who they were prior to it. Knowing what their prior strengths and weaknesses were can help us know how to help them, seeing each child as more than traumatic experience. In this child's case his parents said they had concerns about him even when he was quite young. He was a math genius, doing mathematics on a high school level at age four and scoring in the top ten on a national test at age five. His school was thrilled to have such genius in their midst but his parents saw the downside of this. His obsession with numerical formulas was at times all consuming. They were not concerned that he was autistic, as he had many friends, was very relational, and quite empathic. But they felt there was a concomitant rigidity in him because of the discrepancy between his mental and physical development. They were very eager to have him come and play.

Michael was really quite wonderful and engaged easily in play. But his numerical obsession tinged everything. His initial drawings of himself as a monster were all numerical formulas, although they did have teeth. His initial sand worlds involved dogs being run through labyrinths made up of numerical formulas, especially the formula for Pi. These were drawn in the sand using small gems. The formula's task was always to 'boggle the mind' of the dogs. I asked him if all these mathematical formulas boggled his mind too and he admitted that they did. 'But it's better than the black holes I was obsessed with when I was three,' he said. In his second version of the same world above he added two statues of the god Shiva standing and watching what was happening. He and I and the gods watched while dogs were chased by numerical formulas. His imitation of the dog's barking was very convincing.

For a few sessions he explored a variety of play experiences in which his movement repertoire increased. He found that pounding on a mattress in my office was greatly enhanced if he ran from across the room and then leapt up into the air. He lay down on the same mattress and threw pretend tantrums, eliciting much laughter as well as a freer sense of moving. He enjoyed building and then knocking down tall block towers, often erupting into loud barking as he did so. All of the above was done in the spirit of play and all helped him get out of his head, or at least begin to integrate his physical self with his intellect.

Then I challenged him to a round of 'The Cheating Game', which is a drawing game that I created, useful with both rigid children and timid children. In it, each person draws monsters on different sides of the same piece of paper, separated by a river perhaps. There are three rules to the battle that ensues; you can only draw three monsters, you can only destroy part of one of your opponent's monsters in any turn, and third you have to cheat, i.e. break the first two rules. This child was thrilled with the game. And, not surprisingly perhaps, all of his monsters were mathematical formulas! They were not even vaguely disguised as monsters. Numbers and parentheses and multiplication signs were amassed on his side of the paper and it was apparent that they gave this child joy even as they encumbered him.

Meanwhile, I drew a large dragon on my side that only ate mathematical formulas. I assured him that it could gobble up all of those numbers with one bite. He saw with alarm how I had tricked him into varying his obsession. He would now have to make some figures that were not numbers. But he was also charmed by this trickery. In order to not be destroyed he had to make other monsters which he readily did. I think he was relieved to be free of the obsession, at least for the moment. He drew a large dragon that successfully battled mine. After this, dragons showed up in his sand worlds as the dog provokers instead of numbers and the architecture of the scenes became much more complex as a result.

From the onset Michael left my sessions very stirred up emotionally, despite seeming very happy in his play. He would often weep on the ride home, or speak baby talk. His parents saw this in a positive light as a sign of loosening. They felt his weeping was both grief and relief over the loss of his numerical obsession. They also felt that his intellect, so overly developed at such a young age, had been a hindrance to feeling truly connected to others. The dog phobia rapidly dissolved.

One of his last sand worlds depicted a number of dogs in a very complex series of tunnels that he referred to as a labyrinth. There were no numbers in this world. The dogs were playing and taking baths and resting. Surrounding this world on the rim of the sandbox were numerous dragons that were keeping an eye on the dogs, but otherwise not interfering. They seemed like guardians. Seen from above, the structure of the sand looked like a spinal column or neural dendrites. For me, it seemed that his entire organism had been positively influenced by the play therapy relationship.

In his last visit Michael made one final play scene in which numbers were dressed up as monsters so they couldn't be recognized as numbers. This seemed to be a brilliant compromise on his part. He had maintained his sense of integrity whilst also allowing for subtlety, protection, and the possibility of broadening his frame of reference further, my support and gentle provocation helping him along the way.

Dragon as healer

Eight-year-old Sarah sits by the deep sandbox in my office and creates a world full of dragons. The land itself is littered with jewels forming a mandala pattern. Dozens of dragons sit or play or fight amongst the jewels. In the center of the mandala is a mound with a smaller mound within it and a chalice and a very small dragon sitting on top of this. Lastly, a water dragon emerges from the ocean nearby. This action seems to surprise her even though she made it happen. When she created the mound within the mound it kept reminding me of an image I had seen somewhere. At some point I realized that it looked like an *omphalos*, a structure found in various places in ancient Greece that was meant to depict the navel of the world, used as a symbol of rebirth.

Sarah was sexually molested at the age of three by her father. Her mother had fled with her and her sister, and for a period of time they lived in a remote area by a wild river. She remembered this time as paradise, despite what had come before it. She spoke about it with a sense of reverie. She had begun treatment due to great fearfulness at night and timidity in school, understandable in light of what had happened. She was well liked at school but overly sensitive to the comments and reactions of her peers. At home she felt bullied by her older sister.

She came willingly to play therapy but she was very limited in what she would engage in. Each time she would make very simple worlds in the deep sandbox in my office and she would also draw herself as a monster. None of the other usual avenues of play that benefit abused children were available to her as she rejected all of them. Initially all her sand worlds were rather flat and lifeless. But there were a few bones and jewels in them, hinting at life past and some longing for the future. At first, all of her monster drawings were very small and well-crafted cats. But they were warrior cats.

Despite the seeming deficit of imagery and action, our relationship felt engaged and safe and I found myself gently provoking her to expand her play. I urged her to explore and use the sand's depth and this slowly helped the worlds she made there evolve. I also urged Sarah to let her monsters themselves turn into monsters – furthering their evolution – hoping that, concomitantly, something bigger and more powerful would be born within her own psyche. Week by week the monsters began to get bigger. At some point they grew large fangs. Some of them oozed blood and toxins. Some looked horrified as well as horrifying. These latter monsters of hers greatly disturbed a number of boys who I work with. This was unusual. Most of the many monsters on my office walls are seen by children in a positive light. But Sarah's monsters had a different effect. She was thrilled to know that her monsters were unsettling boys, but she did allow me to remove some of them.

Meanwhile, her use of the sand became deeper and more complex. Then, simultaneously, several things happened. She had a dream in which she had become a golden dragon. In the dream she was walking in her school with a boy who was a friend of hers. And she was suddenly amazed to discover that she could breathe fire! In the dream, she flew around the school with her friend, the challenge being not to set fire to things or other children as she went.

Sarah was ecstatic in the telling of the dream. That same day she had stood up to a girl in school who had been bullying her and the girl backed down in amazement. Then came the world described above, with its image of rebirth and playful power along with the dragon emerging from the river. I thought of the river she had lived by as a child along with what sexual abuse can do to a child's natural life force. It seemed that her life force had reemerged. After she shared the dream and made this world in the sand I asked her if she was still feeling so afraid. She thought about it for some time and then answered simply, 'No'.

One classic image from dragon literature is that of 'a knight in shining armor' battling a fire-breathing dragon, often rescuing a princess from its clutches. Taken literally, there is a significant gendered problem with this classic slice of mythology: girls do not need to be rescued from their dragons. They need to be better connected to them. We can look at this traditional image in terms of the male attempting to free his own feminine side, or to master his own destructive urges. It is important to consider that his feminine side is actually contained within the dragon/princess overlap, so mastery involves dealing with this but not destroying it. Girls often depict dragons as belonging to the central female figure in their sand-play and accompanying narrative. It is often the pet of the princess, perhaps unbeknownst to her royal parents, not her captor. That the girl above *became* a dragon in her dream takes this a step further. The idea of a wounded girl becoming powerful is a common thread in literature. Although girls also struggle with self-regulation, they seem to feel an innate connection to the dragon. The girl mentioned above became a dragon in her dreams to counterbalance what had happened to her. It wasn't possible to change history. But learning how to breathe fire would make it less likely that the abuse would happen again. In the book *Tehanu* by Ursula LeGuin (1990), a girl who has been horribly abused, both sexually and physically, develops the power to turn into a dragon when the need arises. In this capacity she becomes a protector of others and eventually a powerful mage.

Flawed armor

There is a further problem with the image of the 'knight in shining armor'. The heavy metal armor associated with the knight is simply an unwise choice of protection. The dragon's fire could roast the hero imprisoned in his own armor! This conjecture is not superfluous. If our defense system is too rigid it becomes a prison, keeping life energy locked in that is meant to be in a state of movement, expanding and contracting. This armor is the equivalent of holding one's breath, permanently, which results in death.

Wilhelm Reich, a student of Freud and the theorist who first brought the idea of energy to western psychology, saw armoring as one of the main deterrents to emotional health. He believed that muscular rigidity and its concomitant ego rigidity was the cause of neurosis and that it contained within it the history of its origin. In his analytic work he attempted to resolve neurosis by addressing this rigidity or armoring through physical pressure on the musculature and emotional pressure on what he called the patient's 'character' (Reich 1972).

What is brilliant in this schema is the idea that the armoring of both body and ego contains its origin, and therefore may contain its potential resolution. In children it is possible to see more easily the roots of armoring and the gradual development of it in the child's body and personality. It is not yet a 'suit of armor' but simply tensions and their concomitant behaviors. Many children develop armor not just in response to external trauma but also in reaction to their own neurophysiology. There is always both an inner and outer necessity to defend oneself. Life force is its own encumberment, regardless of one's family of origin, one's wiring, or one's personality. We all become armored to some extent out of necessity.

The child can melt this armor through physical and imaginative play. Play, within the context of a safe therapeutic relationship, applies pressure to armor, turning it into a filter.

Dragon as protector, filter vs armor

For many children, in their narrative sand-play, the dragon may be the only thing that can adequately protect the scene's central characters. The kingdom is threatened by a host of zombies and all hope seems lost. Then a dragon or several dragons zoom into the scene and incinerate the zombies. A princess has been abducted and is about to be slain, when again a dragon or host of them swoop in and *voilà!* the problem is solved.

A six-year-old boy with sensory issues began treatment due to daily disruptive behavior both in school and at home. Daniel was obviously very bright but seemed unable to control his body and its impulses. His response to any impulsive action was to make it seem as though he had intended it. In fact he would often enlarge upon his action, yet its origin was clearly a lack of control and not intentional misbehavior. His mother said that he had seemed like a very sensitive child even in utero, strongly reactive to stimuli going on around her. Now at age six he was 'all elbows' much of the time: knocking things over, zooming around, and bumping into people. Of more concern than anything to his parents was his growing identification with 'the bad guys', in stories, movies, or real life. He had been very attached as an infant but this attachment was being undermined by his defensiveness and identification with 'the bad guys', which increased with the birth of two brothers. Testing was later to reveal that Daniel was extremely bright and quite dyslexic, explaining much of the presenting behavior. But by then his defense system had reorganized and he was a more functional child, thanks to dragons.

In our first meeting he spent most of the time creating a very complex narrative in the deep sandbox. There was a castle belonging to a good king and queen. They had a few knights as bodyguards but otherwise they were quite vulnerable to attack. From across the room came a flock of evil guys, vampires, ghosts, and assorted monsters. They chased the king and queen to the top of the highest tower and had them cornered. Daniel looked at me to see what I was thinking. I was thinking, 'I must accept this situation in his play, like it or not. At least for now.' There was a prolonged period in which we both waited somewhat breathlessly to see what might happen. Then Daniel had a large two-headed dragon fly over and slay all the evil ones. The king and queen were free.

He looked at me to see if I understood what had just happened and was satisfied to see that I had. That week his parents reported that he seemed softer, more trusting of them.

Over the next several weeks his sand-play expanded. In the deep sandbox with the castle, the good king and queen remained indoors. Meanwhile the castle itself was filled with dozens of dragons who were there to protect them. They covered the turrets and the surrounding land. In a nearby shallow box lived 'the evil ones', a group of assorted ghosts and vampires. Under the deep sandbox (the sandbox is raised leaving a four-inch space below) was 'the underworld' in which a lone dragon lived with some treasure. And on the other side of the play space on a high stool was 'the land of the dead', which was a graveyard. The complexity of both the architecture and accompanying narrative to these kingdoms was surprising for such a young child. For a few weeks there was no effort by the evil ones to attack. It seemed the dragon force field was working. Meanwhile his parents continued to report a more engaged child at home who was playing better with his brothers and seeming more connected to them. This was combined with moments of regression into rigid defensiveness, but these were shorter in duration than before.

In session four, the same four worlds were created. But this time in the castle there were fewer dragons, and instead a new character, 'the hero', emerged from inside and stood on the battlements. The child then took a break from the storyline and spent some time working with clay, mixing yellow and red and blue into swirls. He then placed these in small clay pots and called them torches. These were placed at various points in the castle. The story then resumed. Up from the underworld came a three-headed dog, scaling first a long ladder, then the walls of the sandbox and then the castle walls. But the dragons and the boy and his hero had anticipated this ascent. The creature was tossed onto one of the torches and it melted. The word 'melted' was mentioned that day many times as if he wanted to make sure that I understood its significance. That the protective fire had shifted from the dragons to torches manned by a human hero felt very significant.

After this, in his sand worlds, the castle became surrounded by an ever-expanding forest. Within the confines of the castle walls the dragons became less central, replaced slowly by animals and then knights. As the trees increased, the animals and dragons decreased. This shift in the castle's defense system, from pure dragons to animals, to humans and trees correlated with a shift in his defenses. And alongside these changes, his parents continued to report a softening (melting) in their son's body and behavior. The forest surrounding the castle is a wonderful example of a living and growing filter, not too rigid and not too porous. A filter regulates what comes in and what goes out, whereas armor does not. A filter helps us know who we are by helping us know who we aren't.

This discriminatory function is so fundamental to being an individual ego, an 'I'. The dragon, in its fire breathing capacity, forces the development of another means of defense. But here, as is so often the case, that firey defense can only be temporary.

The last time I saw Daniel he spent the entire session slowly and carefully drawing a figure that was filled with flowing rainbow energy. Afterwards he asked rather shyly that I put it in a safe place.

Dragon play

When a child creates a dragon-inhabited world, that world is often pivotal. Those worlds are at once the expressed symbol of the child's inner life, *and* contain (in the dragon) the symbol, catalyst, and power for change. The dragon can make those worlds whole, integrated. The dragon's power can then be fought, or utilized as is necessary for the child's movement towards freedom. And they teach us much about conflict resolution. Sarah breathed dragon fire in her dreams and was less afraid of life. Michael used dragons to loosen up an obsession and resolve a phobia. And for Daniel, dragons became guardians that allowed his defense system to re-organize.

In other worlds, a boy places a samurai in the midst of his dragons and the possibility for self-control is present. Or a dragon wakes up when a samurai enters its realm and both the samurai and the child using the samurai must contend with this unbridled power. The dragon gives power to a child whilst also (and often simultaneously) becoming the force that the newly empowered child must defeat. The paradox of this duality is at the root of deep work with children and at the root of all life – establishing balance within the conflicting urges in us, with the riptide-like energy that life-force may entail.

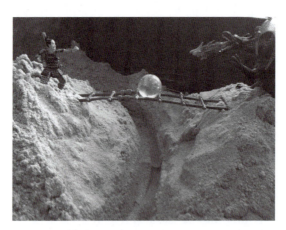

FIGURE 10.2 DRAGON ENVISIONED AS TAOIST MASTER
(CREATED BY AN ADULT MAN IN MID-LIFE WITH A HISTORY OF TRAUMA)

The purpose of playing, aside from the sheer fun of it, amounts to finding and creating oneself and bringing alive the symbols that picture both a reality beyond the self and our experiences of uniting with it (Ulanov 2001). There are a variety of play methods that may facilitate this 'bringing alive' process, especially if they allow for the spontaneous expression of energy embedded in form. The dragon is the ultimate manifestation of this energy and this form. I remain in awe of the image's capacity to help the child form a better and more vibrant relationship to themselves and others.

References

Huxley, L. (1979) *The Dragon*. London: Thames and Hudson.

LeGuin, U. (1990) *Tehanu*. New York: Atheneum.

McCarthy, D. (ed.) (2015) *Deep Play: Exploring the Use of Depth in Psychotherapy with Children*. London: Jessica Kingsley Publishers.

Niles, D. (2013) *Dragons*. Avon, MA: Adams Media.

Reich, W. (1972) *Character Analysis*. New York: Touchstone Books.

Tolkien, J.R.R. (2007) *The Hobbit*. Boston, MA: Houghton Mifflin Harcourt.

Ulanov, A. (2001) *Finding Space: Winnicott, God and Psychic Reality*. Louisville, KY: Westminister John Knox Press.

11

THE LOST AND FOUND

*Helping Children through Trauma Using Neurocellular
Developmental Movement Methods*

KATY DYMOKE

*Each child has the greatest experience and understanding of the unfolding of their
own life's path from the perspective of their soul and spirit. Why have they come
with their special strengths and challenges? What gifts are they offering us as
individuals and humanity as a whole?*

Bonnie Bainbridge Cohen[1]

During my own childhood I grew up as one of five siblings, mostly playing
outdoors and frequently getting 'lost' in the realm of fantasy and play. I have
been a dancer from three years old. Movement has remained an essential aspect
of my embodied life, a source of knowing and sense-making that may challenge
or doubt the literal. In my own movement explorations I have learned, through
experiencing inconsistency within the apparent whole of a unitary body–mind,
that unity is aggregate, illusion. And how, in the ebb and flow of disunity and
dismemberment, we come to experience the inevitability of loss. But I have
also felt how the honest, moment-to-moment experience of that inconsistency
can enable a sense of acceptance and peace. An embodied understanding of
disunity informs and supports others to manage this innate vulnerability
of being human.

My therapeutic work with infants and children integrates principles and
practice from Body-Mind Centering® (BMC®)[2] within a humanistic Dance

---

1   Bainbridge Cohen, B. (2011) 'Offerings from a Body-Mind Centering® perspective and approach
     to working with children with special needs.' El Sobrante: School for Body Mind Centering.
     Page 2 of a handout package for the SPARKS European Commission funded project, Bratislava,
     17–21 September 2014.
2   Body-Mind Centering® and BMC® are the service marks of Bonnie Bainbridge Cohen, used
     with permission.

Movement Psychotherapy framework (DMP). This framework brings influences from consciousness studies and neuroscience together with systems of movement observation (Homann 2010; Levy 1995; Meekums 2002; Sheets-Johnstone 2000, 2010). The fundamental ethos of the BMC approach is likewise integrative, body centred and experiential (Hartley 2005). In BMC, 'though we use the Western anatomical mapping, we are adding meaning to these terms through our experience' (Bainbridge Cohen 2012 [1993], p.2). BMC purposefully applies the sciences of human biology, ontogenetic development, and consciousness studies to educational and therapeutic practice. Core to the approach are specialist skills in movement and touch facilitation and in-depth experiential learning in which we revisit our own childhood development. We can then better support the child through *neurocellular developmental repatterning* (see below) towards the next developmental stage (Bainbridge Cohen 2012; Hartley 2005). We learn to trust in our own bodies when we witness the child move, and move in confluence with her (Burns 2011). When we feel the child's receptivity we facilitate with gentle initiation into new pathways for her to find ease (Burns 2011; Dymoke 2000, 2014; Hartley 1995, 2005; Meekums 2002). This embodied trust, between the therapist and child, infuses the therapeutic relationship as we will explore in the case examples below.

A neurocellular developmental approach
The basic neurocellular patterns

> The Basic [Neurocellular] Patterns are based upon potential patterns of movement inherent in the nervous system from both a phylogenetic (the evolutionary progression through the animal kingdom) and ontogenetic (the developmental progression of the human infant) perspective. These patterns include both prevertebrate and vertebrate movement sequences. (Bainbridge Cohen 2012, p.3)

The human embryo passes through many transformational stages (and levels of systemic organization) akin to prevertebrate creatures, such as the sponge, starfish, and jellyfish. These prevertebrate patterns remain articulate and underlie the more advanced vertebrate patterns. Both phylogenetically and ontogenetically, our prevertebrate patterns are the living foundations of our vertebrate movement. Once the spinal vertebra and the limbs have formed, they articulate their individuated as well as combined reflexive movements in the womb. Our vertebrate patterns include: *spinal*, including the head and tail; *homologous (amphibian)*, symmetrical upper and lower limbs; *homolateral (reptilian)*, separating the right side from the left; and *contralateral*, the oppositional relationship of upper and lower limbs underlying quadruped crawling and bipedal walking (Bainbridge Cohen 2012; Hartley 1995).

The basic neurocellular patterns establish essential pathways supporting the development and survival of the child and are identifiable in observational assessments. The patterns are sequentially dependent and allow for increasingly complex movement. If one pattern is skipped or lacks integration, there is a sense of a missing link in both physical agility and 'mental' plasticity. Bainbridge Cohen encapsulates their integral purpose:

> The development of these patterns in humans parallels the evolutionary development of movement through the animal kingdom. The Basic Neurocellular Patterns are the words of our movement. They are the building blocks for the phrases and sentences of our activities. They also establish a base for our perceptual relationships (including body image and spatial orientation) and for our learning and communication. (Bainbridge Cohen 2001)

Neurocellular developmental repatterning is a process of hands-on facilitation that involves distinguishing and combining the patterns as required to support the child to integrate her movement and proceed with ease to the next developmental stage.

> Development is not a linear process but occurs in overlapping waves with each stage containing elements of the others. Because each previous stage underlies and supports each successive stage, any skipping, interrupting or failing to complete a stage of development can lead to alignm ent movement problems, imbalances within the body systems and problems in perception, sequencing organization, memory and creativity. (Bainbridge Cohen 2012, p.4)

The psychophysical, overlapping, and integrative aspects to the developmental patterns are essential to their application in working with a traumatized infant or child. Through observing the 'imbalances' in each child's movement, we witness the impact of trauma in her responses to stimuli and in her relationships with others (Burns 2011; Rothschild 2000; Totton 2003; Trevarthen et al. 1998). Early trauma will have resulted in vulnerabilities in her healthy developmental trajectory – dysregulation, lack of integration of crucial experience (Levine 2008; Schore 2003; Trevarthen 2005; Trevarthen and Aitken, 1994). Through attending to her neurocellular patterns we can address these vulnerabilities through supporting each child to find her innate internal support (Bainbridge Cohen 2012; Hartley 2005).

Support precedes movement

'Support precedes movement' is a longstanding BMC concept used to emphasize a crucial tenet of healthy development – plant, animal, or human – from a single cell to a growing child. 'Support' is achieved through contact, touch, relating. In this context 'support' is integral to each living organism's basic 'stasis' within its membrane (or skin) – its co-regulated, and therefore balanced, state of health and receptivity – and so, for its vital functioning and development (Bainbridge Cohen 2012; Totton 2003, 2005). 'Support' involves, but implies *more* than, purely physical relationship involving contact and connection. It involves effective and affective relationships, resilience, and responsibility. It is innate to life that one thing supports another with a locus of knowing. One could say support is an innate *a priori* to care giving.

The concept of support is familiar to psychotherapy, where the therapist establishes a 'holding environment' (Aposhyan 2004; Hanna 1988; Winnicott 1990). Contained within this holding environment the client finds stasis, and from there is able to begin to seek out a more unified sense of self that has been lost (Schore 1994; Totton 2015; Varela and Shear 1999). In this context 'stasis' refers to a pre-sensory state of receptivity to incoming stimuli. Stasis provides a basis for mutual engagement in the therapeutic experience. It is a prerequisite for the organized, creative, expressed impulse to move ('motility') and, as such, for potential healing. Elaine Siegel, a pioneer of Dance Movement Therapy (DMT) in America, defines her vision of the power of 'motility':

> as an indicator of developmental levels, as an expressor of internal conflicts, and as a receptor that is imprinted with the reactions to all past and present experiences. Given all these properties along with the fact that it can be influenced, motility is a tool for therapeutic intervention. (Siegel 1984, p.42)

Touch and movement repatterning

In BMC, touch and movement are considered primary, reciprocal, and inseparable (Bainbridge Cohen 1995, 2012). Touching is contingent upon movement and movement involves touching. 'Movement and touch develop simultaneously. Touch is the other side of movement. They are the shadow of each other' (Bainbridge Cohen 1988, p.14).

> Together, movement and touch establish the ground for the development of perception and learning from the other senses… Activity needs to occur before it can be perceived. What we perceive is what we then reproduce or control. How we are touched and moved as infants as well as our 'random movements' underlie our perception of self, our behavior and how we focus on what we will perceive in the future. (Bainbridge Cohen 1994, p.2)

In both BMC and DMP, touch-based practices are valued, accepted, and intelligently safeguarded within professional codes (Caldwell 1997; Dymoke 2014; Hartley 2005; Levy 1995).

The principles of *support precedes movement* and *touch and movement repatterning* are innately reciprocal and require a conducive, receptive environment in which re-organization can take place. It is not for the therapist to unilaterally facilitate change, rather to support the child, with her special strengths, to move through her healing process and to find herself anew, unmasked of the trauma and able to 'move on' (Allen 1979; Bainbridge Cohen 2012). The therapeutic repatterning process is unique to each person, requiring safety and a reciprocal sense of timing – a confluence of movement towards ease – as the following case examples illustrate.

Case examples

The two chosen cases demonstrate the application of facilitative methods from BMC in response to the clinical need of the traumatized child, within a humanistic DMP framework. I start with a pen portrait and a summary of the case assessment session, then a brief analysis of my observations of the therapeutic relationship, and end with the theoretical underpinning for the treatment.

Adrian

I met Adrian as an infant and saw him regularly with his parents over the first 14 months of his life. His birth had been protracted as he was back to back and had a short umbilical cord. He was breast fed and placed on his side to sleep. He was often jumpy, as if startled, and would cry to an extent that worried both parents and tested their coping capacity. Adrian was their first child and his parents were struggling greatly with the unknown nature of his distress.

Summary of initial assessment

My first visit was at home at six weeks old. Adrian was feeding whilst his mother (Ann) and I talked. Adrian's father (John) was at work. Ann felt incompetent for not coping with Adrian's distress and felt defensive towards John. She was concerned about her relationship with John and worried about keeping the family together. I noted her fatigue and how certain elements were lacking in her relational bond with Adrian – a lack of eye contact and vocalizing. I observed signs of stress in her voice and sensed a need for support, inspiration, and reassurance.

After nursing, Ann passed Adrian to me. I noticed low tone in his arms, and his fingers were extended. Resting him belly down across my lap, I placed a hand lightly over his shoulder blade and attended to the almost imperceptible movement of the shoulder blade as he breathed. With very light touch and minute movement I felt an impingement under the shoulder blade.

Adrian's challenge was belly lying. He soon protested if placed on his belly. Contrary to a healthy developmental trajectory, he struggled to bring his arms in and under his shoulders to support his attempts to lift his head. Ann reported frequent, exaggerated startle responses and crying whilst feeding, sleeping, and being held.

Two further assessments, at 8 and 12 weeks, revealed that Adrian was still not lifting his head or turning from side lying onto his back or belly, nor from his back to the side. But he did kick and had full movement of his legs. The apparent disconnection of his arms and brachial area from the rest of his body indicated this area as the potential source of discomfort.

From these initial assessments I developed the following working hypotheses for intervention (these will be explored below): I resolved with Ann and John to support gentle use of his arms and movement relative to his present developmental stage. Regarding the startle response, I considered that a reflexive reaction to the discomfort and residual trauma could be resolved using the modulating reflexive response (which I come to later). Both focus areas would involve gentle touch and movement repatterning.

Observational analysis and intervention [3]

For Adrian, the signs of possible birth trauma were evident. Adrian was experiencing a developmental delay of more than three months in terms of his movement profile assessment. Adrian could lie untroubled on his back but not on his belly or sides, which limits further development of symmetry, sidedness, and asymmetry (Bainbridge Cohen 2012). The weakness of his arms impinged on his ability to push away from the floor in either symmetrical or asymmetrical alignment. However, his limbs and spine were starting to unfold from the deep flexion of the womb, and supported him to lift his head when lying on his side or back (Hartley 2005).

Whilst belly lying his arms lacked motility and integrated movement. I gently positioned his arms so that he could feel (proprioceptively) where his own arms could be supportive to him.

Adrian's response to facilitated movement repatterning was evident following gentle hands on at the shoulder. In supporting ease of movement at

---

3   The observations were made with reference to the BMC Ontogenetic development sheets that are an assessment guide to the four trimesters after birth. These assessments include the senses and perceptual processes, physiological reflexes, and neurocellular developmental patterns.

the shoulder, my touch provided a guide for his proprioception. At the wrist and elbow, support of the same nature facilitated flexion and extension in the painless range. The 'cellular' memory of this repatterned movement will become a resource for Adrian as his body learns to assume purposeful, self-supportive and aligned positions (Bainbridge Cohen 2012). Adrian's affective and tonic state changed, in response to the newly patterned movement experiences, indicating his capacity to rediscover his self-movement.

For the lack of apparent proprioception and tone in Adrian's arms and hands I considered gentle awakening of his reflexive withdrawal response through touch and movement. I started in the early stages by placing my finger in the palm of his hand for him to grasp reflexively. He did so without a startle response, clasping with his fingers and drawing into slight flexion at the elbow. Reflexive withdrawal of his hand invited movement along the pathway of the whole arm to the shoulder and more flexor tone of the whole arm. Later, as part of our interaction I invited gentle traction: Adrian lying supine, me holding both his hands and lifting him up slowly. His head lifted and came to mid-line and he flexed his arms to pull.

At six months old, parallel support from his upper limbs whilst belly lying was improved, but still a challenge. Adrian was still unable to roll over when lying down, but he was crying much less and starting to lift himself up and push up more with his arms in belly lying. He was more relational, communicative, and less distressed. He started to hold his own feet lying on his back. At ten months, Adrian could roll over to one side without protest. In prone, he was able to lift his head with full support from both extended arms and could push to slide backwards on his belly. He had a selection of toys he manipulated in lying and sitting. He could recognize songs and joined with the gestures, sitting up and moving his arms. Ann and John were still reticent and unsure; a lack of interaction between them and Adrian was apparent and he lacked vocal expression.

With the aim of stimulating a more spontaneous playful relationship (Burns 2011; Meekums 2002; Stern 2010; Trevarthen 2005), I proposed more sensory stimuli, singing, vocalizing, speaking, eye contact, and interaction with toys or objects of different colours and sizes. Ann and John welcomed these ideas. As they built their relationship with Adrian and watched as he grew stronger, Ann and John grew in confidence and the love between them returned.

Theoretical underpinning

Adrian's limited movement showed me where he was challenged in relation to the normal ontogenetic profile for his age. Through my support, Adrian discovered the physical and structural support available (but previously not experienced) in his body and began to move with this in relation to his environment (Bartenieff 1980; Meekums 2002; Trevarthen 2005).

At Adrian's developmental stage, learning is unconscious and dependent on touch and movement. Within the BMC touch and repatterning protocol we develop our skills to support others through 'cellular touch', which involves tuning into the tone of the cells of the specific tissues being touched, and from there the body–mind as a whole. The underlying theory from much research in nursing, neuroscience, and somatic fields is that touch is affective and the quality of touch is instrumental in supporting tonic change and so affect regulation (Bainbridge Cohen 1995, 2012; Field 2001; Gallace 2012; Hartley 1995; Juhan 2003; Johnson 2000, 2006). If the tone of the tissues is high with excitement or distress (as when a baby cries) or low due to collapse or non-responsiveness, the therapist responds accordingly with this protocol (Bainbridge Cohen 2012). Trauma can involve chronic patterns of tonic change from either or both extremes – high (fight or flight) or low (shut down and dissociation) (Levine 1997, 2008). Adrian's body presented both patterns at different moments. The affect of my touch was sensed and felt by Adrian. My gentle affective (cellular) touch comforted and modulated down his high tone. Equally, my tone was affected by Adrian's, and awareness of this transference provided a useful indicator of how he was presenting. In so many ways touch is an integral part of the facilitation process and is used reflexively to support affect regulation (Sinason 2006; Totton 2005).

Adrian realized latent movement pathways, finding new vitality in these fresh, supportive patterns (especially in pushing away from the floor with his hands). It is evident how his senses engaged with his purposeful movement so that activity involving his somatic nervous system supported homeostatic regulation of his autonomic nervous system. This tonic shift established his potential to further engage in new experiences and allowed more functional neural pathways to emerge (Bainbridge Cohen 2012).[4]

Neurocellular developmental principles
Belly lying (prone) is considered important for a baby by three months old. She needs to have this platform from where she can to learn to lift her head and use her arms to push away from the floor (Bainbridge Cohen 2012). This motion requires supportive proximal movement from the shoulder, as the head lifts and the baby supports herself on her ribs and lower arms. This early purposeful and organized developmental movement evolves in overlapping phases to bring the child to standing and walking. The infant's development depends

---

4   For more on the cellular communication between nerve cells and target tissues see Bainbridge Cohen (2012, p.175), 'The Autonomic nervous system, an experiential perspective'.

upon neural mapping taking place through sensory-motor processing, which requires the baby to experience being on all sides of the body relative to the earth's surface (Bainbridge Cohen 2012; Burns 2011). New nerve pathways enervate the growing muscular tissues, and the newborn's fluid and reflexive movement integrates within new purposeful movements to eventually *support* the weight of the body to *move* on the earth (Bainbridge Cohen 2002a, 2002b; Sweeney 1998).

The physiological reflexes (and their therapeutic support) have a vital role to play in this fundamentally unconscious patterning process, as witnessed with Adrian, to ensure ease and integrated movement (Bainbridge Cohen 2012). In combination, the stimulation of reflexive responses provides a sense of substance and structural support, enabling movement, and so relationships with the outside world, to become clearer and more effective. In finding the push to support him to leave the floor, with the neurophysiological stimulation this brought, Adrian moved on from the newborn bonded to the earth to the infant moving away with its support (Bainbridge Cohen 2012; Hartley 2005).

Relational dynamics
Early on, Ann talked about her fear of being inadequate as she could not console Adrian. In herself, she coped with this anxiety quite well and responded positively to witnessing my relational handling and play. However, she was fearful of hurting Adrian, and this inhibited and repressed her desire to stimulate him and hampered the development of their bond. But she also realized her fears amplified with John's frustration and this was unhelpful. They both welcomed my reassurance and support and were very able to follow my lead. After the sessions Adrian nursed well and slept, and his startle response settled down. Ann enjoyed watching our interaction and was more relaxed: 'It was good to see you moving fluidly with him. I can do that.' John was happy to develop his own relational bond through play and caring interaction. He gained confidence as Adrian progressed.

In BMC the parents are co-facilitators of their infant's experience. Their empathic relationship with their child provides the base line for movement and transformation to happen (Bainbridge Cohen 2011; Burns 2011). The success of Adrian's therapy was contingent on the inclusion of his parents and on the interpersonal holding of the therapeutic environment by all three adults. This involvement empowered Ann and John in their continued work with the facilitative approach that I modelled (Trevarthen 2005). In reorienting to the strengths that Adrian brought, their relational bond developed in new surprising ways. They introduced relational games such as peek-a-boo and sing-along songs that Adrian loved to do together with them. They used bigger objects, more spacious games, stimulating an opening to a wider field of operation and full-bodied movement interaction.

Chloe

Chloe was attending a special unit in Yorkshire for autistic children. She was seven years old with an assessed mental age of 18 months. Chloe's trauma was due to changes taking place at home. She had responded with defensive and resistant behaviours. During this period her distress at school – due to sensory over-stimulation – was heightened beyond the levels usual for her personal autism presentation. Chloe manifested psycho-neuroimmune reactions with a skin rash, high tone, stiffness, and erratic movement which have all been identified as trauma symptoms (Hartley 2004; Levine 2008; Rothschild 2000). At high levels of anxiety, Chloe had tendencies to hit her head and pull her hair.

I delivered a series of therapy sessions incorporating BMC sensory integration and developmental approaches. The aim was to support Chloe in her self-regulation. Further aims were to nurture Chloe's communication skills and her impulse to relate, and to give support for staff and carers.

Summary of initial assessment
My work with Chloe took place within a small class group with other children and staff present. Our sessions were held in a large room which had climbing bars on the walls and a soft play area. We established different areas for interaction. We started with an open space in which the children could establish a connection to each other and us. We kept talking to a minimum, only sharing necessary information to keep a safe space. We lay or sat in the soft play area and eventually each child found a way to be. Slowly, we negotiated how to accompany them. I modelled interaction using soft balls, movement to music, and body contact. In the soft play space, Chloe and I sat back to back and leant against each other. Eventually we began rocking forward and back in tune with each other. At times I paused to see what would happen, to allow Chloe a space to initiate something new. At times she would wait, at others she would move away. I accepted each response as a positive indication of her ability to relate on her terms. From here on, in our sessions I remained open to enter her world. I held lightly the aim of responding naturally with approaches which would facilitate emotional and homeostatic co-regulation (see below).

Observational analysis and intervention
In that first session Chloe seemed content with me beside her (whilst continuing to engage with her reflection in a mirror) and allowed me to join her and walk with her. Intuitively, I picked up the rhythm of her hand movement. When I

spoke in a rhythm reminiscent of an iambic pentameter – 'Chloe and Katy – looking in the glass'– and repeated it to rhythmic movement of her arm, Chloe smiled. She continued to smile as we walked side by side around the room.

If I stood in front of her, holding her hands, she moved our arms to the beat to mark the rhythm. Chloe would engage with eye contact, smiling at me with her eyes. Sometimes Chloe would take the lead by holding my arm, planting her feet firmly to the rhythm. I accompanied her by walking either backwards in front of her, or at her side. These therapeutic walks could go on for the whole session with only short breaks. Over time Chloe started to murmur sounds as we walked, and shook my arm in anticipation of my voice. Apparently she never usually spoke, nor laughed much.

Chloe and I worked together weekly for six months, initially for half an hour and then, after a few weeks, for an hour. At times, whilst arm in arm and walking, she leant on me for support. I felt intuitively that body pressure could help to ease her aroused state and animated physiological tone. When she was receptive to contact and did not withdraw or protest, I used gentle squeezing and compression down the length of her limbs. I was familiar with working with compression along nerve pathways in the context of mental distress, using fabrics, balls and body-on-body contact.[5] Her self-soothing activity such as frequent oral stimulation (sucking or wanting to put things in her mouth) lessened, indicating that other self-soothing events were effective.

Touch and movement repatterning were integral to our relationship – integral to our contact and synchronized movement. Over time (and deepening connection) Chloe and I shared increased eye contact with body contact and our movement became more sustained and earth bound. The gentle squeeze down her arms got firmer as Chloe stood more calmly and receptively. Bilateral compression from her pelvis into her feet stimulated vocalizing and release of tension – her gait was less rigid and she became more directive of her own movement and mine.

According to her school staff, Chloe was relating and communicating in new ways. In the world we created together, Chloe and I shared a sense of vitality and aliveness. I questioned if her response was an indicator of a more secure relationship and whether I had entered her world or had she entered mine? As she met me openly and took self- directive actions as I did, did this mean that our worlds had merged?

We shared through play with movement, touch, and sound. We established new types of experience, involving many levels of social interaction. Chloe grew able to modulate her mood, and to enter a realm with another person

---

5   See also, Dr Temple Grandin, autistic academic and cattle farmer in the USA who invented a 'cow (body) press' to soothe the cattle and used it herself, www.templegrandin.com

without distress. Staff noted how 'special' our relationship was, which supports this analysis. Improved relationships with staff grew from witnessing us and the many new aspects of Chloe. After two months Chloe's hair grew back, and she was more settled and her skin had cleared.

On the one hand such feedback from carers counteracts practitioner bias, but on the other, it admits its own. The staff and I are not autistic so we see Chloe from our non-autistic perspective. We are not to know for certain whether she is more at ease in her world rather than in this shared one. We may feel her quality of life is improved when we establish a relational bond, as we feel the physical change in that she is calmer and slower. She appears to be processing input more fully so we assume she is 'functioning' more normally. However we should not presume that when left in her own world that her 'normal' is aberrant or *ab*normal. Her distress surfaces when she is required to conform to life in the non-autistic realm, where sensory input levels are intolerably over-stimulating. In our world proximity, motility, and physical contact created a realm that appeared to provide a buffer-zone between her and the external environment. She could breathe and attend to her needs in this intermediary space with the support of another who understands.

Theoretical underpinning
It is well accepted that emotional distress is perceivable, as is the embodiment of emotional regulation (Hartley 2004; Ledoux 2015; Levine 2010; Pert 1997; Schore 1994; Totton 2015). Chloe's disturbed animate state manifested in sympathetic arousal or inertia, and limited motility (Bainbridge Cohen 1995; Kestenberg 1975; Siegel 1984; Stern 2010). Chloe had found a sense of stasis internally (interoceptively) by being able to be fully in her own world without being disrupted or challenged. As she accepted my accompaniment within her world she found a sense of safety and agreement, of being accepted by a cohabitant. Chloe, it appears, was 'less autistic' in our world. If autism is defined by lack of social skills it seemed that Chloe had, to some degree, found them.

To others her arm movements seemed to lack purpose. Yet in *our* world, where we attuned through movement and touch, Chloe's movement responses indicated a self-perceptive and receptive state. The pitch or resonance of this sensory receptive state regulated down her anxiety just as an infant responds to the empathic resonance of her caregiver (Porges 2011; Rothschild 2000; Stern 1985, 2010; Trevarthen 2005). Chloe was connecting and experiencing co-regulation. Movement became purposeful and new ways of functioning reunited her body–mind, and her psycho-neuroimmune symptoms improved.

In our mutual space, Chloe contacted me, leant on me, at times collapsing into my support. In acknowledgement of her yielding, I reciprocated with compression for her to sense and feel her own inner structure, her central core and stability, connecting into the earth through her feet (Hartley 2005). When Chloe was more overtly distressed, it took longer to attune and I had to mirror from a distance or sit on the floor and wait.

By not demanding eye contact, or for her to fulfil a required goal in a specific time, Chloe's defensive responses reduced. She became more self directed and this positive use of her energy grew with assurance when accompanied. With gentle mirroring and positive accompaniment Chloe discovered new levels of self-movement. She now attends to aspects of relationship which she may otherwise have filtered out in haste, or bypassed due to distress (Homann 2010; Lewis 1984; Totton 2015).

In BMC terms, our interaction fulfilled a perceptual repatterning process, which in turn lay down a new neural pathway for further organized impulse:

> If the nervous system displays patterns that are limiting full development, we can go beneath those restrictive patterns to awaken the cellular matrix and thereby stimulate more natural patterns of behaviour to emerge. (Bainbridge Cohen 2011, p.2)

This quote summarizes the BMC therapeutic approach and implies an intervention. But to 'go beneath' requires permission from the 'cellular matrix'. If we do too much too soon the result can be retraumatizing (Bainbridge Cohen 2012; Levine 2010).

Chloe's anxiety levels were aggravated by over-stimulation from her exteroceptive senses. The outside world imposed sensory and relational demands that were not attuned to her functional levels, demands which she was unable to filter or mediate. As a fellow human without her sensitivities, I needed to enter Chloe's world and reciprocate her way of being. I needed to better understand how, with her sensitivities, our world had traumatized her. This immersion enabled a slow journey into understanding and co-regulation; it enabled permission to 'go beneath'.

The body–mind dichotomy reframed in the context of trauma

In the two illustrated cases above, the child's emotional wellbeing is served by providing an embodied experience and a sense of safety and security. In each case, physiological tone and emotional state were modulated reciprocally through touch and movement. This process underlies and precedes the ability to grasp the sense of the experience as conscious thought (Ledoux 2015; Levine 2010) – here, physiological tone and emotional state are 'inseparably-realised' (Sheets-Johnstone 2010, p.110). For an infant or young child, this sense manifests at a physiological level. Her traumatized state can settle *only* if her body can assimilate the tide of affect disturbance (Gallace and Spence 2010; Levine 2010; Porges 2011; Trevarthen 2005). By meeting the child at her specific neurocellular developmental stage we can navigate this tide through rough waters. We physically ride each wave till the storm subsides and the apparent threat to her survival has passed.

From the outside, the traumatized child appears lost and disconnected from others as she struggles to live with unknown powerful feelings. Trauma hijacks the body as a totality (Levine 2008, 2010; Rothschild 2000), disturbing the usual ebb and flow of self-regulation. Thrown into overdrive, the self-regulatory system manifests 'debilitating symptoms' (Levine 2008, p.3) which, if unresolved, compromise the sense of a unitary being. In resolving trauma it is the body–mind totality that is re-established. This healing brings gifts of renewed self-knowing (Levine 2008), renewed capacity and impulse to relate, and renewed vitality. Adrian and Chloe experienced all of these elements.

In embracing the unknown within the terrain of the body, with its emotional storms and gentle mists, the terrain becomes a landscape of darkness and light that we can explore, mark out, name, and move in. By embracing emotional trauma as an innate alarm system, left unattended and on full volume, we come to understand how to enter that shared landscape and offer support and care for the traumatized child. We enter directly into the child's zone of desperation, bringing safety, acceptance, gentle guidance through touch, making time for healing, for the 'story' to unfurl (Marz and Lindy 2010). With trust in our capacity to inhabit this landscape with greater ease, we become more than ourselves in the company of others.

References

Allen, F.H. (1979) *Psychotherapy with Children.* Lincoln, NE and London: University of Nebraska Press.

Aposhyan, S. (2004) *Body–Mind Psychotherapy: Principles, Techniques and Practical Applications.* New York: W.W. Norton.

Bainbridge Cohen, B. (1988) 'Touch and Movement. Study Guide.' *Senses and Perception 1.* El Sobrante: School for Body–Mind Centering.

Bainbrige Cohen, B. (1994) *Cellular Consciousness. The Embodiment Process.* El Sobrante: School for Body–Mind Centering.

Bainbridge Cohen, B. (1995) *The Evolutionary Origins of Movement. The Basic Neurological Patterns.* Course manual. El Sobrante: School for Body–Mind Centering.

Bainbridge Cohen, B. (2001) *Basic Neurocellular Patterns.* Available at www.bodymindcentering.com/course/basic-neurological-patterns-bnp, accessed on 14 February 2016.

Bainbridge Cohen, B. (2002a) 'Fetal Movement.' In IDME course notebook. El Sobrante: School for Body–Mind Centering.

Bainbridge Cohen, B. (2002b) 'IDME Underlying Questions.' In IDME course notebook. El Sobrante: School for Body–Mind Centering.

Bainbridge Cohen, B. (2011) 'Offerings from a Body-Mind Centering® perspective and approach to working with children with special needs.' Page 2 of a handout package for the SPARKS

European Commission funded project, Bratislava, Slovakia, September 17–21, 2014. El Sobrante: School for Body Mind Centering.

Bainbridge Cohen, B. (2012 [1993]) *Sensing Feeling and Action: The Experiential Anatomy of Body–Mind Centering.* Northampton: Contact Editions.

Bartenieff, I. (1980) *Body Movement: Coping with the Environment.* London: Routledge.

Burns, C. (2011) 'The Active Role of the Baby in Birthing.' In G. Miller, P. Ethridge, and K. Tarlow Morgan (eds) *Exploring Body–Mind Centering. An Anthology of Experience and Method.* Berkeley, CA: North Atlantic Books.

Caldwell, C. (1997) *Getting in Touch: The Guide to New Body-Centered Therapies.* Wheaton, IL: Theosophical Publishing House.

Dymoke, K. (2000) 'Touch, a Touchy Subject.' In P. Grennland (ed.) *What Dancers Do That Other Health Workers Don't.* Leeds: Jabadao.

Dymoke, K. (2014) 'Contact improvisation, the non-eroticized touch in an "art-sport".' Special edition – Contact [and] improvisation. *Journal of Dance and Somatic Practice 6*, 2, 205–218.

Field, T. (2001) *Touch.* Cambridge, MA: MIT Press.

Gallace, A. (2012) 'Living with touch.' *The Psychologist 25*, 896–899.

Gallace, A. and Spence, C. (2010) 'The science of interpersonal touch: an overview.' *Neurosciences and Biobehavioural Reviews 34*, 2, 249–259.

Hanna, T. (1988) *Somatics: Reawakening the Mind's Control of Movement, Flexibility, and Health.* Cambridge, MA: Da Capo Press.

Hartley, L. (1995) *Wisdom of the Body Moving.* Berkeley, CA: North Atlantic Books.

Hartley, L. (2004) *Somatic Psychology, Body, Mind and Meaning.* London/Philadelphia: Whurr.

Hartley, L. (2005) 'Embodying the Sense of Self. Body–Mind Centering® and Authentic Movement.' In N. Totton (ed.) *New Dimensions in Body Psychotherapy.* Maidenhead: Open University Press.

Homann, K.B. (2010) 'Embodied concepts of neurobiology in dance/movement therapy practice.' *American Journal of Dance Therapy 32*, 80–99.

Johnson, D.H. (2000) 'Intricate Tactile Sensitivity: A Key Variable in Western Integrative Bodywork.' *Progress in Brain Research 122*, 479–490.

Johnson, D.H. (2006) 'The Primacy of Experiential Practices in Body Psychotherapy.' In G. Marlock and H. Weiss (eds) *Handbook of Body Psychotherapy.* Stuttgart: Schattauer.

Juhan, D. (2003) *Job's Body: A Handbook for Body Workers.* New York: Station Hill Press.

Kestenberg, J. (1975) *Children and Parents: Psychoanalytic Studies of Development.* New York: Jason Aronson.

Ledoux, J. (2015) *Anxious: The Modern Mind in the Age of Anxiety.* London: Oneworld.

Levine, P. (1997) *Waking the Tiger: Healing Trauma.* Berkeley, CA: North Atlantic Books.

Levine, P. (2008) *Healing Trauma.* Boulder, CA: Sounds True Inc.

Levine, P. (2010) *In an Unspoken Voice.* Berkeley, CA: North Atlantic Books.

Levy, F. J. (ed.) (1995) *Dance and Other Expressive Art Therapies: When Words Are Not Enough.* New York/London: Routledge.

Lewis, P. (1984) *Theoretical Approaches in Dance Movement Therapy.* Volume 2. Dubuque, IA: Kendall/Hunt Publishing Company.

Marz, E. and Lindy J. (2010) 'Exploring The Trauma Membrane Concept.' In E. Martz (ed.) *Trauma Rehabilitation after War and Conflict: Community and Individual Perspectives.* New York: Springer.

Meekums, B. (2002) *Dance Movement Therapy.* London: Sage.

Pert, C. (1997) *Molecules of Emotion: Why You Feel the Way You Feel.* New York: Scribner.

Porges, S. (2011) *The Polyvagal Theory: Neurophysiological Foundations of Emotions, Attachment, Communication and Self-regulation.* New York: W.W. Norton.

Rothschild, B. (2000) *The Body Remembers: The Psychophysiology of Trauma and Trauma Treatment.* New York: Norton.

Schore, A. (1994) *Affect Regulation and the Origin of the Self: The Neurobiology of Emotional Development.* Hove: Lawrence Erlbaum.

Schore, A. (2003) *Affect Dysregulation and Disorders of the Self.* New York/London: W.W. Norton.

Sheets-Johnstone, M. (2000) 'Kinetic tactile-kinesthetic bodies: ontological foundations of apprenticeship learning.' *Human Studies 23*, 4, 343–370.

Sheets-Johnstone, M. (2010) 'Kinesthetic experience: understanding movement inside and out.' *Body Movement and Dance in Psychotherapy 5*, 2, 111–127.

Siegel, E.V. (1984) *Dance-Movement Therapy, Mirror of Our Selves: The Psychoanalytic Approach.* New York: Human Sciences Press.

Sinason, V. (2006) 'No Touch Please – We're British Psychodynamic Practitioners.' In G. Galton (ed.) *Touch Papers: Dialogues on Touch in the Psychoanalytic Space.* London: Karnac Books.

Stern, D.N. (1985) *The Interpersonal World of the Infant.* New York: Basic Books.

Stern, D.N. (2010) *Forms of Vitality: Exploring Dynamic Experience in Psychology, the Arts, Psychotherapy and Development.* Oxford: Oxford University Press.

Sweeney, J. (1998) *Basic Concepts in Embryology: A Student's Survival Guide.* New York: McGraw-Hill.

Totton, N. (2003) *Body Psychotherapy: An Introduction.* Maidenhead/Philadelphia, PA: Open University Press.

Totton, N. (ed.) (2005) *New Dimensions in Body Psychotherapy.* Maidenhead: Open University Press.

Totton, N. (2015) *Embodied Relating: The Ground of Psychotherapy.* London: Karnac Books.

Trevarthen, C. (2005) 'Stepping Away from the Mirror: Pride and Shame in Adventures of Companionship: Reflections on the Nature and Emotional Needs of Infant Intersubjectivity.' In C.S. Carter, L. Ahnert, K.E. Grossman, S. Hardy *et al.* (eds) *Attachment and Bonding: A New Synthesis. Dahlem Workshop Report 92.* Cambridge, MA: MIT Press.

Trevarthen, C. and Aitken, K.J. (1994) 'Brain development, infant communication, and empathy disorders: intrinsic factors in child mental health.' *Development and Psychopathology 6*, 4, 597–633.

Trevarthen, C., Aitken, K., Papoudi, D. and Robarts, J. (eds) (1998) *Children with Autism: Diagnosis and Interventions to Meet Their Needs.* London: Jessica Kingsley Publishers.

Varela, F. and Shear, J. (eds) (1999) *The View from Within.* Thorverton: Imprint Academic.

Winnicott, D.W. (1990) *The Maturational Process and the Facilitating Environment.* London: Karnac Books.

12

RELATING WHEN RELATING IS HARD

Working with Aggressive Children in Child Centered Play Therapy

DEE C. RAY

As I walked down the hall, I could see her in the distance. She was screaming, flailing her body between the wall and the teacher beside her. She was surrounded by three adults, all attempting to hold her still while trying not to physically hurt her. All three adults expressed their anger and frustration through raised voices, stern tones, and physical tension. I could hear her shouting, 'But I don't want to be red, I want to be green.' Other children were starting to come out into the hallway while teachers quickly rushed them back into their classrooms. 'I don't want to be red, I want to be green.' The male principal, over six foot three inches and 200 pounds, came out of his office and walked toward her. She screamed louder, 'I don't want to be red, I want to be green.' As I came closer, I heard an adult, 'You did not listen, you have to be red.' Another adult, 'I told you that you were going to be red if you didn't follow the rules.' 'But I don't want to be red, I want to be green.' Another adult, 'I told you over and over, you never listen.' The principal reached out his hand and firmly said, 'Come with me.' The little five-year-old girl with pigtails in her hair, who stood less than four feet tall and weighed 40 pounds, took his hand and walked calmly with him back to his office. I met Nia in the principal's office and asked if she wanted to go to the playroom.

Nia was hesitant but curious. It was the first time we met. As we entered the playroom, I made the introduction, 'In here is the playroom, and you can play with the toys in lots of the ways you like' (Landreth 2012, p.184). She walked over to the toy animals and with one movement of her arm, she knocked every animal off the shelf. She looked at me and said, 'There,' as if to say, 'What are you going to do about that?' I responded, 'You wanted those all off the shelf. You're wondering what I think about that.' She seemed confused. She moved to the doll house, looked closely at a doll, and threw it across the room. She continued this process until she had thrown each item out of the doll house.

Nia: You have to clean that up.

Me: You wanted to make a mess for me to clean up.

Nia: Yep! You have to.

Me: You're telling me just what you want me to do.

Nia: Yep! You have to do what I say.

Me: You want to be in charge of me.

She then set up a play scene in which she was the teacher and I was a little girl. She wrote the rules on the board, mostly a mixture of unintelligible letters.

Nia: These are the rules and you have to follow them. If you don't follow them, I'll move your card to red.

Me: So, I really need to follow the rules or I'll be in trouble.

Nia: Yes, and you are trying but they're really hard to follow.

Me: You're letting me know that it'll be super hard to follow all the rules.

Nia: But you really want to.

Me: I'm going to try hard to follow the rules but it's going to be hard.

Nia: See, you already messed up. You were supposed to raise your hand before you said anything. That's an orange.

Me: I already made a mistake. Now, I'm in trouble.

Nia: Yep. You're really sad.

Me: (In a whisper) How do I show I'm sad?

Nia: (In a whisper) You cry.

Me: (Crying softly) I'm so sad.

Nia: No! Louder. Cry louder.

Me: (In a louder voice) I'm so sad.

Nia: (In a teacher tone) You need to be quiet. You're already on orange and next you're going to be on red. *(Whispers to me in her own voice)* Keep crying!

Me: (Continuing to cry) I'm so, so sad.

Nia: (In a teacher tone) I told you. Now you're on red. You need to be quiet. Now, just get out! *(Changes her tone to her own voice)* You don't really have to get out. You want to cook dinner together?

And so began my relationship with Nia, a young girl who had been described by the school staff as aggressive, violent, impulsive, uncontrollable, and lacking ability to be in relationship. Aggression expressed by children is often perceived by others as a disability, a set of isolated behaviors to be eradicated, or an innate defect of children who will eventually succumb to criminal behavior. Yet, in my experience, aggression is a communication tool used by children to get unexpressed needs met. Early in development, young children use aggression to express their desires due to a lack of verbal skills. Toddlers and preschoolers often grab the toys they want, reach for food when they are hungry, and push others out of their way. As they grow older, most children gain verbal skills to learn to communicate what they need from others. In nurturing environments, children learn that their words can be used to get needs met rather than aggressive acts. Yet, in other environments, children learn that aggressive acts are the primary way or, sometimes, the only way to meet needs. The use of aggression by most children is not a conscious effort to hurt others. It is a way of being, outside of personal awareness, that children experience as their means of moving through or surviving in the world. When children continue to experience the environment as hostile and unresponsive to personal needs, they will continue to use aggression as a means of survival or a method to meet basic human needs for connection.

In child-centered play therapy (CCPT), the therapeutic relationship is based on the philosophy of Carl Rogers (1989) who believed that humans are holistic organisms, working toward thoughts, feelings, and behaviors that are self-enhancing. Rogers (1989) stated that a person's:

> deepest characteristics tend toward development, differentiation, cooperative relationships; whose life tends fundamentally to move from dependence to independence; whose impulses tend naturally to harmonize into a complex and changing pattern of self-regulation; whose total character is such as to tend to preserve and enhance himself and his species, and perhaps to move it toward its further evolution. (pp.404–405)

From the child-centered perspective, aggressive acts expressed by children are behaviors that are perceived by the child as self-enhancing, as moving toward actualization. Aggression may be inspired by the inability to cope with environment or an attempt to establish a social connection in the only way that is responded to by adults, however negatively (Ray 2011). Following the use of aggression, however, children often experience incongruence because their actions do not necessarily result in a feeling of self-enhancement or personal contentment.

In the case of Nia, our first interaction revealed that she was willing to become highly aggressive to meet her needs. The incident in the hallway was a result of an interaction in which she wanted to talk with another child in the classroom. Her lack of skills to connect to others in the context of strict school rules was confusing for her. She desired to follow the rules but she more strongly desired to connect to other people. When she was met with a restriction (the teacher stating that she could not talk with the other classmate), she acted in a way to meet her needs. She continued to talk, expressing the need openly. The reaction of the teacher to move her behavior 'color' to red was perceived by Nia as a denial of her need, a direct interruption to having her need for connection met. As per her pattern, she attempted to then have her need for relationship met through a more familiar route, an aggressive interaction with the teacher and other adults. In this interaction, as she increased her aggression, the adults increased their contact which had been non-existent prior to the event. Hence, even though she received negative physical and emotional attention from adults, she experienced a connection that she so desperately needed. Although adults experienced feeling disconnected from Nia, *she* experienced the human contact that was most familiar to her and met the primary need for relationship. The end result of the hallway interaction was frustration and anger on the part of the adults, who questioned Nia's ability to be a 'normal' member of society. It was confusion for Nia, who simultaneously experienced a sense of connected relationship *and* a sense of disconnection from her own feelings and those of others. Her confusion about how to 'be' in relationship was apparent in her play. Nia entered our relationship by initiating what she expected to be an aggressive interaction between us. Because I responded to her in a reflective way and accepted her need to connect to me through aggression, she initially experienced dissonance and confusion about how to authentically connect with me. Often, children who struggle with connection will reach out using their most effective coping skill to date, aggressive acts of contact.

The therapeutic relationship

In establishing the therapeutic relationship with a child, I seek to provide an environment that offers the child an opportunity to express herself through the language of play. The playroom is organized with diverse toys and materials, provides open space, and is a confidential location (Landreth 2012; Ray 2011). Play materials allow for nurturing, expressive, realistic, symbolic, and aggressive play. The playroom itself sends the message that all feelings are accepted and valued. Within the playroom, I embody the child-centered qualities necessary to foster a therapeutic relationship: genuineness, unconditional positive regard, and empathic understanding (Rogers 1957). In being genuine, I am authentically myself within the relationship. In holding unconditional positive regard, I experience a full acceptance and prizing of the child. In empathic understanding, I seek to experience the child's world from her perspective. These qualities of connection help foster an environment of understanding and acceptance. In CCPT, the goal for children who are aggressive is to facilitate the expression of the needs behind the aggression (Ray 2011). It is only within the context of a relationship in which the child feels valued, accepted, and understood that there is a willingness to explore different ways to get needs met. In the case of Nia, within the playroom, she began to play out her struggle to follow rules and her desire to feel connected once she felt accepted and understood by me.

Aggressive children are often confused regarding their own needs and behaviors. Because they have sought to fulfill their needs through aggression, they equate their needs and desires with a self-perception of 'being wrong' or hurting others. This confusion results in a belief that their basic needs are problematic and unworthy. Nia equated her need to connect with another child to breaking the classroom rules. This resulted in her belief that something was innately wrong with *her*, not with her behavior. By the time aggressive children are referred for play therapy, they have experienced this confusion between need and aggressive acts so many times that they are unable to distinguish between the two, as evidenced by using aggression as an automatic reaction to expressing feeling or desire (Ray 2011). When the child is confronted with rules that restrict needs and subsequently feels misunderstood for having such a need, the typical reaction is to rigidly hold to familiar behaviors. The great irony of effective child therapy is that the more children feel understood and accepted in their current rigid ways of meeting their needs, the more they feel free to explore alternative courses of action. When I accurately conveyed my understanding of Nia ('You want to be in charge of me'), she began to fully express her world-view through the teacher–child play-scene. She allowed me further into her world to understand what happens for her when she tries to navigate her needs within the context of restrictions.

In our second session, Nia came into the room and immediately began screaming and pointing at the toy snake that was across the room.

Me: You're really scared.

Nia continues to scream, forming no words, but still pointing.

Me: You're really, really scared of that one.

Nia: (Stops screaming, paces around the room far from the snake) What's it doing in here? Get it out of here.

Me: Oh, you really don't like that one. You want it gone.

Nia: It's ugly. It's mean.

Me: So, you don't like it because it's ugly and mean.

Nia: (Reaches out her hand to me) You come with me. Stand up and come with me.

Me: (I take her hand and stand up) You want us to go together.

Nia leads us closer to the snake whilst holding onto my hand. She stops a couple of times to step backward, looks at me, and then moves forward again. We move within touching distance of the snake.

Nia: You touch it. *(I reach out my hand to touch the snake)* You pet it. *(I pet it).* Aren't you scared?

Me: You think I might be scared but you still want me to pet it.

Nia reaches out her hand to touch the snake and pulls back, then reaches out again. She touches my hand whilst my hand is on the snake.

Me: (Whispering) You really wanted to touch it. You wanted us to do this together.

Nia: (She touches the snake directly) He's…she's not that bad *(The shift in the gender of pronoun is not a typo here! Nia's unconscious language usage represents a common occurrence for many children in the play therapy room)*

Me: She seemed bad but she's not really.

Nia: (Picks up snake, petting it) Everyone thinks she's scary but she's not. She's really nice.

Me: Others don't really understand her but you know she's nice.

Nia: She is ugly but underneath she's pretty. *(Flips snake over to show belly)*

Me: It seems confusing. She looks one way but she's really another. She's pretty. You know that.

For the next eight sessions, Nia chose to play with the snake at some point in each session. She continued to say that others think the snake is mean and that the snake sometimes does mean things. Then she began to nurture the snake by feeding it with a bottle and petting it. She made a bed for it and covered it when she left the playroom so that it would be safe. She verbalized that the snake needed to be hidden because others think it is bad. She wanted to protect the snake.

Nia's play with the snake seemed to reveal how she viewed herself and how she perceived other people viewed her. There was no need for me to interpret Nia's play. At the age of five, Nia appeared to have an accurate understanding of how others saw her. I did not need to explain how her behaviors push people away. I did not need to direct her in methods to help people like her more. She used these sessions to fully explore what it meant for her and her relationships that others saw her as mean. She also tapped into a gentle, nurturing part of herself. From this place she was able to nurture and take care of the snake that no one else liked. But she needed a partner. She chose me to be with her through this exploration. I believe that my ability to be fully present and accepting of her was critical to her choice to allow me to be a part of her process. Once we approached the snake together and I conveyed my nurturing for the snake, I believe she felt that I could accept her too.

Aggression within the relationship

When working with children who are aggressive, aggression within the therapeutic relationship is common and expected. The relationship provides acceptance and understanding but it also initiates new, confusing feelings for the child. When the adult does not respond as expected, children may become perplexed by unfamiliar interactions and the meaning of those interactions. The child may rigidly hold to old behaviors to elicit familiar reactions. After all, aggressive acts have brought them into relationships with others. Without those acts, they may fear losing these tentative relationships that are meeting basic needs of connection. Therapists who choose to work with aggressive children need to be prepared for holding steady with therapeutic conditions when a child is operating aggressively.

For Nia, she acted aggressively toward me in her first nine sessions. The following is one example of a typical interaction in which Nia engaged in aggressive acts toward me.

> Nia: (Seeing that the sand in the sandbox had clumped together) You need to come down here and fix this sand.
>
> Me: It sounds like you're angry about the sand and you want me to fix it.
>
> Nia: (In angry tone) I said you need to come here now and fix this.
>
> Me: You're angry with me. Tell me what you want me to do.
>
> Nia: (Yells) Fix it!

Me: You want me to fix the sand. I'm not sure how to fix it. You can tell me how to fix it.

Nia: (Stands up with handful of sand) I said fix it!

Me: Nia, you are really angry with me but I'm not for throwing sand at. You can throw sand at the sandbox.

Nia threw the handful of sand at me.

Me: Oh…that got in my eyes and hurt *(As I wiped sand from my face)* Nia, I'm not for throwing sand at. You can tell me how to fix the sand.

Nia: You're stupid.

Me: You think I'm stupid because I don't know how to fix the sand. You want me to feel bad.

Nia: No, you're just stupid.

Me: You're really frustrated with me and want to call me names.

Nia: Shut up.

Me: (Whisper) You want me to be quiet.

Nia played in the sand quietly for another minute and then stood up. She asked if I wanted to be her mom and cook for her.

In this scenario, Nia uses aggression as a way to control her relationship with me. She begins by directing me in a harsh tone. When I responded calmly to her direction, she raised her voice. When I still responded to her in a calm and caring way, she moved to further aggression by throwing sand at me. As I set the limit, she follows but then uses insulting language. Nia progressed through her usual aggressive behaviors from bossiness, to threatening, to throwing, to name-calling in an effort to experience the expected response. These acts were her repertoire of coping skills to deal with feeling competent in a relationship. Up to this point, adults in her life responded by raising their voices or using punishment to subdue her aggression. When I did not react with anger or attempts to control her behavior, she moved to another coping skill. By the end of the interaction, none of her coping skills had elicited the expected reaction, leaving her to experience relationship in a new way.

Throughout these interactions in which Nia engaged in aggressive acts, I held the firm belief that she was capable of developing new coping skills, capable of engaging in a relationship that would be truly self-enhancing for her, and capable of regulating her emotions. My responses intentionally sent the message that I believed in her and her ability to find a way to meet her needs and be in relationship. I reflected her feelings by noting her anger and frustration. I reflected her intentions of wanting me to fix what she did not like and wanting to hurt me. I presented her option to tell me how to do what she wanted. I genuinely admitted that I was limited in knowing how to fix the sand. And I offered her alternatives to her behaviors such as throwing the sand in the sandbox or telling me how to fix the sand. During this interaction, I held unconditional positive regard for Nia whilst trying empathically to understand her perspective. I sent the non-verbal message that I was with her even when things are tough between us. However, I am not a therapeutic robot who responds accurately to interactions that prompt my own feelings of frustration or anger. In this interaction, I responded genuinely with my reaction to having sand thrown in my eyes. I expressed that I was hurt but followed my expression of hurt with an attempt to continue to be in relationship with Nia. I provided her with another way to be in relationship rather than the reactionary models she had previously experienced, allowing her the experience of tapping into her own being to access what was needed to be in a self-enhancing relationship.

The following is another interaction that occurred later in our relationship. Nia set up a play-scene in which I was the mother and she was the child. She wanted us to cook a meal together for our friends. She used the sand and available water to make the meal. She ran out of water and was frustrated about not having enough water.

Nia: I need more water for the soup.

Me: It looks like you're out of water for the soup we're making.

Nia: (Frustrated tone) Go get me more water.

Me: You'd like to have more water but there is no more water. You can pretend to have water.

Nia: (Pleading tone) Can I please have more water?

Me: You really want more water but there is no more water. You're frustrated.

Nia: I don't know how to make the soup without more water.

Me: It's really tough to figure it out. You're thinking hard.

Nia: (Excited tone) Oh, I can move the water from the pie we made.

Me: You thought of a whole new way to fix the problem and have more water.

Nia: Yep! You just have to keep thinking.

Me: You know that if you keep thinking you can figure it out.

In these later interactions, Nia started to experiment with different behaviors when she had a need. She started with her usual way of directing others to get what she wanted. When the limit was set she moved to another coping skill of pleading, which was new for her. After finding pleading to be ineffective, she moved to creative problem-solving by taking time to think through the problem and the need. By allowing her the freedom to express her needs and providing her with empathic understanding, Nia was free to facilitate her own creativity, discovering new ways to meet her needs. She was able to meet her need and remain in connection with me.

Children who act aggressively may be overly reactive to external stimuli, even responding negatively to praise and reward. External positive reinforcement may be seen as insincere or as a therapist's attempt to manipulate the child. The child may experience praise as incongruent with her internal sense of self and may respond with further negative action. Alternatively, the child may be hungry for praise (to battle feelings of discouragement) yet short-lived external positive reinforcement is no match for the intense feelings of internalized insignificance. It is important for us as therapists to truly understand how praise and reward represent one side of a coin, the other side comprising criticism and punishment. Praise and reward naturally and inevitably imply criticism and punishment. The person who praises also has the power to denigrate, and so praise, used unwisely, will apply an ineffective hierarchical structure to the therapy relationship. Given this understanding, how can we find ways to encourage aggressive children in their exploration and ability to develop positive coping skills?

My unconditional positive regard for Nia was held by a genuine belief that she could figure out how to meet her needs. As play therapist, my regard and prizing of the child is expressed through an encouragement process integrated throughout the relationship. Through truly listening and recognizing the child's world, I send an implicit message that the child is worthy. Through connectedness and encouragement in the relationship (fostered by physically and verbally matching the different modes and levels of the child's communication) I send the message that the child's way of perceiving the world is valuable. Through recognizing the child's struggles and attempting to be with the child during such struggles, instead of trying to 'fix' the problem, I demonstrate that the child is capable. Instead of saying, 'You did a good job of thinking of another way', which implies approval and externalized reward, I respond with encouragement, 'You were thinking of a lot of different ways to do that', which recognizes the child's ability to figure out new ways of coping. The child is then able to internalize these types of responses and, as such, begin to experience feeling competent and creative in making self-enhancing decisions. In the previous excerpt from Nia's session, Nia demonstrates a growing sense of her own capability to generalize her experiences in the playroom and beyond.

Her statement 'You just have to keep thinking' represents her capacity to connect her new coping skill, developed in the playroom, to the idea that she could possibly use this skill outside of the playroom in her everyday life.

Setting limits

When a child acts aggressively within the therapeutic relationship, positive regard and empathic understanding are necessary for the relationship to thrive and to facilitate growth in the child. However, these particular conditions flourish *only* in a safe and structured relationship. Limits are necessary for effective therapeutic relationships. Because CCPT values the need for expression in a permissive relationship, limits are set only when needed and only to provide safety for the child, therapist, and room (Axline 1947). Landreth (2012) presented the ACT structure of limit-setting that works well for children who are aggressive. In ACT, the therapist *A*cknowledges the feeling, *C*ommunicates the definitive limit, and *T*argets an alternative. Because relationship is the basis of CCPT, the therapist first acknowledges the feeling of the child, such as 'You are frustrated…', 'You are angry…', or 'You are excited…'. Acknowledging the feeling helps the child feel understood and valued by the therapist. The second step of ACT is for the therapist to set a limit that clearly defines the unacceptable behavior such as 'I'm not for hitting', 'The puppets aren't for cutting', or 'Your head is not for banging'. Because young children often have difficulty thinking in the moment of ways to expend their negative energy, the therapist provides an alternative to help with expression, such as 'You can hit the pillow', 'You can tear the paper', or 'You can throw the ball'. In session, the ACT method is used in one response such as 'You are frustrated with me, but I'm not for hitting. You can hit the doll.'

In ACT, the child's feeling is acknowledged and valued, which is paramount to facilitating the therapeutic relationship. In addition, ACT sends the choice to act back to the child. The therapist is not responsible for 'making' the child act in a certain way. The therapist states the behavior that is inappropriate and returns responsibility back to the child to follow or, in some cases, not follow the limit. The CCPT therapist believes that the child has the ability to regulate their own emotions and behavior, the ability to act in a way that is most beneficial for their self-enhancement. In the earlier scenario with Nia, seeing her intention to throw sand at me, I used the limit, 'Nia, you are really angry with me but I'm not for throwing sand at. You can throw sand at the sandbox.' Through this response, I reflected Nia's feelings about me but set a limit on her behavior. It was her choice to follow the limit. In that particular scenario, Nia chose not to follow the limit and threw the sand at me. I responded by setting the limit again. I also expressed an authentic feeling response that I had been hurt. At that point, she chose to follow the limit. In school, Nia learned that if she did not control her behavior, an adult would step in to control it for her. Nia knew that if she was physically aggressive, an adult would hold her or restrain her until she stopped being aggressive. For so many children, this adult response teaches them that they are incapable of regulating their own behaviors. They become dependent on others for regulation and experience themselves as incapable of making decisions that are self-enhancing. In play therapy, the therapist believes in the child's capacity to make decisions that enhance self and others. Nia demonstrated that when she was provided with a response in which the therapist was caring and believed in her abilities, she could follow the limit. She experienced her strength in positive decision-making, getting her needs met whilst being in relationship. Additionally, Nia experienced a way of relating in which I expressed an authentic reaction to her aggressive behavior while also expressing a desire to stay connected with her. I believe that Nia integrated the experience of an adult accepting and caring for her, whilst being vulnerable with her, into how she sought to meet her own needs. She truly understood that I would be alongside her no matter what.

ACT also provides structure for the therapist so that the therapist feels safe within the relationship. Although CCPT relationships are permissive, they are not an 'anything goes' environment. The therapist uses ACT to establish safety in the relationship and in the environment so that both the child and the therapist can feel secure as they journey through therapy together. When Nia threw sand at me, I set the limit so that I would feel safe with her. I believed that she would eventually choose a behavior that benefited both of us and would allow us to be in relationship together.

ACT is an effective strategy for limit-setting by which children typically learn to regulate their actions. However, there are times that children have difficulty responding to limits appropriately and will increase their levels of aggression in the playroom. Decision-making regarding use of strategies such as repeated ACT limit-setting, choice-giving, and ending the session is discussed in CCPT literature (Landreth 2012; Ray 2011). When therapists work with highly aggressive children, review of the literature and supervision/consultation are recommended to engage in effective and practical limit-setting that maintain the therapeutic relationship.

Therapist reaction to aggression

Working with aggressive children is challenging to the therapist as a person. Professional skills are integral to therapeutic success but I have found that each therapist's holistic health (her 'way of being') is the salient ingredient in an effective therapeutic relationship. Children who are aggressive will often engage in name-calling, insults, and attempts to physically hurt the therapist. It is natural for a therapist to feel drained, incompetent, and/or angry when working with certain children. Because the therapist seeks to provide an environment of care with a high level of personal genuineness, the child's frequent rejection of the therapist may trigger feelings of ineffectiveness, helplessness, or hurt. When engaging in relationships with children who are aggressive, therapists benefit from being in their own consultation relationships in order to process their experiences in therapy and their own personal reactions.

Additionally, therapists may be impacted by belief systems that hinder their work with aggressive children. In a previous publication on working with aggressive children from a CCPT perspective (Ray 2011), I noted beliefs that are common to play therapists and pose obstacles to working with this population.

1. My job is to make children feel better.

2. Each time I see a child, he/she must feel better than when we started.

3. Children should follow rules.

4. Children should follow rules with minimal disruption.

5. If children do not follow rules, it is my job to enforce the rules.

6. I have the power to control a child's behavior.

7. If I do not control a child's behavior, I am ineffective/a failure.

These beliefs are common to play therapists because they are common to most adults. Culturally, adults view children from these perspectives and hold a rigid view regarding the need for children to be happy and submissive to adults. These particular beliefs contradict the values within CCPT in which the therapist–child relationship is seen as vehicle for full expression, regard, and empathic understanding. An aggressive child is conceptualized as a child who uses aggression to express feelings or meet needs. In CCPT, the therapist focuses on how to develop a relationship that allows the child to express feelings and needs in a self-enhancing way. The focus is not on the aggression or stopping the behavior. In CCPT, the therapist knows that the aggressive behavior will fade when the child has developed better coping skills. Because aggressive acts are common in play therapy, a therapist's potential belief that a child should be calm, follow rules, or be pleasant will actively interfere with the relationship. When new play therapists enter the field, I often explore their personal beliefs regarding children and how these beliefs will impact their work with children.

A personal reflection on working with aggressive children

In my own development as a therapist, I initially struggled with some of my belief systems regarding working with children. Three that were prevalent for me were:

1. I should never be angry with a child.

2. I should like all children all the time.

3. If I am kind to children, they will/should return my kindness with kindness.

These beliefs became problematic as I began to specialize with children who were aggressive. Children referred for play therapy who present with aggression can be cruel, hurtful, and vengeful directly toward the therapist. As therapy became more intense and the child more expressive, I would experience moments of personal incongruence. As a child attempted to punch me, I might react with a smile while I responded, 'I'm not for hitting.' In these moments, I experienced inner conflict, consisting of feeling anger yet chastising myself for feeling anger, resulting in a belief that I was an incompetent therapist. For me, this type of inner turmoil went even deeper and I would conclude that beyond not being a competent therapist, there must be something wrong with me as a person. Personal therapy to work on my own feelings of self-worth and how these feelings impact my personal and professional relationships was invaluable to me. Through therapy, I learned that my beliefs about not being angry with children and holding myself to a standard of having to like all children was directly related to my own need to be accepted by, and pleasing to, others. Being myself is risky in relationships because being human means that I have human feelings that include positive and negative feelings toward others, even children. I learned to accept that when a child tries to hurt me, I feel hurt. When a child is unkind, I feel hurt. And sometimes my anger emerges from my hurt.

When I internally accepted more of my own feelings, I experienced less anger and hurt in session with children. I began to separate a child's need to hurt me from my need to not to be hurt or rejected. When I integrated this awareness into my work, I could fully experience the child without the barrier of my own internal conflicts. I was able to be fully in the child's world and see why it was important for the child to hurt me. My empathic understanding, my ability to be with the child in the moment, increased to a great degree.

Another benefit of this self-work was I became able to genuinely express myself to the child in the moment. I was not afraid of my hurt or my anger so I could use it therapeutically to connect with the child as a fellow human. Hence, I regularly share my immediate reactions of hurt as they occur in the playroom. Common phrases for me in working with aggressive children are 'You really wanted to hurt me and you did', 'You are trying to figure out the meanest thing to say to me', 'You want me to feel bad', 'That hurt'. As I have become more accepting of myself and genuine in my expression, children respond in a way that allows me deeper into their worlds. They are often open about their intentions, 'You should be hurt, just like me', 'You shouldn't be hurt, I can take it so should you'. These moments lead to connecting relational points where the child feels that I truly understand what is happening for them.

In addition to personal therapy, I rely on processing sessions with colleagues. Although I have been a play therapist for 20 years, I still learn a great deal from consulting with trusted colleagues about my clients and moments in session. There are some sessions in which I might set limits for an entire 45 minutes, never feeling connected to the child. At these times, I value being able to talk about my feelings about the child and the session with someone who knows me well. Sometimes, I will start with a statement like, 'I'm really angry with this kid…'. Through consultation, I work through what is happening for me in this relationship and why my feelings are strong. I have come to believe that any strong negative feeling I have toward a child probably has more to do with something happening within me internally than something about the child. Consultation helps me to figure out how to move into being therapeutically focused on the child and when I need to do more self-care.

I also engage in regular internal exercises to prepare myself to facilitate therapy with children who are intensely aggressive. I will take a few minutes before session to think about the child and be mindful about what might occur in the coming session. I will attempt to empathically attune myself with the child by seeing the world through his eyes before the session. I engage in unconditional positive regard exercises by reminding myself that the child can do this work, the child can figure out how to engage in self-enhancing ways of being if I am fully available to him, and that the child is an amazing person in coming as far as he has come. I might practice certain expected limits or responses in my head to see if they feel true to me yet therapeutic for the child. This type of mindfulness directly before session helps to focus me therapeutically on the needs of the child, and less on my reaction to the child.

To summarize my personal reflections on this work: *I spend time working on me so that I can be therapeutic for the child.* I am not aware of an easier route or techniques that increase my effectiveness in relationship that do not involve my own personal work. As therapists engage in practice with clients who require a great deal of personal resources, self-exploration, supervision, and consultation are critical to effectiveness.

The case of Nia

I was asked to see Nia in play therapy in the middle of her kindergarten school year. Her teacher was frustrated with her behavior, which was disruptive to Nia's own learning as well as the education of other children in her class. Nia was loud, demanding, and threw tantrums when she did not get her way. The incident in the hallway on the first day I met her was a frequent weekly occurrence. The teacher had attempted several behavioral methods to improve Nia's behavior but Nia appeared unresponsive to praise and rewards, as well as consequences. Play therapy was a last resort prior to the next step of sending Nia to an alternative school for children with behavioral problems. Nia's mother reluctantly agreed to Nia's participation in play therapy with the clear stipulation that she would not have to attend any sessions or be involved. Nia's mother was a single mother of three children and worked two jobs.

Nia's therapy sessions were held in the school twice a week during the school day, 30 minutes per session. I limit sessions to 30 minutes in school settings due to school timetabling limitations. Nia quickly fell into a play pattern in which she always engaged in play with the snake at some time in the session and then engaged in mother–daughter play with me. I have previously described the snake play in which Nia grew to nurture the mean and ugly snake who was actually nice and only wanted to be liked. In the mother–child play, Nia was highly verbal and alternated between playing the mother and playing the child. In her mother–daughter play, Nia verbalized details about her home life. Her infant brother died within the last year and Nia re-enacted the funeral several times in which she played the mother who cried and screamed out in pain. In some sessions, she played out the mother–daughter dressing to go on dates. She often chose cooking meals together as her most frequent relational play. In the initial mother–daughter play, Nia chose to be the mother.

Nia: Let's make dinner.

Me: You want us to make dinner together.

Nia: You make the soup and I'll make the cake.

Me: You're giving each of us a job.

Nia: (Hands me the bowl and spoon) You're doing it all wrong. Here, let me show you. (She grabs the bowl and spoon from me) See, you do it like this. (Gives me back the bowl and spoon)

Me: You needed to show me. I just wasn't doing it right.

Nia: (Yells) No, what are you doing? You're doing it wrong again. What's wrong with you? Give it to me.

Me: You're mad at me. I keep doing it wrong.

Nia: Why can't you do anything right?

Me: I'm doing it all wrong.

Nia: You *always* do it wrong.

In early sessions, interactions in which Nia (as the mother) yelled at me (as the daughter) were frequent. As the daughter, I made mistakes and most everything I did was wrong. Nia was relentless in her criticism and her tone was harsh. Following our eighth session, we walked down the hall back to her classroom.

Nia: You're really nice.

Me: You want me to know that you like me. I like you too.

Nia: Can I come live with you?

Me: You think I'm so nice that you want to live with me.

Nia: Do you have toys at home?

Me: I don't have many toys.

Nia: Why not?

Me: My kids are all grown up so I gave most of my toys away.

Nia: You didn't have to give them away. I could play with them.

Me: You would like it if we spent time together and played together.

Nia: I like you.

Me: I like you too.

In the following, ninth session, Nia initiated mother–daughter play in which she was the mother.

Nia: (Starts to mix water and sand in a bowl) Now, I'm going to show you how to make soup.

Me: You're showing me just how to do it.

Nia: (Hands me the bowl and spoon) Now, you do it.

Me: (Start to mix) You decided it's my turn.

Nia: (Soft tone) You're doing it wrong.

Me: You're letting me keep doing it even though it's wrong.

Nia: That's OK. You can do it that way.

Me: So, even though I'm doing it wrong, you decided that would be OK.

Nia: Sometimes we do things wrong.

Me: Yep, I guess sometimes we do things wrong and it's still OK.

In this interaction, Nia began to show self-acceptance in relationship with her mother. Even at the age of five, she had an awareness that she does not know how to do things correctly but that should be OK. She began to offer nurturance to herself. I believe that Nia experienced a softness in our relationship, a feeling that she is accepted and worthy for who she is, not what she does. She was able to transfer this acceptance to provide unconditional positive self-regard. As she grew in her acceptance of self, she grew in her compassion to others, experiencing less of a need to control or make aggressive contact with others. Following 14 play therapy sessions, Nia's teacher reported that she had not thrown a tantrum in over two weeks and was following limits in the classroom. The teacher also described Nia as more flexible when things did not go her way. Because behavioral problems had decreased, Nia's teacher felt more positive and Nia's classmates engaged with her more.

In Nia's case, behavioral changes were evident quickly after seven weeks of twice-weekly sessions. However, in many cases, especially when children present with high levels of aggression, therapy can be expected to take much longer. In play therapy, results from meta-analyses indicate that children who participate in play therapy reach optimal effects at approximately 35–40 sessions (Bratton *et al.* 2005). The trajectory of CCPT shows that children experience some measurable effects following 11 sessions but that behavioral/relational/ emotional problems continue to improve up to 40 sessions (Ray 2008). The play therapy experience is unique for each child, and hence there is no way to predict exactly how long therapy will be needed for a child to experience herself as worthy, capable, and creative in engaging in enhancing ways of being in the world.

Conclusion

Children who are aggressive present as an especially challenging population for child-centered play therapy. Aggression is a natural behavior within the trajectory of child development. However, some children fail to move beyond acts of aggression when attempting to get their needs met, and fail to progress developmentally towards verbalization and problem-solving as positive alternatives. These children engage in verbally and/or physically aggressive acts of a magnitude that impairs their relationships with adults and peers.

In order for these children to develop positive coping skills for meeting their needs, aggressive children need to experience a relationship in which a therapist allows for full expression of need whilst noting limits on behaviors. Acts of aggression frequently offer potential interference to the warmth and nurturance experienced in quality therapeutic relationships. Although the CCPT therapist seeks to initiate and sustain a relationship marked by genuineness, unconditional positive regard, and empathic understanding, these conditions may be impacted by a child's expression of aggression. Aggression can be felt to directly contradict the essential conditions of effective relationships. The CCPT therapist facilitates a relationship in which the therapist sends a very particular message: that the child is valued, worthy, and capable. It is through this relationship that the child experiences self as capable and engages in creative, self-enhancing ways to meet their needs for connection and relationship.

References

Axline, V. (1947) *Play Therapy.* New York: Ballantine.

Bratton, S., Ray, D., Rhine, T. and Jones, L. (2005) 'The efficacy of play therapy with children: a meta-analytic review of treatment outcomes.' *Professional Psychology: Research and Practice 36,* 376–390.

Landreth, G. (2012) *Play Therapy: The Art of the Relationship* (3rd edn) New York: Routledge.

Ray, D. (2008) 'Impact of play therapy on parent–child relationship stress in a mental health clinic setting.' *British Journal of Guidance and Counselling 36,* 165–187.

Ray, D. (2011) *Advanced Play Therapy: Essential Conditions, Knowledge, and Skills for Child Practice.* New York: Routledge.

Rogers, C. (1957) 'The necessary and sufficient conditions of therapeutic personality change.' *Journal of Consulting Psychology 21,* 2, 95–103.

Rogers, C. (1989) *The Carl Rogers Reader.* New York: Houghton Mifflin.

13

THE RHYTHMS OF AN OILY CART SHOW

Theatre for Young People with Complex Learning Disabilities

TIM WEBB

I sometimes feel that my son is not 'present', that he is just being carried along in the world. During TUBE I felt that he was very much 'present', engaged and interested. I think the performance was too compelling for him to miss! Magic stuff! You really 'get' our kids – thank you.

R.D., parent, of the Oily Cart show TUBE, in the version
for young people on the Autism Spectrum

In the beginning

Best to confess from the start that no one in the Oily Cart is a therapist. What we do is theatre not therapy. To be precise we are a theatre company that creates work for two kinds of audience: very young children, between the ages of six months and six years, and young people from 3 to 19 years old classified as having Profound and Multiple Learning Disabilities (PMLD) or an Autistic Spectrum Condition (ASC).

The company began life in 1981 when Max Reinhardt, Amanda Webb and Tim Webb came together with the specific aim of creating theatre for children under the age of five. At that time theatre created for such young children was rare but by using a wide variety of theatrical languages including amazing visuals, puppetry, live music and the active participation of our audiences we successfully engaged audiences in nurseries, playgroups, one o'clock clubs and the like.

A turning point came in 1988 when we were invited to a West London school for Severe Learning Disabilities (SLD) to perform for young people ranging from three to nineteen years. Up to this point we had considered that the key characteristic of our theatre was that it was age-appropriate. We used themes, language and design aimed specifically at a particular age range and so we questioned how a show made for the under fives could be suitable for an 18- or 19-year-old. We reasoned that, whatever his or her cognitive abilities, an 18-year-old would have a considerably different view of themselves and the world around them than a five-year-old. So rather than performing a show made for a very different audience we asked if we could spend a week in the school, observing and joining in with work and play, with the aim of developing a piece of theatre appropriate to the needs of these older students.

We learned a great deal in that week. It quickly became clear that the range of personalities and abilities to be found in that school of a hundred pupils was vast. On the one hand there were the senior classes containing young adults who were mobile and articulate and would go on to lead reasonably independent lives. On the other there were people with complex sensory and cognitive impairments who needed assistance with the most basic activities and who would continue to need this individual attention for the rest of their lives.

We realized that the enormous range of personalities and abilities in this audience would require that we use many different channels of communication. Seeing and hearing are the dominant senses in most forms of theatre. Audiences generally sit at one end of the room watching and listening to performers who move around, talk and sing at the other. Many of the young people in this Special School had impaired vision or impaired hearing or both. Theatre for them could not rely on the seeing and hearing staples of orthodox theatre.

The teachers also told us of the cognitive impairments which affected many of the school population. We were told of:

- processing delays that meant those affected would need extra time to appreciate a scene, event or character

- poor short-term memory in some of the pupils with the result that they would not remember at the end of a performance what had happened at the beginning

- lack of understanding of causation and so difficulty in comprehending that a particular action was likely to have a specific outcome.

We came to realize that for some of these young people we needed to create a form of theatre that did not depend on the most treasured principles of the stage and storytelling. In some instances we would have to make theatre for people who lived in the moment, neither remembering what had come before nor anticipating what might come next. Most drama introduces characters and dilemmas at the start of the show and during the course of the action we see the characters develop and the dilemmas resolved. The theatre for many in our intended audience could not be like that.

Fortunately, the week that had prompted so many questions also provided a few answers. Several teachers had suggested we attempt something longer than the traditional 45 minutes to one hour running time for a children's theatre piece.

We ourselves had come to the conclusion that because of the huge ability range in the school we would need to create discrete units of performance, each one suited to the requirements of different groups of young people. The spectrum of requirements ran from individuals who were mobile, articulate and able to anticipate some sort of independent living, through to those with multiple impairments, little if any verbal language and who required assistance with most everyday activities.

Although we believed that these discrete pieces of performance each aimed at a different ability level were essential, we also planned on bringing the whole school together at one or two points to reinforce a sense of community and to assert the value of theatre as a shared experience.

Above all, the week had taught us that our theatre needed to be multi-sensory. It would not get us very far if was only accessible via the eyes and the ears. There would be a significant number in our Special Schools' audiences for whom seeing and hearing were not accessible channels. We should introduce textures, smells, tastes into our work, and in particular we should find ways of addressing the vestibular and proprioceptive senses (sometime rolled together as 'the kinaesthetic sense') by which the body is aware of its own parts in relation to one another and of its position and volition relative to the world around.

We were introduced to the world of prioritizing kinaesthetic experience when a group of teachers showed how they 'hammocked' students. They would place an ex-navy hammock on floor, help a student to lie down on it, then lift them a short way into the air and swing and bounce them to and fro. For some students the process was slow and gentle; for others it was extremely vigorous. All the students we observed being hammocked were clearly delighted and we knew that we must add hammocking or something similarly kinaesthetic to our repertory of multi-sensory stimuli.

Box of socks

Based on this short but productive period of research we rehearsed and made a show, *Box of Socks*, and organized a short tour to Special Schools in the London area. It embodied as many of the things we had learned during the research period as we could fit in.

To begin with *Box of Socks* lasted for a whole school day. We were already challenging ideas of the duration of performance. The cast were three aliens from outer space, one of whom had several sock puppet offspring. The offspring, and the title of the show, came via a generous donation of socks from The Sock Shop.

The first the young people saw of us was when they all assembled in the school hall to find a smoking spaceship, from which we aliens emerged coughing and spluttering. From that point on the whole school was our venue. We went from classroom to classroom, from gym to art room to dining hall, interacting with the students as we found them. We joined in with their activities and communicated with them using the language that they used, sometimes highly verbal, at others practically mute. Our aim was to make theatre as interactive as possible.

Of course, because we came from outer space, we knew nothing of life on earth. Every single person in the school knew more than we did. I believe that many of the students found this empowering. 'Why are you making marks on the white stuff?' enquired one of us. 'It's writing,' came the reply. 'Why are you putting solids in that hole in your head?' I asked. 'I'm eating my dinner,' was the answer.

In the afternoon the aliens invited the whole school into the hall to celebrate their visit to Earth. There was an intergalactic magic show and a disco featuring such universally famous stars as Fela Kuti and Kylie Minogue. Some of the senior students helped with the food shopping for the party and were appalled and delighted when one of the aliens charged into the cake shop calling for 'meat!' and the butcher's demanding 'cake!'.

So although we began and ended with a gathering in the school hall, involving some sitting and watching, but also including eating, drinking and dancing, in between we expanded from an expected location of performance (the hall) into a promenade using the whole school. What's more, by taking each group of students as we found them and responding to the activities in which they were involved and to their suggestions, we encouraged them to become co-creators of the piece. There was the opportunity for everyone's voice, using words or not, to be heard.

Box of Socks was very well received on its first tour of Special Schools and we quickly began to get other bookings. The show incorporated in embryonic form many of the tropes that were to feature in much of our work for people with complex disabilities. But we had a lot more to learn and plenty of productions and audiences from which to learn it. Each year since 1988 we have created at least one new production for young people with complex disabilities. Much of what we have learned from these experiences might fall under the heading of *The rhythms of relating.*

The rhythms of an Oily Cart performance: Music and song

Music plays an essential role in every Oily Cart production for young people with complex learning disabilities. There are several reasons why we might be defined as a music theatre company. Even our name, which we borrowed and mangled, from the D'Oyly Carte Company, the original producers of the Gilbert and Sullivan operas, points to the centrality of music in our work.

Max Reinhardt,[1] one of the three co-founders of the company, sometime performer and full-time Music Director, not only brings many musical influences from around the world into our work, he also brings many international musicians.[2] We bring these musicians from different backgrounds into the company partly to reflect the diverse society in which we live but also because they are highly skilled improvisers who can respond directly to the requirements and the interventions of the audience.

But the first and best reason for having Max Reinhardt's wonderful music played by such skilled musicians is that music is the single most effective medium that we have at our disposal. A great many of the young people we work with are responsive to music – finding a way to dance to a groovy tune or becoming quiet and contemplative as they listen to something legato and in a minor key.

But the role of music, and especially rhythm, in our work goes further than that.

Low pitched sounds

For both PMLD and ASC audiences we have found that bass instruments are particularly effective and over the years we have returned again and again to bass clef instruments. Different shows have involved the double bass, the bass clarinet, the tuba and large percussion instruments of our own design made of gas and water pipe and made for us by a specialist instrument-maker called Jamie Linwood.

These low-pitched instruments are particularly effective for those in our audiences who are hearing impaired. The bass sounds operate at a level where they are as much felt as heard and can communicate with people with little or no hearing. For the show *Drum*, 2011 and 2012, which existed in three versions – one for children under two years, another for those with PMLD and a third for those on the autism spectrum – we used a one-and-a-half-metre diameter drum. Audience members would take it in turn to lie on this while

---

1   Also a world music DJ and one of the presenters of BBC Radio Three's *Late Junction*.

2   In our current production, *Light Show*, we have the Australian virtuoso double bass player Adam Storey. In our 2014 to 2015 piece, *The Bounce*, we featured Maya Youssef, a brilliant Syrian kanun player. Numerous jazz players have passed through the ranks, including Dutch cellist Ernst Reijsiger, trumpeter Byron Wallen, and flute and sax player Finn Peters.

we drummed around them, carefully adjusting the intensity of the drumming to suit their reactions. This is a variation on the idea of resonance boards, or hollow resonating boxes or platforms used to help hearing impaired people perceive sounds. The rhythmic low-pitched sounds of the drum engaged young people from all three of our audience categories and it was wonderful to see 6- to 12-month-old babies bouncing up and down on the drum skin. Teenagers on the spectrum could barely be prised from the drum head.

Music in support of verbal communication

We definitely ration the amount of verbal language in any Oily Cart show for PLMD and ASC audiences. We often set a word limit of 30 to 40 words and that is more than ample. We also use an even more limited quantity of Makaton and sometimes PECS (Picture Exchange Communication System) to support the spoken words that we use. But for the Oily Cart the most effective support for words in general is music.

Many, in our PMLD audiences especially, will not understand or use more than a handful of words and we feel that if such a limited vocabulary is channelled through a song or chant then it will communicate more effectively than if merely spoken. Song allows us to use a great deal of repetition of the lyric, and a good deal of emphasis on particular parts of the lyric in a way which does not seem forced and can be highly entertaining. In regular speech, repetition and emphasis can quickly begin to appear teacherly, hectoring or just boring. Repeat and emphasize in a song and most of the time it's fun. An Oily maxim might be 'Why just say it if you can sing it?'

Name songs

Towards the end of any production for young people with PLMD/ASC we perform the 'Name Songs'. In a Name Song each young person in the audience is sung a song in which the only lyric will be her or his own name. We make the assumption that for any young person with limited vocabulary, that vocabulary will at least contain their own name. For the Name Song we recycle melodies that have occurred earlier in the show, based on the overture principle that if you've already heard a song, then it will sound sweeter the second time around. As we sing the Name Song to each of the young people we project his or her image onto a live video screen, or sometimes use a reflection in a mirror. The image can be seen by everyone in the room and the young person becomes the focus of everyone's attention and love for the duration of that song. We have had many wonderful reactions. Often the young person will smile or pull a funny face but you can see they have awareness that they are part of a group and are amongst friends. That is very satisfying. Of course some participants remain indifferent to their Name Songs and others can appear bashful, even embarrassed. This is where the Oily Cart style of interactive performance comes into its own. If something is being well received we will do will do it longer and stronger. But if something is clearly causing discomfort we will withdraw it and even switch to something else.

Our primary goal with this form of performance is to engage and communicate with each young individual by finding a language or languages that we share. But secondarily, our aim is to help all the young people in the audience become aware that they are together, participating in a shared experience. Achieving this second goal is much less common than with the first. But if it is going to happen it most often happens during the Name Songs.

Even if the young person being sung to does nothing to indicate awareness of the people around them, in Special School hall performances especially, something wonderful can and does happen on a regular basis. At the back of the hall we will frequently see the dinner ladies, the bus drivers, the office staff and passing teachers listening to the Name Songs and watching the images on the video screen. This impromptu audience is generally smiling and quietly commenting on what they can see and hear. They are so delighted to see a child they all know responding in this novel setting and there is a real sense of the school as a caring community.

The Jazz Structure in an Oily Cart performance

Even when nothing that could conventionally be described as music is going on in an Oily Cart PLMD/ASC show, the action is very much governed by certain rhythms. For example we have found that both ASC and PMLD audiences generally respond better to close-up work once we have succeeded in gaining their confidence. Three-quarters of an Oily Cart production is spent with the performers sitting or standing beside the participants and working with them at a distance of less than a metre. This proximity is an essential component of the Oily style of interactive performance. Such close-up performance is not scripted and consists of the performer freely improvising according to the reactions of the participant. At its most straightforward an interaction like this could involve the performer fanning the participant and using verbal language, facial expression, vocalizations or whatever works to find if the young person wants something more, less or completely different. In these close-up sections of the show every participant's experience will be unique. Someone might prefer energetic fanning. Someone else might prefer the gentlest of breezes. A third young person might want nothing to do with this fanning and indicate that they would prefer a repeat of the spraying with the mister, so why not go back to that?

Personalized, improvised interaction is a key part of any Oily Cart show. But as I discussed earlier, we also have the objective of making our theatre a social experience for our participants. We also need to have some control over the length of each section in a show and of the show itself. Nowadays a typical Oily Cart session will last just under the hour.

To reconcile these different objectives we work to what we refer to as the 'Jazz Structure' of an Oily Cart performance. This enables us to intersperse a shared, group experience with one-to-one improvisation within a performance and keep the whole thing to an acceptable running time.

In a show like TUBE, 2013, which came in three versions, one for ASC, one for PMLD and one for the under-twos, the cast consisted of three performers (our musician George and two others), supported by a stage manager. They performed to an audience of six young people with a disability who were each accompanied by an adult (a teacher or family member).

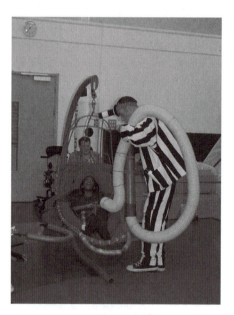

FIGURE 13.1 OILY CART PRODUCTION TUBE, 2013[3]

As TUBE began, our performers each introduced themselves to a pair of young people, finding out their names and the names of the accompanying adults before going on to demonstrate how the adults could make the suspended seating swing, bounce and twist. It was all unscripted and informal and all

3   The musician, percussionist and jazz drummer George Panda played two instruments made specifically for this show out of plastic drainage pipe. This kind of instrument is sometimes called a 'boom-bam', sometimes a 'bat phone'. For us the key was that the instrument was made from tubes, as was everything in the show – whether seen, heard, felt or smelt.

three performers would have to find a style of address that was suited to the young people they found themselves with. In the 'Jazz Structure', as we call a section of this nature, there are 'solos', because each performer is working independently with just one or two of the participants.

To move from a close-up moment like this, George would begin to play and bring all the performers together for a tightly rehearsed and choreographed ensemble moment. The audience would shift focus to what all the performers were now doing and how their fellow participants were reacting. This section in the Jazz Structure is called the 'ensemble'. The jazz analogy comes from the fact that in many forms of jazz, from the big bands of the 30s and 40s to the small group jazz of the 50s and 60s onwards, a jazz piece often begins with an arranged section with all members of the band playing together. This is followed by a series of sections in which the musicians improvise independently through to a coda that is again arranged. Sometimes there are short ensemble passages, or riffs, punctuating the series of solos.

This pattern: ensemble opening – solos – riff – solos – riff – solos – riff – solos – coda is a regularly used Oily Cart template, enabling us to incorporate freely improvised one-to-one sections into a structure that can be enjoyed by the whole audience.

The Breath Pause

There is another rhythmic element present in many of the recent Oily Cart productions for PMLD/ASC audiences and one that is usually associated with the Jazz Structure. This is what we call the 'Breath Pause'. While the playing of a new theme will often introduce a passage of close-up 'solo' work, these solo passages will frequently end with the performers becoming quite still, looking at one another, and breathing a deep sigh. This sigh is followed by a pause before the musician will again begin playing to cue the next solo section.

Often, in the pause following the sigh, participants, especially those in a PMLD performance, will utter small sounds. When this happens it seems to me that they are taking the opportunity to comment on the action. There is no way to be certain of that but these Breath Pause moments do ensure that the participants have time in which they can add their own contribution to the music of the piece.

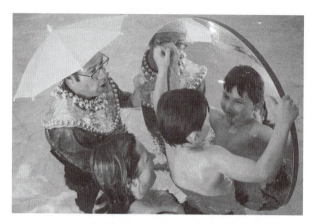

FIGURE 13.2 OILY CART PRODUCTION *POOL PIECE*, 2008 AND 2009

We first became aware of the importance of punctuating a show with these moments of stillness and silence during the development of the show *Pool Piece* (2008 and 2009). *Pool Piece* was one of our shows that take place in the hydrotherapy pools of Special Schools. Normally the size of the hydro pools restricts the size of our audiences to two young people with PMLD or ASC, together with two accompanying adults. But for part of our development period we had the use of an especially large pool and some extra time. As a part of this exploratory phase we decided to work with a population group that held something in common with our PMLD/ASC audiences, namely they made little or no use of verbal language. This group was a 20-strong baby and toddler group, all of whom were said to be developmentally typical.

We prepared a session for this new audience in a similar manner to our PMLD/ASC hydrotherapy shows. To the accompaniment of live singing and music, played on instruments taken from a Javanese gamelan, we took our audiences on a journey around the pool. We explored chiming buoys floating on the water, fountains and spray curtains from above, and bubbles from below.

For all the versions of *Pool Piece* we used a wonderful orchestral gong to punctuate the action. It was fascinating to see the speed with which the developmentally typical babies and toddlers reacted to the gong. The heads of these under-twos whipped instantaneously to the exact location of the gong on the poolside. The reaction of the young people in the PMLD sessions was very different. Their heads turned slowly and uncertainly as you might expect, but then, as the complex sound of the gong faded away something wonderful happened: one or even both of the young people in the water would utter vocal sounds. From that moment on we began to leave spaces and silences in our performances to give the young people the opportunity to join in. In subsequent performances of *Pool Piece* we referred to this as the 'gong moment' and this evolved over the course of several shows into the Breath Pause.

Rhythm to give an event significance

The Breath Pauses are just one of the means whereby we punctuate the action of the show with moments of stillness and silence. One reason for freezing the action in this way is that it powerfully focuses the attention of our PMLD and ASC audiences. If we are about to introduce a significant prop – say, a fan – into the action, we find that the young people are more likely to notice and appreciate the event if it happens when there is no other sound or activity to distract them.

Moments of quiet and stillness are useful for all of us to do some processing and reflection without distraction. This might be especially significant for people with PMLD and ASC for whom there may well be barriers affecting information processing.

Introducing an event in stages

Another common Oily Cart technique is to introduce a new object or a new event in stages. For example, in our show for PMLD/ASC *Blue* (2006 and 2007), we would use back-projected video on a large screen when we wanted to bring a new object into the action. At one point in the show a character hauled on a large trunk in which there was an old-fashioned type of water pump, operated by a pull-up, push-down handle. Before the pump was opened we heard, for a few seconds, the sound of running water. Then a video image of running water appeared on screen. Finally the lid of the trunk was thrown open, the pump hauled upright, and the handle operated by the performers to pump out lots of water. (The water was actually being circulated in and out of the pump by an electric motor.)

Introducing a new event in this way – first the sound, then the image, then the real thing – enables us to address the participants via different senses in turn and allows plenty of processing time. It also encourages the accompanying adults to talk to their companions about what might be coming up next. As the sound cue comes up, you will hear questions like, 'What's that sound?' and 'Can you hear that?' from the adults. The repeated sound/image/real-thing pattern also helps build a sense of anticipation in the audience.

Comic timing

There is another sort of rhythm at work in any Oily Cart show and that is the kind commonly referred to as 'comic timing'. Theorizing about comedy is a thankless business. The very act of theorizing mostly drains the fun out of the comedy and as a director of performers who often have to do comedy business I find that the more I have to explain how and why something might be funny, the less funny it gets. Some performers, however, and plenty of other people too, seem to have a built-in sense of how to be funny. They have a way of delivering a line or making a move that gets a laugh. Sometimes it has to do with the pacing, the placing of the stresses and a build-up to an ending which, when it comes, comes unexpectedly. On the other hand it can be about the build-up of a pattern of events or words. You have a rhythmic sense of how the pattern is developing but then, surprisingly, it does not conclude at the moment you expect…it goes on and on beyond the point where you were thinking it simply had to end. In either case it's definitely about rhythm; you are working with a repeating pattern and bringing it to a climax that is either all too expected or a big surprise.

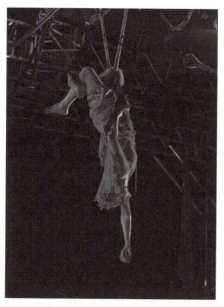

FIGURE 13.3 OILY CART PRODUCTION *SOMETHING IN THE AIR*, 2009–2012

There was a piece of effective comic business for PMLD/ASC audiences in our show *Something in The Air* (2009–2012). In this production six young people and six accompanying adults were winched up to two metres into the air, on an aerialists' flying rig. The specially designed seating for the audience could swing, bounce and spin as it hung from the rig. The brilliant aerial company Ockham's Razor flew amongst our suspended audience. When the trapeze artist swung the seats were also made to swing; when the aerial hoop artist span, all the seats twisted too; and when the bungee artist bounced, the seats bounced along with her. It was spectacular and it was beautiful. But the introduction to the bungee sequence was also comic and clearly laugh-out-loud funny for the PMLD/ASC young people participating.

It began with the bungee artist Tina Koch dropping a tennis ball-sized red ball from the top of the rig. The only stage direction was that no one in the cast was to touch the ball until it had finished bouncing and rolling. This could be quite frustrating. Just when you might have thought that ball had finally come to a halt it would start rolling again and for no apparent reason. Finally, the cast picked up the ball and danced with it for a short while.

Next came a red football. After a lengthy pause, when Tina simply held the ball still high above the audience, building up suspense, she let it fall it and bounce till again it was quite still. Then once more the cast could dance with it.

The process was repeated with a hefty gymnastic red ball. This was held aloft for an even longer time before being dropped and rolled around for an unfeasibly long time before it could be picked up and danced with. Finally, Tina, clad in red naturally, launched herself from the rig and bounced every which way on her bungees.

It was when the gymnastic ball entered the sequence that the laughs began. This grew to a peak when Tina appeared hanging from the rig, curled up into a ball and hung for an age before launching into space.

So, you see, it is difficult to theorize about comedy. Perhaps you just had to be there. But on so many occasions during the tours of *Something in The Air* I heard the laughter, and each time I wondered about the fact that many of the young people who joined in with that laughter were classified as having PMLD. Yet what they were laughing at was the development of a pattern or a rhythm that they had been able to perceive, although they were supposed to have all sorts of difficulties with processing and cognition. But then I am always being surprised by how these young people defy expectation and challenge the labels hung on them.

Playing with time

Many other rhythms of performance still remain for us to explore. That first Oily Cart show for audiences with Special Needs *Box of Socks*, from 1988, lasted a whole day and took place all over the school and the surrounding area. Much of our work since then has consisted of shorter performances, around an hour in length and played in school halls and classrooms, theatres, arts centres and the like. The reasoning behind this is mostly economic. But whenever we have had the chance to branch out from this pattern the results have been intriguing.

When we performed the PMLD/ASC show *Blue* at the Manchester International Festival of 2007 the festival commission enabled us to create two additional characters to the ones featured in the official touring version. These new characters were embedded – one in a Severe Learning Disability SLD) school, the other in a school specifically for young people on the autism spectrum – for the full week leading up to the show. Our aim was to prepare the young people in the two Special Schools for a visit to the theatre where they would participate in a performance of *Blue*.

From the beginnings of our work for PMLD/ASC audiences one difficulty has been has been that some young people, especially those on the autism spectrum, become anxious at the prospect of visiting unfamiliar places and meeting new people. Obviously a theatre visit is not the most inviting prospect for such a group. But over the years we have devised strategies for overcoming any apprehension. Nowadays we post online 'Social Stories' that describe, with plenty of illustration, what happens when you visit a theatre or a theatre company comes to you. The young people can see in advance how they will journey to the theatre, or how their school hall will be transformed and how the actors will look and behave. The Social Stories make it clear to our audiences that they have options. That it is OK to laugh at a character they think is funny. That they can choose to join with various activities if they like, but that they do not have to join in if that is what they prefer. This sort of Social Story preparatory work, in print, online, does seem to assuage anxiety and yet we have learned from experience that the most effective kind of preparation is that which happens over a longer time and is experienced rather than viewed in print or on screen. At the Oily Cart we are great believers in shows that begin long before they start and continue long after they have ended.

So to prepare for *Blue* in 2007 in Manchester we launched our brand new, embedded characters.

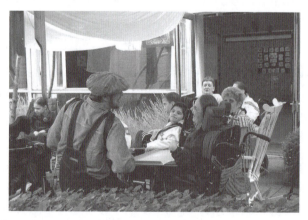

Figure 13.4 Oily Cart production *Blue*, 2007–2008

The characters in this show were passengers waiting at a railway station. Each one had a piece of luggage containing the thing that was most precious to them in the world. One character's luggage contained music, another's the night sky, and a third, as I mentioned earlier, a trunk filled with water. The young people who came along to see the show were asked to bring their own bag containing what was most precious to them. But their preparation for the theatre had begun several days before that when one day, quite without warning, they arrived at school to find a shack had been erected in the playground. The shack was well equipped with a well from which water could be pumped, a small cooker, a washing line, pots of herbs for cooking and a little bed. And someone was living in there.

The direction to the embedded performers was to have as little as possible to do with the young people for the first day or so. In the specialist autism school this had the effect of generating great curiosity. Over the next couple of days the students came to the shack and joined in with the singing and dancing, cooking and eating, washing the clothes and hanging them out to dry. The students also began to invite their unexpected guests into the classrooms, IT and art rooms, and the dining halls to show them the life of the school. By the third day even those students who had initially kept well away from the shack began to make contact. Finding that a guest had been, apparently, *sleeping* in the school turned out to be particularly fascinating.

When the time came for everyone to go with their new friends to the theatre to join in the *Blue* show the confidence of the young people from the autism school in particular was massive. The students had thought about what they most valued to carry in their luggage, and when they arrived at the theatre several of them actually embraced the characters on stage. The stories they had heard from their guests in the shacks had made the people they were now meeting at the theatre seem like old friends. A couple of the teachers from the autism school were in tears as they watched their young people joyfully taking part in this extraordinary encounter.

We want to explore this kind of extended performance much further. I am especially eager to investigate a performance rhythm that extends through the school day, overnight and on into the next and following days. The more time we can spend with the young people the greater their confidence becomes and the more they feel that the world being created around them by the performers is one in which they truly belong. Then the young people will offer their own ideas and become, even more, the co-creators of an Oily Cart wonderland.

Harry experienced *The Bounce* this afternoon. Rarely can I take my son into a situation so suited to his needs, seemingly designed exclusively for his pleasure. Not only was he able to participate but he got so very much out of it. It was as though something in him was touched and ignited; he was washed over by *The Bounce's* magic. This was an absolute pleasure for me too. My face is still aching from simultaneously smiling and holding back the tears.

Parent, of the Oily Cart production The Bounce, 2015

Fred's disability often means that he is always being asked to conform or work hard to fit into a social norm that is not suited to him and so he struggles but as soon as we walked into the space, Fred's differences were embraced and even celebrated. I felt like we were in a bubble of Fred's world and it was just magical. It was a stark contrast to the harsh world outside. I found the whole experience very emotional to watch and the Oily Cart Company have reminded me how wonderful my son is and we should be encouraging people to accept his differences rather then make him 'fit in'.

Parent, of the Oily Cart production The Bounce, 2015

14

A MEANINGFUL JOURNEY

Including Parents in Interactive Music Therapy
with Emotionally Neglected Children

STINE LINDAHL JACOBSEN

Working with children and families at risk within the field of child protection is a challenging and emotionally straining task. Family dynamics are complex, and when working with children individually the family of the child is always part of therapy, regardless of whether they participate in the sessions or not.

For every at risk child referred to therapy, we must consider many aspects before entering into therapy and forming an alliance with the child and the family. In some cases it is simply clear that therapy is contraindicated. When a child's home life is defined by *current* physical/emotional abuse or neglect, it most likely will be ineffectual, possibly unethical, to work with that child in therapy. A metaphor for the ineffectual nature of such input would be: an alcoholic remains sober for one hour a week to engage in addiction counseling, but continues to drink for the other 167 hours of the week. What could that one hour of therapy hope to achieve? And unethical? Amongst many aims, music therapy tries to support the child to feel safe enough to work with defense mechanisms and to feel safe enough to become vulnerable. If there is literally no safety (or no movement towards the development of safety) in that child's family life, how can it be ethical to invite the child into that vulnerability? The defense mechanisms are necessary coping strategies in the child. Without them, the child might not survive (Jacobsen and Killén 2015; Killén 2012; Robarts 2014). In these cases of current trauma, systemic work with the whole family in its wider social context is needed prior to any consideration of individual therapy.

And even when we consider therapy to be a positive possibility, the picture often remains blurred, the decisions complex. Often we cannot be certain about whether or not there is an adult offering enough current stability in the child's life. An emotionally neglected child has a lot of unmet needs and if I, as therapist, start to meet these needs as the only reliable adult in this child's world how will it affect the child when therapy stops? How big is the risk that the feeling of neglect will be intensified in the child when the therapist takes a holiday or the therapy ends? Are the benefits big enough to serve as counterweights to the possible side effects of therapy?

These are tough questions that most likely only can be answered individually in each case for each child going into therapy. It is a clear sign of positive potential if at least one of the child's parents/caregivers is willing to engage in the therapy process. If that adult is engaged, the hope is that a stable attachment base can be built, re-established, or developed for the child. For me, including parents in the therapy process is a central and necessary part of working with vulnerable children.

As a young music therapist I did not fully understand the importance of working with the whole family when working with vulnerable children and children at risk. This chapter is about my personal journey in discovering the value and benefits of including parents when working with emotionally neglected children and trying to secure their healthy development. The chapter includes two case vignettes to illustrate my thoughts on the clinical application of including parents in the music therapy process.

Emotionally neglected children

Emotional neglect is here understood as resulting from parents' inability to engage themselves with their child in an emotionally positive manner. Often parents are unaware of neglecting their children. Most parents love their children but might not know how to show it. Often children do experience joy and love but in a sporadic, insubstantial, and ambiguous manner which often results in contradictory feelings: lack of self-worth, feeling unwanted, just not sure *how* to feel. These children only feel they are worth something when they meet their parents' expectations or needs and are likely to develop a negative and distorted self-image together with very low self-esteem. And their parents' expectations or needs are often ambiguous, ambivalent, and emotionally confusing.

Modern attachment theory explains how a child's early experiences of emotional communication can be regulated or dysregulated within interaction, resulting in secure or insecure attachments (Schore and Schore 2008). Neglected children are more likely to develop anxious and insecure attachments to their caregivers and some also suffer from disorganized attachment behavior (Hildyard and Wolfe 2002). Attachment is a critical component in the development of right-brain receptivity and in the regulation of a healthy sense of self, including the dynamic regulation of internal states and external relationships (Schore and Schore 2008). As such, emotionally neglected children are likely to suffer from a wide range of physiological, emotional, and behavioral regulatory difficulties.

Neglected children all experience contradictory emotions – their longing for love and attention, combined with continual experiences of rejection, simultaneously draw them towards, and push them away from, parents and the entire outside world (Killén 2005). In an attempt to idealize the parent, many neglected children often take responsibility for the neglecting and abusing behavior of the parent. The children become the carrier of guilt, and there are no limits in their efforts to stay loyal towards the parent (Killén 2005).

Some emotionally neglected children will also experience depression, and this often will be evident in their capacity to play. Many of these children do not play much, or play in a stereotyped way (Irgens-Møller and Bjerg 2004; Killén 2005). Traumatic experiences can make play less spontaneous, more destructive, more immature, less motivated, and more compulsive. Many of these children are caught in an inescapable theme, and their way of playing lacks life and free improvisation. Emotionally neglected children who are somehow better able to cope can, as an exception, develop special creative abilities where they express themselves and their inner world through creative mediums (Irgens-Møller and Bjerg 2004; Killén 2005; Robarts 2014).

Research indicates that the particular parental environment of a neglected child – defined by inattentive, unpredictable, insensitive, unavailable, and misattuned parental capacity – increases the risk of diminished cortisol response and long-lasting down-regulation of the neurotrophic system, which can lead to anxiety, stress, and depression (Carpenter et al. 2009; Elzinga et al. 2011). Emotional neglect can cause severe cognitive and academic deficits, social withdrawal, limited peer interaction, and increased internalizing (Young, Lennie and Minnis 2011). After the findings of an international survey of clinicians, a new distinct diagnosis of Developmental Trauma Disorder was proposed to reflect the complex psychiatric challenges of emotionally neglected children (Ford et al. 2013).

Attunement and emotional communication

A parent's ability to self-regulate (including recognizing and experiencing a wide range of emotions, as well as cognitively understanding the mental state and the needs of their child) is necessary for the healthy development of every child. Stern (2000) describes the necessary intersubjective experiences needed within a parent–child dyad for the child to develop a robust emotional self. These processes include the parents' affective attunement towards the infant. Stern describes how caregivers imitate the infant *and* vary the repetition of the imitation in order to keep the infant interested and maintain her attention.

The repetition over a specific theme is of particular appeal to the infant, who tends to organize the world by looking for invariants. Through exploration and play, and interplay with nonverbal sounds, the infant learns about complex behavior and comes to recognize and regard specific behavioral features more than others. Thus, infants are taught to identify the invariant features in interpersonal behavior (Stern 2000).

When a parent displays affective attunement, she is letting her infant know that its emotions are recognized and that those emotions are shared by the parent. In his book *Forms of Vitality*, Stern (2010) described these emotional connections as, 'moments of meetings', where the relationship changes and moves into a deeper level of intersubjectivity. The variation of the theme in affect attunement is an important aspect of successfully communicating the emotional quality of the infant's state of mind. The infant's expressive state is 'matched' by her parent, but 'matched' in a modality different from the infant's initial expression. To correspond correctly with the child, the parent uses different affect attunement mechanisms or nonverbal forms of vitality including movement, force, space, intention/directionality, and time (Stern 2010).

Interpersonal interaction relies predominantly on nonverbal channels of communication. Verbal language is an insufficient medium for expressing quality, intensity, and nuance of emotion (Mandal and Ambady 2004). The ability to send and receive *nonverbal* messages is an important part of our capacity to communicate, both nonverbally *and* verbally (Knapp and Hall 2009). Conversational structure relies on nonverbal negotiations in which communicative timing and turn-taking are explored and developed. These nonverbal cues can consist of facial expression, body language, and prosody. Turn-taking is a jointly negotiated, complicated process, and it can easily fail. According to Knapp and Hall (2009), sometimes two nonverbal signals can contradict one another, turns can overlap each other, or cues can be missed. In this vulnerable process, feelings can be falsified if parents misinterpret or miss the nonverbal emotional/intentional signals from their child. Nonverbal communication skills are thus essential in supporting the development of both self-regulation and nonverbal communication skills in the child. Supporting a child in developing the ability to self-regulate emotion, thus becoming emotional stable, is one of the core aspects of parental capacity. Self-regulation is mainly developed in early childhood through sensitive interaction between mother and infant. These early experiences are crucial to healthy child development and highly relevant when working with emotionally neglected children, either alone or together with their parents (Jacobsen 2016).

Music therapy with emotionally neglected children

Two factors explain the considerable lack of literature concerning music therapy with emotionally neglected children: The 'label' *emotional neglect* is used primarily in a social service context; music therapists are not commonly employed within this area. Certain music therapy literature does, however, describe the general needs and characteristics of emotionally disturbed children including those who develop attachment disorders (Robarts 2014) and those who suffer complex trauma (Hussey *et al.* 2007). Effect studies of music therapy with children with psychopathology including behavioral, developmental, and emotional disorders indicate that music therapy is an effective intervention (Gold, Voracek and Wigram 2004). More studies are currently underway which are needed to provide empirical evidence for the use of music therapy with children with both behavioral and emotional problems (Porter *et al.* 2012).

Trevarthen and Malloch (2000) outline the essential nature of music therapy as 'an intimate way of communicating impulses of the self that creates benefits by transforming an active and intimate relationship with a therapist' (p.5). Human communication is built on the musical qualities of interacting rhythm, tone, tempi, pitch, timbre, and intensity – and it is through sensitive attunement within this realm of 'communicative musicality' (Malloch and Trevarthen 2009) that music therapists build and work with relationships. Music therapists try, through musical interplay and attuned emotional communication, to develop self-regulatory and attachment capacities in vulnerable children. In this way, music therapy aims to restore or repair central developmental milestones (Robarts 2014).

Most children are drawn to music and, despite the hesitancy towards relating to others often displayed by emotionally neglected children, developing a meaningful relation with the therapist through music is often possible. Emotionally disturbed children often find it difficult to engage in direct and/ or spoken language experiences of their painful past. Music can offer a way to circumvent anxious patterning and re-traumatizing habits, offering a direct, nonverbal modality in which victimized children can move towards a safe expression of early traumatic events:

> Music is an ideal way to help these children self-regulate and soothe as it creates a middle ground between over-arousal and numbness and helps the child to experience a state of stability... The immediate success that children experience in the music therapy setting can provide a boost to self-esteem and create a successful, non-threatening environment in which the therapist can help the child to decrease symptoms of arousal or disinhibition. (Hussey and Layman 2003, p.2)

Kolind (2008) suggests that music therapy, especially improvised singing, creates a safe frame for the emotionally neglected child. This safety enables the child to express otherwise defended nonverbal features of her inner self (Kolind 2008); more so because musical–poetic features (specifically) provide the child with natural emotion–language bridges – tools with which to feel, associate, and reflect, and then later on, to verbalize and combine sentences (Kolind 2008). This bridge-building, in a safe environment, enables child and therapist together to re-vision the child's traumatic narrative in new, healthy, creative ways (Hughes 2000).

Music therapy with families

We know that parental attunement is crucial to healthy child development – consistent experiences, over time, of synchronous playful interaction are central to attachment and the development of a child's robust sense of self. Including parents in therapy, to aid in the healthy development of emotionally neglected children, is highly relevant, ethical, and effective (Jacobsen and Thompson 2016; Killén 2005; Stern 2000). Musical interaction between family members facilitates quality social interaction. Music is a powerful medium to use in any attempt to bring parents and children together because music facilitates play and the inherently communicative functions of play (Jacobsen and Thompson 2016). Through musical play, interaction occurs naturally and spontaneously. Parents and their child in music therapy can re-engage in early developmental forms of nonverbal interaction and experience these intimate connections in a new way. Music therapy can facilitate, for the parent and child together, the experience of shared timing, rhythm, pulse, melody, and pitch, all of which are natural elements of the early bonding process (Davies 2008; Drake 2008; Jacobsen, McKinney and Holck 2014; Johns 2012; Salkeld 2008; Trevarthen and Malloch 2000; Trondalen and Skårderud 2007). In an age-appropriate and mutually enjoyable form the parent and child can strengthen their joint attention, interplay with turns, attunement, synchronization, and imitation (Holck 2011; Trolldalen 1997).

Music is an accessible medium for parents (Abad and Williams 2007; Bull 2008; Horvat and O'Neill 2008; Howden 2008; Oldfield 2006a, 2006b). Several studies describe how parents find it reassuring to participate in music therapy with their child because they can freely express themselves and share deeper feelings *both* consciously and unconsciously without verbal discussion (Davies 2008; Hasler 2008; Howden 2008, Oldfield 2006a).

Music therapy is considered particularly relevant in the assessment of parent–child interaction (Jacobsen and McKinney 2015). Analysis of musical interaction can elucidate family interaction patterns, symptoms of dysfunction, family interpersonal skills, and nonverbal communication skills. Music therapy assessment can also indicate parents' ability to meet the child's needs as well as their ability to communicate with the child (Jacobsen and Killén 2015; Molyneux 2008; Oldfield and Flower 2008).

Case vignettes

To illustrate my journey towards acknowledging the value of including parents in music therapy, three cases are presented here within the field of work with vulnerable children. The first case is early on in my career and retains a strong focus on child work alone. The second is more recent and illustrates work within a family therapy setting.

Pernille and Julie

Early on in my career, I worked with a seven-year-old girl Pernille and her mother Julie. Pernille and Julie lived at a family care centre together with Pernille's younger sister. Pernille's father had physically abused Julie, and Pernille had witnessed some of these dramatic events. The young family had been through much and were to some degree traumatized from their experiences. Julie was scared, immature, and had always had difficulties setting aside her own needs in favor of the needs of her children. Pernille presented with a level of insecure attachment behavior. The family was referred to music therapy because Pernille loved to sing and because mother and daughter needed positive experiences together in order to be able to possibly build new healthier interaction patterns. After the initial assessment period the common goal that Julie and I could agree on was to give Pernille a good experience and to give Pernille the opportunity to express her inner feelings in a safe place. At this point Julie was not ready to include her own parenting skills as part of the focus in therapy.

The sessions were mostly led by me as I introduced exercises and games to the family. I tried hard to empower Pernille and Julie by letting them own their time together but this continued to be a challenge throughout their sessions. However, both mother and daughter engaged in the sessions by improvising and interacting through the music. They talked together about song lyrics and the experience of sharing songs. Pernille and Julie were enjoying the experience of being able to interact in a healthy and trusting manner.

At one point Pernille expressed how she loved a song called 'Waking up in the Night' and that she wanted to sing it to her mother. Pernille explained how the lyrics reminded her of her father, whom she missed, even though she knew it was difficult for Julie to talk about him. Pernille sang the song full heartedly while I accompanied her on the piano. Julie listened in silence next to Pernille.

Waking up in the Night

Are you lying alone
I hope you are
Dreaming a few dreams I like
Will I forget you
Will you forget me
Were we from the past
is everything over now
I wonder if you feel like me
Waking up in the night

Woken by a dream
I miss to talk to you
I miss to hold you
It has been raining on my window
Droplets on my cheek
Uh, I would do anything
Do anything to go back

Afterwards Julie gently acknowledged that Pernille missed her father and that she was proud of how Pernille sang with her own strong voice. It made her very proud of her daughter and also helped them both remember good times they shared in the past. Singing the song together was a way of remembering and sharing complex emotions without either Pernille or Julie being confronted with feelings of guilt, shame, and remorse.

Pernille and Julie seemed to improve in their capacity to interact, despite the fact that Julie still had not referred to her own parental abilities at any point in the therapy process even though I tried to respectfully address this many times. Julie, however, began to be able to set aside her own needs when trying to meet Pernille's need for expressing herself freely. This development enabled mother and daughter to enjoy many positive moments together. The small (but powerful) changes in Julie's parenting skills were not conscious to her. As such, it was a challenge for me to find a way to let Julie be empowered by her progress as she did not fully own it. Finally it made sense to me that maybe Julie did not need to know about these changes – the family would benefit regardless. The focus Julie and I had initially agreed on was to support Pernille's healthy emotional development. But the sessions also strengthened the family bond and improved Julie's parenting skills. As a therapist I could feel my natural tendency towards meeting Pernille's need for affirmation and warmth, but I needed to hold back and give Julie a chance to be there for her daughter. I learned to focus on facilitating the interaction between mother and daughter, even though the 'focus' was on the child's emotional development.

Anton and Lars

Several years later another family – Anton (8 years) and Lars (26 years) – were referred to music therapy because Anton was not thriving in school and found it difficult to be with the other children. Anton wanted to be in charge all the time, which also made it difficult for teachers to guide and support him. Lars was a lone parent, had a full-time job, and was very busy during the week. Gradually, as Anton grew older it was getting more and more difficult for Lars to cope with the situation. The small family had moved a lot due to Lars' struggle to provide for the family financially. Lars fully acknowledged that Anton was not happy or thriving as he should. Despite acknowledging the problem it was hard for Lars to find a solution as he did not really know how to handle Anton. Both Anton and Lars had a bad temper, so their communication often ended in quarrels or conflicts where Anton would walk away in anger and frustration. But they also clearly cared for one another.

In our early assessment sessions, Lars told me that he and Anton would like to play music together and have a good time, because this was rare and difficult for them in everyday life. I suggested that they could try to explore ways to be together in the music, so they could find a new and better way to be together. Lars told me that Anton tended to focus on his own musical expression. Lars did not, however, see how his own lack of clear and engaging expression or behavior played a role in the fact that Anton did not seek his father in musical play. For Anton and Lars activities in the music therapy session consisted of well-known songs and communication exercises with an improvisational approach. They were engaged and willing to try out different things, such as free improvisations with simple headlines including, 'Today I'm mad' or 'Breakfast at our place'. There were rarely many words or reflections between father and son, but clearly a desire to experiment and express.

One day, in the midst of a chaotic and unbridled improvisation with Anton on drums, Lars piano and me on Spanish guitar, something very special happened. After a lot of noise and powerful expression, suddenly Lars and Anton found each other in a slow powerful pulse. It happened unconsciously without words, but the timing was sublime, and in that moment Lars and Anton looked at each other out of sheer surprise at their unfamiliar synchronization. This experience was a catalyst for positive change whereby father and son began to play together as a musical partnership. Through musical support and activities suggested by me, the dyad experienced how they could find each other in the music. For example, through turn-taking in improvisation, Lars and Anton practiced imitation and becoming finely aware of each other's emotional expression. In another more challenging exercise, Anton and Lars were encouraged to make a synchronous switch in the quality of their music without using words or verbal exchange. The music could go from very loud to very quiet or very fast to very slow. Again, they had to open to each other's expressions and adapt their own expression to the other. When asked about their experiences, they would explain that it was nice, that they could feel each other more, and that they felt closer to each other. This improved depth of connection also continued at home. They had started to use music at home by listening and dancing to rock music together, and sometimes Lars would also sing a little lullaby for Anton. Things started to improve in school as well. Anton had begun to develop patience and understanding in his interactions with his peers. He was now more capable of relinquishing control and letting others make decisions.

Still, however, there was no real change in everyday life regarding arguments or solving conflicts. One day Anton spontaneously exclaimed how nice it was that he and Lars never argued in music therapy. I asked them both why they thought this was the case. Lars answered that it must be because of the different setting; in music therapy there are clearly specific tasks and there is enough time to do them. Anton agreed and said, 'In here I know what to do.' I asked Anton if he sometimes doubts what to do at home. He replied, 'Sometimes.' Lars explained that he doesn't always know what to do when Anton gets angry but that he would like to get better at it. Anton explained that he also wanted things to get better. After this little talk Anton and Lars continued playing with the nonverbal music therapy activities.

In the concurrent conversations with me, Lars also wondered out loud why things were so much easier within the music therapy setting. I asked what he thought was different and he pointed to the fact that there were clear agreements and boundaries in music therapy. Then, on his own initiative, Lars suggested he would try to have more clear agreements and boundaries at home as well. After this conversation, I invited Lars and Anton to start taking turns in deciding the activities in therapy. My aim was for them to try out, and practice, how to define settings, create boundaries, and make choices on their own. They agreed to this change and between them they started to lead the sessions more. Sometimes both Lars and Anton would suggest activities that were impossible to get working, but each time they would solve and adjust with little guidance from me. Their shared progress, and the quality of the therapy environment, now meant that conflict resolution could be experimental, playful, and fun. Gradually, father and son came to suggest musical activities that would well work for both of them. Towards the end of therapy Lars talked about how he tried to have clearer agreements and boundaries at home – 'agreements that work for both of us'. Anton explained how they still sometimes had fights but that he no longer got angry and walked away.

Lise and Helle

Around the same time as working with Anton and Lars I was introduced to Lise, a four-year-old girl, and her 23-year-old mother Helle. The family had been referred to the family care center where I was employed because Lise's kindergarten was concerned and had notified children's social services. When Lise was around other children she 'acted out' and it was extremely difficult to get her to comply with the requirements of the usual kindergarten day. Helle acknowledged the problem and also acknowledged that she had a responsibility as a mother to improve her parenting skills. Helle asked for help and wanted to make things better for her child. Helle had had a difficult upbringing herself without much support from her parents. She was unemployed and had stopped going to school after 10th grade (16 years old).

In our initial assessment it became clear that Helle was extremely passive in her interaction with her daughter. She noticed everything Lise did, both good and bad, but she hardly reacted at all. When we began a little musical exploration, Helle was only minimally engaged. She hesitated often and searched for my guidance. Lise enjoyed herself but was mostly in her own world, not really expecting interaction with Helle or me. She gave her mother instructions but did not discuss anything with her. However, the assessment also showed evidence of a good emotional bond between Helle and Lise. When confronted with the results from the assessment, Helle displayed self-insight and positive motivation towards going into treatment. I showed Helle video clips from our assessment sessions. Together, we agreed that Helle would work on her clear expression as a parent: on her guidance and positive affirmation of Lise.

Our sessions involved structured exercises (with a focus on social and collaborative skills) and free improvisations (with a focus on emotional bonding within balanced dialogues). To begin with Lise and Helle chose from a series of activities – each with the aim of supporting mother and daughter to listen to each other, to take instructions on board, and to play with different relational dynamics.

The turn-taking exercise especially received a lot of attention throughout the sessions. This exercise had a very simple structure: player one starts playing, player one stops playing, player two starts playing, etc. However, for this family it was very difficult to create a dynamic dialogue with flow. Initially, when it was her turn, Lise explored the instruments with much expression and beautiful melodies and forgot the context she was in. She played for more than a minute on her two xylophones and clearly had fun doing it. She did not expect to interact or to be interrupted. When Helle played on her tambourine her rhythmical phrases were unvaried in dynamics and lacked vitality. After 19 seconds Lise interrupted Helle and started to play again, without Helle giving the turn back to Lise. They then both stopped and Helle gave the turn willingly to Lise verbally.

Throughout the sessions, I tried to model the possibility of short and dynamic turns. I was attempting to support Lise and Helle to become more acutely aware of each other – to tune into the nonverbal communication signs available within musical play including clear musical ending, rhythmical body language, and facial expression. Sometimes Lise and Helle were able to imitate me and create a flow in the dialogue, but on a bad day all collapsed and Lise withdrew into her own world. After such a session, Helle and I sat and talked. She told me how she knew she needed to change her approach with Lise at home. She explained, 'I need to make decisions and stick to them.' Her experiences within our sessions had become an embodied metaphor for Helle. She told me that she needed to 'not play the triangle' any more at home (the triangle left her feeling quite subdued and weak in musical interaction). Helle said that she had to play louder and with more purpose, 'I have to mean it.' All of this made sense to Helle, but it was difficult for her to put into practice.

So we continued to work with improvisation and collaboration exercises in our music therapy sessions and slowly Helle and Lise's interactions started to change. Lise started to seek Helle in the music, as Helle's expressions were getting clearer and had more vitality and variation. Lise started to listen to Helle, imitate her. and simply look in her direction. This progress seemed to give Helle a much-needed boost in confidence. Helle naturally started to direct her nonverbal musical expressions towards her daughter by inviting her in, playing with more vitality and keeping her daughter interested. Helle was no longer passive. She gave her daughter positive affirmation, through verbal praise and nonverbally within the music by following Lise very closely and very clearly. Near the end of the 12 sessions Lise and Helle were using spontaneous turn-taking and turn-giving in the free improvisations and there were no more mechanical monologues between them. Helle's confidence was growing at home too. Lise and Helle's relationship was now based on a much more healthy balance. Lise was getting better at following demands and expecting a dialogue with her mother. Helle was getting better at providing that dialogue and setting supportive boundaries. In kindergarten Lise was getting along much better with the other children and she was more willing to meet demands.

Discussion

When working with families, I need to be conscious and clear about the many roles I take on as music therapist. In part, this is due to the risk of forming a deeper alliance with certain family members and not others. And partly because of the risk of disempowering the family as a whole, by being considered the 'expert'. At times I will assume the role of systemic advisor, individual therapist, dyadic therapist, directive practitioner, person-centered practitioner, family support, clinical expert. The key for me is to be conscious about the role I have assumed and to be conscious that I can shift fluidly between roles in order to meet the changing needs of the family whilst continually working towards the aims for therapy. If I am not aware of my role or that I am shifting between roles, it can be quite confusing and chaotic for the family. There is no single 'best' stance, but rather a 'best fit' for each unique family and context. Reflective practice is vital, and many different approaches can have therapeutic value. The opportunities for different roles are diverse and plentiful. Music making within music therapy is especially powerful. When making music the family system can become more flexible and open to change, thereby giving the music therapist a range of possible ways to work towards the family's goals (Jacobsen and Thompson 2016).

As a music therapist, to create a relational bond with a vulnerable child in therapy is a powerful and satisfying experience. But to facilitate this process happening between child and parent – where ideally it should have happened in the first place – is a unique privilege to experience. The underlying theoretical perspective of enabling emotional connection and strengthening communicative musicality remains the same in both approaches – but the clinical approach is somewhat different. Having employed both approaches, when working with emotionally neglected children (and in most cases of vulnerable child work), I would always strongly advise including parents directly in therapy if possible. Dyadic work can empower families to reach their own potential. We have the chance to plant strong seeds that in turn can grow into beautiful trees capable of surviving even the harshest winters.

References

Abad, V. and Williams, K. (2007) 'Early music therapy: reporting on a 3-year project to address needs with at-risk families.' *Music Therapy Perspectives 25*, 52–58.

Bull, R. (2008) 'Autism and the Family: Group Music Therapy with Mothers and Children.' In A. Oldfield and C. Flower (eds) *Music Therapy with Children and their Families*. London: Jessica Kingsley Publishers.

Carpenter, L.L., Tyrka, A.R., Ross, N.S., Khoury, L., Anderson, G.M. and Price, L.H. (2009) 'Effect of childhood emotional abuse and age on cortisol responsivity in adulthood.' *Biological Psychiatry 66*, 69–75.

Davies, E. (2008) 'It's a Family Affair: Music Therapy for Children and their Families at a Psychiatric Unit.' In A. Oldfield and C. Flower (eds) *Music Therapy with Children and Their Families*. London: Jessica Kingsley Publishers.

Drake, T. (2008) 'Back to Basics: Community-based Music Therapy for Vulnerable Young Children and Their Parents.' In A. Oldfield and C. Flower (eds) *Music Therapy with Children and Their Families*. London: Jessica Kingsley Publishers.

Elzinga, B.M., Molendijk, M.L., Oude Voshaar, R.C., Bus, B.A., *et al.* (2011) 'The impact of childhood abuse and recent stess on serum brain-derived neurotrophic factor and the moderating role of BDNF Val66Met.' *Psychopharmacology 214*, 319–328.

Ford, J.D., Grasso, D., Greene, C., Levine, J., Spinazzola, J. and van der Kolk, B. (2013) 'Clinical significance of a proposed developmental trauma disorder diagnosis: results of an international survey of clinicians.' *The Journal of Clinical Psychiatry 74*, 8, 841–849.

Gold, C., Voracek, M. and Wigram, T. (2004) 'Effects of music therapy for children and adolescents with psychopathology: a meta-analysis.' *Journal of Child Psychology and Psychiatry 45*, 1054–1063.

Hasler, J. (2008) 'A Piece of the Puzzle: Music Therapy with Looked-after Teenagers and Their Carers.' In A. Oldfield and C. Flower (eds) *Music Therapy with Children and Their Families*. London: Jessica Kingsley Publishers.

Hildyard, K. and Wolfe, D. (2002) 'Child neglect: developmental issues and outcomes.' *Child Abuse & Neglect 26*, 679–695.

Holck, U. (2011) 'Det tidlige samspil og musikterapi.' [Early interplay and music therapy] *Livsbladet 05*, 11–15.

Horvat, J. and O'Neill, N. (2008) 'Who Is the Therapy for? Involving a Parent or Carer in Their Child's Music Therapy.' In A. Oldfield and C. Flower (eds) *Music Therapy with Children and Their Families*. London: Jessica Kingsley Publishers.

Howden, S. (2008) 'Music Therapy with Traumatized Children and Their Families in Mainstream Primary Schools.' In A. Oldfield and C. Flower (eds) *Music Therapy with Children and Their Families*. London: Jessica Kingsley Publishers.

Hughes, D. (2000) *Facilitating Developmental Attachment: The Road to Emotional Recovery and Behavioural Change in Foster and Adopted Children*. Lanham, MD: Rowman & Littlefield Publishers.

Hussey, D. and Layman, D. (2003) 'Music therapy with emotionally disturbed children.' *Psychiatric Times 20*, 6, 86–99.

Hussey, D., Reed, A., Layman, D. and Pasiali, V. (2007) 'Music therapy and complex trauma: a protocol for developing social reciprocity.' *Residential Treatment for Children and Youth 24*, 1, 111–129.

Irgens-Møller, I. and Bjerg, M. (2004) 'Positiv relationserfaring for børn i musikterapi.' [Positive experience of relation for children in music therapy] *Dansk Musikterapi 1*, 2, 4–14.

Jacobsen, S.L. (2016) 'Child Protection: Music Therapy with Families and Emotionally Neglected Children.' In S.L. Jacobsen and G. Thompson (eds) *Music Therapy with Families: Clinical Approaches and Theoretical Perspectives*. London: Jessica Kingsley Publishers.

Jacobsen, S.L. and Killén, K. (2015) 'Clinical application of music therapy assessment within the field of child protection.' *Nordic Journal of Music Therapy 24*, 2, 148–166.

Jacobsen, S.L. and McKinney, C. (2015) 'A music therapy tool for assessing parent–child interaction in cases of emotional neglect.' *Journal of Child and Family Studies 24*, 7, 2164–2173.

Jacobsen, S.L. and Thompson, G. (2016) 'Working with Families: Emerging Characteristics.' In S.L. Jacobsen and G. Thompson (eds) *Music Therapy with Families: Clinical Approaches and Theoretical Perspectives*. London: Jessica Kingsley Publishers.

Jacobsen, S.L., McKinney, C.H. and Holck, U. (2014) 'Effects of a dyadic music therapy intervention on parent–child interaction, parent stress, and parent–child relationship in families with emotionally neglected children: a randomized controlled trial.' *Journal of Music Therapy 51*, 4, 310–332.

Johns, U.T. (2012) Vitalitetsformer i Musikk [Vitality Forms in Music]. Skriftserie fra Senter for musikk og helse. NMH-publikasjoner 2012: 3. Oslo: Norges musikkhøgskole.

Killén, K. (2005) 'Omsorgssvigt er alles ansvar.' [Neglect and abuse are everybody's responsibilty] Kbh, DK: Hans Reitzel Forlag.

Killén, K. (2012) 'Barndommen varer i generationer. Forebyggelse af omsorgssvigt.' [Childhood goes on for generations. Presention of neglect and abuse] Copenhagen: Hans Reitzels Forlag.

Knapp, M. and Hall J. (2009) *Nonverbal Communication in Human Interaction*. (International edn) Boston, MA: Wadsworth Cengage Learning.

Kolind, I. (2008) 'Improviseret sang. En kvalitativ empirisk "single-case" analyse af fænomenet improviseret sang med fokus på terapeutiske kvaliteter og intrapsykiske processer – i musikterapi med et omsorgssvigtet barn.' [Improvised song focusing on therapeutic qualities and intrapsychic processes in music therapy with an emotionally neglected child. Unpublished Master's Thesis, Aalborg University, Denmark.

Malloch, S. and Trevarthen, C. (2009) *Communicative Musicality: Exploring the Basis of Human Companionship*. Oxford: Oxford University Press.

Mandal, M.K. and Ambady, N. (2004) 'Laterality of facial expressions of emotion: universal and culture-specific influences.' *Behavioural Neurology 15*, 1–2, 23–34.

Molyneux, C. (2008) 'Music Therapy as Part of a Multidisciplinary Family Assessment Process.' In K. Twyford and T. Watson (eds) *Integrated Team Working*. London: Jessica Kingsley Publishers.

Oldfield, A. (2006a) *Interactive Music Therapy in Child and Family Psychiatry*. London: Jessica Kingsley Publishers.

Oldfield, A. (2006b) *Interactive Music Therapy: A Positive Approach*. London: Jessica Kingsley Publishers.

Oldfield, A. and Flower C. (2008) *Music Therapy with Children and Their Families*. London: Jessica Kingsley Publishers.

Porter, S., Holmes, V., McLaughlin, K., Lynn, F. *et al.* (2012) 'Music in mind, a randomized controlled trial of music therapy for young people with behavioural and emotional problems: study protocol.' *Journal of Advanced Nursing 68*, 2349–2358.

Robarts, J. (2014) 'Music Therapy with Children with Developmental Trauma Disorder.' In C.A. Malchiodi and D.A. Crenshaw (eds) *Creative Arts and Play Therapy for Attachment Problems*. New York: Guilford Press.

Salkeld, C. (2008) 'Music Therapy After Adoption.' In A. Oldfield and C. Flower (eds) *Music Therapy with Children and Their Families*. London: Jessica Kingsley Publishers.

Schore, J. and Schore, A. (2008) 'Modern attachment theory: the central role of affect regulation in development and treatment.' *Clinical Social Work Journal 36*, 9, 9–20.

Stern, D. (2000) *The Interpersonal World of the Infant*. New York: Basic Books.

Stern, D. (2010) 'The issue of vitality.' *Nordic Journal of Music Therapy 19*, 2, 88–102.

Trevarthen, C. and Malloch, S. (2000) 'The dance of wellbeing: defining the musical therapeutic effect.' *Nordic Journal of Music Therapy 9*, 2, 3–17.

Trondalen, G. (1997) 'Music therapy and interplay: a music therapy project with mothers and children elucidated through the concept of "appreciative recognition".' *Nordic Journal of Music Therapy 6*, 1, 14–27.

Trondalen, G. and Skårderud, F. (2007) 'Playing with affects…and the importance of "affect attunement".' *Nordic Journal of Music Therapy 16*, 2, 100–111.

Young, R., Lennie, S. and Minnis, H. (2011) 'Children's perception of parental emotional neglect and control and psychopathology.' *Journal of Child Psychology and Psychiatry 52*, 889–897.

15

NOISE, TIME AND LISTENING

Enabling Children to Express Themselves through Music

HUGH NANKIVELL AND SARAH BUTLER

This collaboration is between two curious adults, one an experienced Early Years Foundation Stage leader and the other a professional musician/composer. Our chapter describes a method we have developed together over the last eight years sharing and learning from our experiences observing, listening, playing and discussing the explorations of three- to five-year-old children.

Initially, we write about the way we structure our early years sessions. These sessions can be divided up into four distinct (but overlapping) sections: Provocation, Exploration, Sharing and Analysis. They involve what we define as a combination of 'roundabout' and 'traffic light' activities. We then present case studies of children who have each followed their own individual musical journey. We describe how these children respond to a range of provocations and then detail how we react to the children's explorations and journeys. We conclude by discussing the roles that we, as adults, play in allowing children to express themselves through music. We question to what degree adults value the importance of listening, allowing time and the acceptance of noise and how much this impacts upon musical play, creativity and development of learning in the classroom.

Provocation

What is a provocation? In this context it is a deliberate and thoughtful decision made and presented by an adult at the start of a session and is designed to extend the ideas of the children. The provocation can be very short (e.g. showing an instrument or singing a song) or can be slightly longer (e.g. telling a story with music or showing a film). The length of a provocation will depend on how the group responds to it. The provocation and the exploration usually merge one into the other without clear demarcation.

We use the term 'traffic light' to describe the process we use within the initial stages of the provocation. If you analyse traffic movement at traffic lights from above, it is easy to get a grasp on the flow, speed and direction of traffic – you can say that north–south is moving (green light) while east–west is stationary (red light). For us, 'traffic light' indicates that an external observer can see and hear what is going on in the whole group and immediately get a grasp of who is leading, who is following and what material is being looked at (see Figure 15.1).

What is the adult's role in provocation? When we begin a session we might have an idea as to where it might lead, but the key is that we are completely open to following what emerges.

Exploration

Provocation moves smoothly into exploration. This is the time when children lead and are playing, exploring and experimenting with ideas that emerge (or not) from the provocation. This is usually the longest period of time in the session. It can quite easily feel as if we are not doing anything at all.

What is the adult's role in exploration? We have learned to resist the urge to lead in the exploration. It is our role to follow the children's individual journeys, to listen to them, understand their thinking and to support the learning that is emerging.

The exploration time is a 'roundabout' session. By this we mean that an external observer might find it difficult to immediately comprehend what is going on, because there will be a multitude of activities all simultaneously happening independently in the same room. It may well be noisy and initially appear chaotic to the outsider, because everyone is learning at their own speed. We call this roundabout learning because of the way that, when you analyse road roundabouts from above, it is difficult to explain exactly what is going on at any one moment. Drivers are making their own decisions as to when to stop and when to go depending on the movement of other vehicles. The dynamic of roundabouts is a fluid and constantly evolving process.

The end of exploration involves an immediate reflection on what has taken place and we quickly make decisions on the learning we want to present in the sharing.

Sharing

Sharing involves presenting material that has emerged and offering it to the group. This might mean asking a young person or group to perform something they have been making. It might be that we show a film or play an audio recording of them playing/creating. It might be that we sing or play a version of it ourselves. Or we might teach something that has been created by an individual or small group to the whole class group. In this way an idea, an invention, a creation is validated and amplified for everyone to see. This is again back to 'traffic light' time, where one person – the adult – is making the decisions and is holding and controlling the session.

Analysis

All the way through the provocation/exploration/sharing journey we analyse children's learning. However, we need a separate time to engage in a detailed reflection (a thoughtful analysis) on what has occurred during each session. With each other, and sometimes other adults, we look back at footage (audio, visual, notes written) and compare notes. This analytical process builds up a rapport, a trust and a collaboration and this leads to the next stage of the process. In this way, we often get the opportunity to see learning from different perspectives. The openness within this sharing allows us to then create the next provocation, and so the whole system is cyclical.

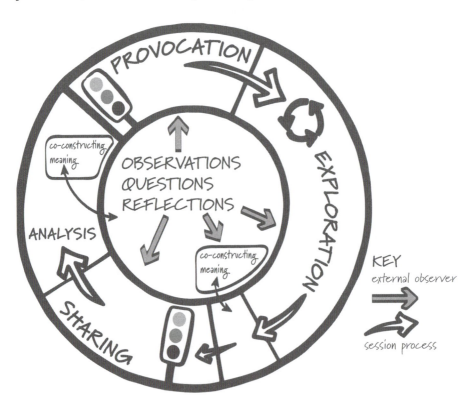

FIGURE 15.1 THE CYCLE OF PROVOCATION/EXPLORATION/SHARING/ANALYSIS

Case studies

We have written nine short stories of individual children who we have worked and played with in three different Early Years settings. The children are all four or five years old. The stories vary in length and detail, but we have structured them all in a similar way in order to demonstrate:

- the importance of the early years music session structure

- the relationships that can develop between adults and children

- the importance, in many different ways, of allowing noise, time and listening to impact upon those relationships and the individual learning journey.

We have simplified the process we followed in the case studies so that the sequence of events can be easily understood. However, we are aware of many other elements and considerations in the complex four-point cyclical process that we have not described; these include collaborative partnership, flexibility using professional knowledge, understanding of child development, psychology, musical composition, arrangement and conducting, and the interest in continual reflection.

Ethan

Ethan at age four was very interested in taking things apart and putting them back together again as his way of exploring and understanding the world.

Each week, whenever Hugh brought an instrument into the classroom, Ethan closely observed how he set up and prepared the instruments for the provocation. For instance, Ethan noted how Hugh tuned the guitars and ukuleles, and he also noticed how the glockenspiels and xylophones were set up. (Most weeks Hugh had to put all the notes on, as they were usually all off when the xylophones were collected from the cupboard.) Ethan often seemed less interested in the adult-led provocation itself (e.g. a song, a form of notation, a film, a recording) but was always interested in the mechanics of the actual instruments.

Once the provocation was over (or sometimes as it merged into the exploration) Ethan set to work with the guitars and ukuleles to take the strings off and look inside the sound hole and investigate the winding mechanism of the guitar. With the xylophone and glockenspiel he took off all the notes and tried to fit them all into the frame/box along with whatever else he could fit into it. One session he spent the entire time filling the box with unit blocks. It seemed clear that Ethan was not going to make any 'music' until he had explored and investigated the object that makes the sound. One week Ethan explored all the things that he could play with the cello bow including the guitar and his shoes.

For several days Ethan was really interested in using a toy stethoscope from the doctor's kit. On one occasion he explored playing the drum with a stick, while wearing the stethoscope and holding the end of it on the drum skin. Each time he was shocked by the sound but continued to experiment. He put the end underneath the drum and was experimenting with sound in a similar way to a recording engineer when setting up the microphones for a recording.

It seemed that Ethan really needed time to explore and discover sound for himself and, as adults in this context, we needed to give him that time. In the 18 months we worked with him, he never seemed especially interested in conventional music-making within the group, but was fascinated by how the instrumental machines worked and the mechanics of sound. It felt very important to us that we should give him that time and that space to explore his creativity.

We continually asked ourselves, what is Ethan trying to tell us and are we really listening? Ethan challenged our thinking because he did not fit the stereotype of a musical child, and indeed he may never be conventionally musical. But it is our role to support whatever musical results come from the provocations. If we demonstrated and discussed with Ethan the technical aspects of musical instruments, he became interested and engaged. Who knows where this may lead?

Megan

Megan, aged four, was a quiet member of her class. She had a visual impairment and kept her coat on much of the time. She enjoyed the songs and the different instruments that were brought in to the class but had not shown any particular musical engagement in the first term of Hugh's work at the school.

One week in the second term, Hugh brought in a couple of old violins from the school cupboard and found a half-size cello. He took these instruments in for the group to use as the provocation that week, alongside a new visitor who brought with him, and played, the double bass.

Megan immediately wanted one of the violins, and thereafter tried to keep a hold of it for much of the session. She became upset whenever it was parted from her. With the violin, Megan's music-making blossomed. She played the violin all the time (in a very scratchy way, that was quite 'noisy' for some, especially the other adults in the room). This was the starting point for Megan's proactive involvement in the music-making. The violin was her trigger. After observing the way that the music leaders sometimes wrote down music and then placed it on the music stand, Megan started to explore music by composing long notated solo violin pieces (see Figure 15.2). Her comfort and confidence in these bold, and supremely confidently played, nascent improvised violin sonatas were always a joy to observe.

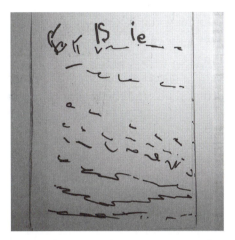

FIGURE 15.2 PAGE 1 OF MEGAN'S 24-PAGE 'VIOLIN SONG BOOK'

We encouraged Megan by praising her creative explorations on the violin. Her experimentation later extended to more original playing on other instruments including the keyboard (where she discovered how to play it using her hands, arms and legs). She continued to play the violin each week and was given one by her parents for her birthday at the end of the term.

Jason

Jason, aged four and at the start of his schooling, was obsessed by dinosaurs and other animals. He was a child who clearly enjoyed using language to express thought and he initially seemed captivated by music as a mode of expression to validate his knowledge and love of dinosaurs. He made up many pieces of music, using instruments, words and drawings. He would continually talk and create stories as he explored the new instruments. Hugh's initial provocation of a dinosaur dance song resonated with Jason and he instantly connected with Hugh and musical exploration.

One week Jason had composed a song about an owl. The following week Hugh suggested that he sing it again and that we record it and had brought in the computer and a microphone. On this second week there was a recorder in the classroom, brought in by another child in the class. Jason wanted to play the recorder. During the exploration time, Jason taught Hugh the Owl song. Jason then told Hugh to sing it and also play the ukulele while Jason played the recorder and conducted them both.

Then together, they played the song for quite a long time as a duet. While this was being sung some children entered the room and began moving to the music. When the music stopped Jason observed some of the children still moving. So he then clearly explained that we would play a game (like musical statues) and he, as performing conductor, would stop and watch which of the dancers did not stop with the music. He led this game for quite a while, and again later in the sharing.

Jason continued this musical enthusiasm as he explored song-writing, arranging and conducting skills, and used music as a means of directing both adults and peers.

Lewis

Lewis was a four-year-old who enjoyed ordered and quiet activities. He was sensitive to noise and his class teacher understood this and responded to his needs. He enjoyed organized sound evidenced prior to Hugh's arrival with the class, through singing existing songs and nursery rhymes with the whole class.

The first session with Lewis's class involved getting out a box of instruments and allowing all the children to choose one and play with it. After a while they exchanged instruments and continued their, mainly loud, explorations.

Initially Lewis could not cope with the apparent chaos of this dramatic increase in noise. He expressed this disquiet with screaming and tears and becoming red-faced and upset.[1] We gently supported Lewis in his distress by reassuring him that it was OK, and making sure that another adult spent time with him in one-to-one support to build his confidence. We had regular discussions with the class teacher about this sensitivity. Gradually, as he became more familiar with the routine, things did change for Lewis, and the tears and disquiet reduced until, by the end of the third week, they completely vanished. The group adjusted and the loud volume generally decreased. At the same time Lewis began to engage with sound on his own and in partnerships with others. In his own time, Lewis had found his confidence and remained an integral, creative and enthusiastic member of the group. This adjustment process is not about being child led, but is instead about responding to the child's needs.

One week, in the second term of working with Lewis's class, Hugh sang the song 'London's Burning' to the group as a provocation. The group later began writing their own songs and Lewis came up with a new song, 'Scotland's

---

1   On rare occasions, some children with specific needs resulting in specific hypersensitivities (for instance, autism or significant developmental trauma) may find the collective musical environment too much to cope with. In these rare instances, the child's needs will lead the way to a solution – possibly with the child leaving the group for an alternative activity. But this was not the case with Lewis, and is not the case for most children who show some initial discomfort.

Burning'. We encouraged this, and in the sharing we all sang it together. The following week many other 'burning' songs emerged including 'Paignton's Burning' and 'Paignton Zoo's Burning'.

Lewis had transformed from someone fearful of loud noises, with no apparent experience of being a creative musician, to becoming an enthusiastic music leader within the group, coming up with songs, melodies, lyrics, notation, structural ideas and much more.

Alex

Four-year-old Alex had gained great confidence during nursery and upon starting reception began to show his outgoing personality to his familiar peers. During his time in nursery Alex would create stages out of hollow blocks and listen to different CDs he could self-select. He also loved to explore instruments and had an assured sense of rhythm.

For the first week of term, Hugh had composed a song about the brand new school building that Alex's school had moved into. Hugh sang it to the group at the start of the session and the group joined in with singing, body percussion and then instruments.

Alex had a drum and played it for the ten minutes or so while we sang the song. As we repeated the song, and added extra verses, Alex then began to improvise. It was immediately clear that he:

- was really steady

- could play cadences (he realized the end was coming up and played with the ending)

- was very sensitive – never too loud, shifted tempo with us, and was a real accompanist

- was happy to play a supportive role and did not want to stop playing.

Later that afternoon we sang this song for the school music coordinator, performing whispered and loud verses. Alex accompanied sensitively. One of the class teachers explained how she had also observed Alex's sensitive musical accompanying.

Alex always wanted to play in any group, and loved being part of a band. He formed his own band which he named 'We Go Rockin' with his class friends Cathy and Hugh. He is a musical glue that is needed in these kind of situations. Most bands need a steady rhythm player and Alex seems to know this and fits that role perfectly.

A few weeks later, Hugh brought a large chromatic xylophone (containing both black and white notes) to Alex's school. Hugh brought it in as it was an ideal accompanying instrument for a song begun the week earlier about rain.

Alex was clearly interested in playing the xylophone and, along with some other children, improvised on it confidently both solo and in duets and trios. Later in the afternoon, after asking them if they were interested, we took Alex and Cathy to a quiet space to record them. They each played a short xylophone solo while we all listened. We recorded them and they listened back on headphones. Sarah then suggested that they play a duet together. They agreed and sat side by side behind the xylophone and started to play (see Figure 15.3). Generally Alex was leading, but they both had moments of copying each other and trying different techniques (sliding up and down – glissandi, crossing over hands with sticks, etc.). They seemed to be fully focused on their playing; both faces were full of concentration and occasional smiles. The music was flowing and went on for 14 minutes. Time restriction came into effect and unfortunately we had to stop the children playing. The week after Alex played his long duet with Cathy, he wrote a song (his first) with Hugh.

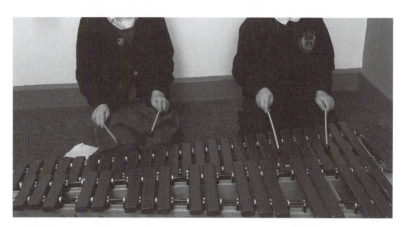

FIGURE 15.3 ALEX AND CATHY PLAYING THEIR LONG XYLOPHONE DUET

We believe that it is important to listen to a child and then give them time and support to allow them to explore their musicality both alone and in a group. Considering the Alex and Cathy duet, we asked ourselves: if we hadn't been time restricted, how long would they both have continued playing? Who would have stopped first? Would we have seen anything else from each child? Where else might we see this musical confidence flourish?

Cathy

Cathy, aged four, was silent and often very cautious of new visitors into the nursery setting. She didn't speak and would stay next to familiar adults.

On first meeting Hugh, Cathy sat at the edge of the group next to a familiar adult, without engaging in the use of instruments or vocal sound. However, to our delight, the music and exploration of sound appeared to totally captivate Cathy and when asked if she would like to join in she nodded and sat within the group allowing the familiar adult to move away.

Cathy demonstrated she had the ability to hear the beat and keep in time with the music and seemed to really enjoy playing music in different groups of people (both with adults and children). She played and smiled a lot, but still spoke very little.

Halfway through the second term, Hugh taped out a large white sheet of paper on the floor (approximately 2 metres by 3 metres) and put out instruments and pens together at the start of the session.

Cathy first began to talk to Hugh on this occasion when she began drawing around the bottom of her drum, making many circles on the paper. Hugh began to write in the letters 'D r u m' every time Cathy drew a new circle (see Figure 15.4). After a short break from this interaction, when Hugh returned a few minutes later, Cathy was also writing the letters 'D r u m' inside the circles. Hugh began counting the circles, Cathy joined in (she drew over 30 drums that afternoon) and they were soon counting together.

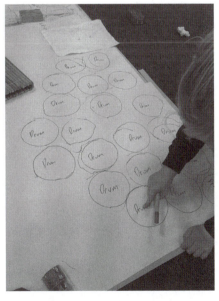

FIGURE 15.4 CATHY DRAWING AND COUNTING THE DRUMS

The following week Cathy played her extended xylophone duet (see Alexander's story above) and the week after that wrote an extended Christmas song with Hugh:

> *Father Christmas on the sleigh*
> *Coming to my front room*
> *Then he got stuck in the chimney*
> *The children pushed him out*
> *Then he put the presents down near the Christmas tree.*
> *Father Christmas on the sleigh*
> *Then he got stuck near the door*
> *'Cause the door was locked*
> *Then I opened the door*
> *Then he put the presents down near the Christmas tree.*
> *Father Christmas on the sleigh*
> *Then he got stuck on the roof*
> *He climbed up the ladder and the ladder fell down*
> *People rescued him*
> *Then he put the presents down near the Christmas tree.*

We know children need to be allowed the opportunity to exchange ideas and explore experiences that make them feel happier to voice their thinking to others, so they truly have a chance to be heard. Cathy's journey through our project has allowed her to demonstrate her views and reflections on her experiences. Cathy's confidence developed not only in her own musical skill but also in her ability to talk to others and express her thinking through words and music.

Emily

Emily was a four-year-old girl who spent a lot of her time in nursery, and at the start of reception engaged with adults in discussions. She loved to create her own imaginary storybooks using pictures and words. When Hugh first met her she confidently sang all the time and made up her own songs.

One week Hugh brought a music stand in as part of the provocation. It was unpacked, put up, some sheet music placed onto it and then Hugh performed this music to the group. This provocation had an immediate impact on the group. The children seemed to understand that the music stand had a power (whoever has the music stand controls the stage) and also that the act of creating some form of notated music was one way forward.

In the exploration session that day, many children began creating songs and pieces by writing, drawing and scribbling music down and then placing that music on the music stand and playing it. Emily was a leader in this respect and moved quickly (over a few weeks) from scribbled wavy lines to written-out lyrics for songs and then on to words for singing and drawings of instruments that are needed to accompany those words. In this way, Emily increased her songwriting capacity and developed a relatively sophisticated notational system for her songs. Her creative ingenuity influenced others in the group.

One week during the exploration time, Emily composed a song called, 'Bobl Is My Friend'. She wrote the words out for the song and then sang it to us. It was clear that it was a fixed composition with a defined melody line and structure to the lyrics (three lines, each one repeated).

> *Bobl is my friend*
> *Bobl is my friend*
> *This is Bobl's song*
> *This is Bobl's song*
> *La la la la la*
> *La la la la la*

There is a quality about this repeated lyrical structure that revealed something about Emily's status and thinking process. Within the classroom there had been some battles about friendships as the four-year-olds struggled to assert themselves and work out their position in the social fabric of the group. Emily did not have many clear friends, but what she did have was music. This song explains that position and tells us that she does have a friend and it is Bobl, and that her friend has a song, that she sings, and this is how it goes 'la la la la la'. This is an unusually confident song.

Hugh recorded Emily singing the song in the (noisy) classroom on the video camera and then asked Sarah if we could take Emily outside the classroom in order to record her in the quiet of the corridor. Hugh had his laptop with a multi-track recording programme already set up on it and recorded Emily on 'track one' singing her Bobl song. She sang it and we then played it back to her on headphones. While she was listening back she began to sing again. So we recorded her on track 2, while she was listening to track one. Emily started exploring and developing and changing the music. She then added a third and fourth and fifth layer on top of her own voice. She sang higher and in a squeaky voice, she extended the song and harmonized with her own voice. Eventually we explained, reluctantly, that we could do only one more overdub recording (track 6). What happened this time was that Emily continued long after the other five tracks had finished. She knew this was the last track to be added and so wanted to make the most of it. She transposed her voice, repeated and extended sections and went on for about a minute longer than the other tracks. She finished with a cadence and then, just to emphasize the point, sang the words 'It's finished.'

This extended vocal arrangement of her song is an extraordinary piece of music. We have played the recording to many adults and most have been astonished at her confidence, her facility and her adventurousness. This 15-minute session that we had with Emily in the corridor then led onto a whole range of unexpected outcomes for Emily, for us, and for the whole class.

Hugh gave the six-track recording to a musician colleague who made two remixes of her voice using beats and other instruments. The following week we played one of these to the group as the provocation. Some of the children started dancing around enjoying the beats and having fun, laughing and enjoying themselves. This was great for Emily's status in the class.

Hugh took the Bobl song off on a journey, determined to share it with as many other people as possible and to see what they thought of the song. Hugh was interested to provoke groups through hearing this song and so to value the output of a four-year-old girl on the same playing field as an adult's compositional attempts.

The legacy of the Bobl song is that:

- Emily's subsequent songs became more complex and developed

- Emily now (aged eight) still composes songs

- there were many other performances of the Bobl song including with 60 adults at the Colston Hall in Bristol; by a group of gifted and talented teenagers at a music residential; and a public performance with over one hundred performers at Dartington Arts Centre

- the rest of the class began writing far more songs

- a simple song (three lines, four notes) written by a four-year-old can be relevant outside of her immediate peer group.

Louisa

Louisa was a confident and articulate five-year-old girl who had always spent a lot of time engaged in long narrative interactions with adults and her peers. Prior to meeting Hugh she would love to create stages, dramas and act out songs from her favourite pop band One Direction.

At the start of the second week Hugh sang two songs to the group. (Louisa had not been present at the first session.) He sang them his introductory 'Hello' welcome song which he had sung the previous week, and he also sang an improvised song about the day, the weather and travelling to school. This was inspired by an interest in narrative songs we observed from the previous week.

As the exploration time began, Louisa immediately began singing and creating. She sang to Hugh a long 'Camping Trip' song (two minutes in total). She clearly had an idea about the structure and began by accompanying herself on the ukulele. Halfway through she put down the ukulele and picked up the guiro at a significant moment, when she sang words about time passing. She then proceeded to go back to the ukulele for the ending of the piece.

The idea that you might use different instruments to orchestrate different moments in a story was beautifully demonstrated here.

In the third session, Louisa had a ukulele and some shakers and when asked how she could play them together she answered, 'I play them at different times.' In her new song Louisa said that the ukulele could be for 'please' and the shakers for 'thank you'. This awareness and need to use different sounds for different words is another clear understanding of orchestration denoting differences.

In the fourth session there were two examples of further clear and strong connections that Louisa has with different sounds. After she had sung her song, 'Cakes and Magnifying Glasses for Friends', Hugh asked her, 'Why did you use the sticks?' Louisa's answer was, 'Because I needed the stick sound!' Later, Hugh had this little conversation with her about the story she had been telling.

Hugh: If you could play an instrument [in this story] what would you play?

Louisa: I would play the fish-shaped tambourine.

Hugh: Why?

Louisa: Because it sounds like fairies.

Later in the same session, Louisa sang/told a story involving many ideas and props (police cars, fairies, dinosaurs, trains and more). Hugh spoke to her when she had finished her multi-faceted story:

Hugh: What is the difference between speaking and singing in a story?

Louisa: It makes a difference to my voice, 'cause your voice might not be the same as their voice.

Hugh: What do you mean?

Louisa: 'Cause their voices have a different tone.

Then she demonstrated the difference between a fairy voice and a policeman voice and explained that 'they change their voice in capital letters'.

We were really struck by Louisa's use of the word 'tone' and later found it had been used that morning by her class teacher when describing different voices in a story. The teacher had also explained that capital letters or large coloured letters or different fonts in a story can be used to denote different effects. Louisa is able to hear something, grasp what it means and then usefully incorporate it into her own life almost immediately. Listening to Louisa's immediate responses, with regard to what the music and story needs in terms of accompaniment and instrumental support, feels really important.

In six sessions during the summer term we observed Louisa composing/improvising at least 11 named songs/pieces. These were:

'A Place To Go In The Summer'

'Camping Trip'

'Loud Soft Loud Soft'

'The Magic Word'

'I Had A Shower Before I Went Downstairs'

'Fire Alarm'

'Gems For Friends'

'Cave Gems From The Mine'

'Cakes and Magnifying Glasses For Friends'

'Sports Day'

'Clapping and Stamping'

As a songwriter and composer Hugh was very interested to listen to all of Louisa's songs. He paid attention to them and observed what Louisa was doing with her song writing, to try and place it and reference it. Louisa demonstrated that she was a wonderfully developed composer and has a clear understanding of:

- orchestration
- cadence in music
- the difference in impact between speaking and singing in a story
- the idea of scoring/notating a song for herself and others.

By the last week of the term, Louisa had created a score of a piece for Hugh to perform ('Clapping and Stamping') without her involvement, just like a composition commission (see Figure 15.5).

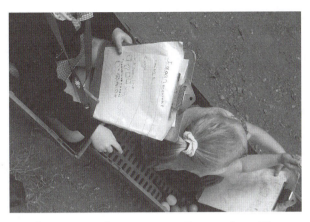

FIGURE 15.5 LOUISA'S SCORE FOR 'CLAPPING AND DANCING' FOR HUGH TO PLAY

Isabella

Isabella started nursery at age four with a strong love of language and an understanding of how to use words to create narratives and use descriptive recall. She would often be found in the role-play area constructing stories or songs on a block stage prior to Hugh's arrival at the school.

Hugh seemed to inspire Isabella immediately. On Hugh's first day at her school, as the children arrived for the afternoon, Isabella found him singing along with his guitar and immediately engaged. In that first session, Hugh sang a brand new song and encouraged the creation of new songs from the group.

Within the exploration time of that first session, we observed Isabella in a wonderful stand-off, a kind of simultaneous battle of the bands, two duets squaring up to each other and playing at the same time. Isabella and another girl were singing an original song written by Isabella. They also had a music stand on the floor with the 'music' by Isabella on it. The opposite pair were singing a nursery rhyme. The two duets squared off at each other singing and playing loudly. At one point they stopped and a boy from the other duet moved towards Isabella:

Boy: Do you want to play 'Baa Baa Black Sheep'?

Isabella: (Said nothing and shook her head)

Boy: What do you want to sing?

Isabella: Our song

Boy: (Seems perplexed and asks her again)

Isabella: (Says nothing, but holds her ground and then starts singing again and the boy walks off to find someone else)

This little encounter says a lot about Isabella and her confidence in her own creative expression and her willingness to try new things. Isabella's confidence in her thinking was also demonstrated through 'The Listening Game', a game she initiated a few weeks later with the following rules:

The Listening Game
Someone plays music,
Everyone else is in another place,
And then we listened,
And if we have heard it,
We come running out.

Isabella completely engaged when creating melodies, songs, musical games and playing instruments. She moved with the music, she motivated others and she worked in collaboration. She truly 'played' music. During term one, at the end of our music sessions when we shared some of our music for peers and parents, she always wanted to perform and was clearly leading and enjoying that role.

We notated her conversations, wrote out her songs and game rules and shared these with each other, other staff, Isabella's parents and the children. In this way we were building up a picture of Isabella's modes of thinking and supporting her by demonstrating our detailed listening and interest in her creativity.

In term two, week three, Isabella worked with a small group from her class. Together they went on a musical tour of their new school. This was a provocation to see how they would respond to different parts of their new building through song. Isabella redirected the tour so she could incorporate a spontaneous concert, inviting the adults she passed to be part of the audience. This tour, along with three instant concerts lasted the entire afternoon. The provocations for the next two weeks were a direct response to Isabella's engagement with the organization, design and planning surrounding the music that happens in a concert.

Isabella would often use whatever materials were near her to create the props for her shows, including parachutes, stones, hollow blocks and more. During one extended session, the week after the school tour, Isabella was clear she wanted to create a show for other people. Autumnal leaves and flowers were placed with care along a wooden bench and sticks were pulled out of hedges with the support of a peer to create the edge of her stage.

Isabella had a clear plan regarding the development of her concerts, (this was everything surrounding the music – the stage design, the poster, a proposed concert tour of local houses, etc.) but did not yet have the ability to express her musical thinking. Every time she was asked if she was ready to create her song or music she would redirect the comment as she found more items to decorate and adorn her theatre. She would echo and add to Hugh's songs but she was clearly not ready to share her musical ideas in this situation. We needed to be open, patient, curious and wait.

The direction a child takes needs to be followed with care and consideration or their thinking and ideas can easily be lost, redirected or misinterpreted. Isabella spent the first term of the music project creating and making up songs to express her feelings, interests and friendships. However, in the second term of the music project this line of thinking changed completely. By close observation and engagement with Isabella over a period of time we were able to see how she explored music through a completely new approach. Isabella sees music as a whole, containing the process and all the potential products. Her way of relating these elements was complicated by *our expectation* that there would be music composed and rehearsed prior to a performance.

We questioned, and continue to question, what was Isabella trying to tell us? Are we just following our own previous pattern of thinking when considering what is needed in a show. For Hugh it seemed obvious that for a show you need some music first of all, but for Isabella this is not evident. Isabella's journey has gone from making a lot of music, to becoming obsessed with the mechanics of putting on a show and exercising control. It has been a learning journey for us to see how our provocations can lead in many directions other than those we might be expecting.

How adults' responses allow children to express themselves through music

Throughout the time we have spent together on these creative music projects several things have emerged that have helped us to understand the dynamics of a session and how we can best support the children. We need to allow there to be noise, we need to listen closely to each child, we need to allow time to build relationships, and we need time to share and explore our different responses as an Early Years leader and musician.

Noise

What is noise? 'Unwanted sound' is quite a common definition. So 'music' for one person is 'noise' for someone else. In fact, this perceptual dichotomy is quite common. Think about a train carriage full of seeping headphone beats when you are trying to concentrate.

In many classroom musical explorations there is a lot of sound, and for some in the room this is going to be 'noise'. Children are talking, singing, shouting, playing instruments, interacting with each other in different groupings all at the same time. When adults provide musical instruments for children to play, there needs to be a concomitant acceptance that they are going to need to fully explore their instruments. They are going to find ways to play them, and this will require all kinds of investigations, including loud playing.

Often the first period of play with instruments does not entail much listening to each other. But here we observe individuals exploring sounds and objects. We believe that this 'noisy' situation is important because it is only through experiencing loud volumes and overlapping sounds that children are able to:

- rationalize what it is that they feel about those sounds, volumes and the instruments which help them to create them

- work out how to adjust their sound

- learn how to share the space as a group.

During a 'noisy' exploration we notice how the children work in their own selected space individually, in pairs or in small groups. The children find ways in which they can refine their own hearing by focusing their attention on their own explorations. It is often the adult or the child who is not fully engaged who finds the noise overwhelming.

The overall volume usually does settle down as the children gradually begin to self-regulate. But, in addition, we have also learned that if we fully focus our attention on one person or activity then we seem to ignore (or are better able to cope with) the surrounding noise.

Time

We have to allow time for things to emerge, develop and naturally finish. Genuine learning can only happen when there is time for it. So how do we reduce the dominance of the clock and make sure there is time for the session to run comfortably? How do we give enough time to each person who requires it?

The provocation-exploration-sharing-analysis model enables us to be flexible, to run each session with as little time pressure as possible. We have also learned that it takes a number of weeks of interacting and listening to individual children in order to begin to piece together a map of their learning. It feels important to us that we are flexible in our use of time, both within each session and over a term or more.

The prospect of being able to give individual time to each child in a group can sometimes seem overwhelming, but it is both essential and possible over a long period. We have learned how to select groups, and then discuss changing them each week by carefully gauging what has happened in each session for the individual and within the group dynamic. In order to foster each child's creativity, we might need to recruit additional strategies, approaches and adults. It takes time to find out these things. We need to allow time to really explore what it is the children are doing, and this might take one week, or might take a whole year.

Listening

We know the importance of adults listening to children, but we keep asking ourselves, what do we really mean by listening? Since we have been working together we have discovered that there are many different ways to listen that include more than just the ears. It is vital that we listen to children, not to mark off the next criterion in a prescribed model of developmental learning, but to understand their thoughts, questions and ideas. If we all spend more time listening and watching we will become aware of hidden learning that is taking place. By watching each learner as they develop and create interactions, make enquiries and examine ways that they can illustrate their ideas, we start to find ways to connect with their thinking.

Children can tell us important things through their actions and we can learn from them about their mode of learning, their thinking and how to support them – but only if we listen to them. We notice the importance of mimetic echoing sounds and actions of children (in language use, visual art, music, etc.) and how this allows them to gain confidence and ownership of their ideas. Attuned listening will validate the importance of their thinking during these periods of exploration. Over time the adult develops as a facilitator in the child's thinking through his or her skill in listening to the child's 'voice'. This journey of exploration continues as children start to feel accepted, and their thinking is valued. We have noticed how the children's opinions and beliefs develop as they move towards exploring a range of sounds which are used to express an idea, share experiences or tell a story.

Relationships

For us, the relationship between adult and child is initially developed through the trust established by the familiar adult (Sarah) and the subsequent introduction of Hugh to the group. The familiarity of a welcome song binds the group into a weekly meeting routine. Over time, confidence and joint understanding develop further as the children have their thoughts and actions validated. This validation occurs through an echoing, or a re-presentation of their words or actions into music.

By allowing children the chance to be heard through listening, time and noise we are giving them freedom to work things out themselves and make their own connections and decisions. Each child's story is different and individual. When working with children we understand the importance of valuing strengths and differences. The documented cases illustrate how, over time, the children's learning becomes broader and deeper as they reflect and challenge their own views on the world and their relationships.

The process of exploration and enquiry using music has allowed us to support the children in their construction of stories, in expressing thoughts and feelings, and in having a sense of belonging and exploring what matters to them. Music has been a significant tool when representing and exploring their ideas or common themes in their lives: their experiences, love of mummy or family, friendships, power and dominance of others. This musical means of exploring ideas is of high value and appears to open wider thinking across a broader range of materials and modes.

We have found that when the children's learning is observed from our often differing viewpoints (as an educationalist and musician) it has allowed us to develop a rich interpretation through comparison and contrast. Establishing a collaborative approach needs time to develop. It has taken us a long time to get to this place where we feel comfortable in being open, and can share our pedagogic and musical thoughts on what we observe and are relaxed in sharing a diversity of ideas. We are both curious and have listened to each other and have allowed the noise to subside so that we can think.

We continue to question how we can work towards giving all children this full opportunity to explore creativity in their classes. We need to find a way in which each child is free and never hindered, stopped or redirected during the process of creative exploration.

16

A VOYAGE INTO THE SEASCAPE

Dramatherapy in Schools

PENNY MCFARLANE

Marianna was in her element. Soft swathes of blue-green material floated behind her as she turned and twirled with almost balletic-type movements. Her performance was hypnotic, at least to the 20 or so of us adults and children, watching. She was, she informed us, a water princess and she had laid out the room with more blue-green material and black to represent the rocks of an underwater world. We, the audience, were enticed into it, spellbound, and all the more so because we knew, on some level, that she was trying to tell us something of utmost importance. As we were all gathered there, with the aim over a weekend to help children and their families come to terms with the loss of a much loved family member, we knew that Marianna's show had something to do with the death of her mother.

Marianna's aunt was at first intrigued and then very tearful. 'My sister loved the sea,' she explained. 'Before she died she often took the children to the beach to watch the waves and, just at the end, she told Marianna that she would always be there, with her, in the droplets of water which made up the sea, the rain or a rainbow.'

Marianna, eyes shining, finished her performance to huge applause. Hitherto withdrawn, seeming to internalize her grief, she became, according to her aunt, a different person after the weekend. In the, often haphazard, process of grief she had been through the stages of denial and anger, but had, for some time, been stuck in a refusal to accept. By becoming the water princess she had somehow assimilated and absorbed her mother's memory. Her mother could now, always, be part of her and we had been witnesses to this fact, this truth.

Alida Gersie, renowned in the therapy world for her storytelling work, suggests that 'the acknowledgement of death is paramount to the full awakening of the person to adult maturity, symbolically portrayed in myth, legend and fairy tale' (Gersie 1991, p.16). A change in mind and behaviour is much more likely to be brought about through the absorption of metaphorical content rather than direct communication since this is the province of the 'right brain', which is able to grasp holistically complex relationships, patterns and structures. This, through the gift of her imagination, is what appeared to have happened to Marianna.

This ability to grasp complex relationships, patterns and structures holistically is fundamental to the effective practice of dramatherapy. Marianna chose the sea as her metaphor for explaining how the essence of her mother could be contained and live on in the individual droplets of water.

This chapter will endeavour to use the same metaphor to describe how the various and differing aspects and issues of relating to children through the medium of dramatherapy can be brought together to create a healing energy which is effective, sustainable and, most importantly, 'more than the sum of its parts'. As well as exploring various models of dramatherapeutic intervention, difficulties in and examples of the practice, it will look at how allowing and interacting with the 'flow' of children's play is an integral part of this healing energy. Additionally it will discuss how, by alternately and appropriately employing 'directive' and 'non-directive' techniques, the dramatherapist can relate to the children she supports in a way that is effective, safe and containable through the 'ebb and flow' of these rhythms. It will also consider how metaphor can act as an 'anchor' through which the child can safely process and, if necessary, rewrite the narrative of trauma.

Historically, of course, drama as a healing art form is not a new concept. The catharsis of the ancient Greek tragedies left their audiences purged of emotion. As Sue Jennings reminds us, 'dramatic ritual which can establish individual and social identity has existed for millennia in some form or other' (Jennings et al. 1994, p.1). However, it was only in the second half of the 20th century that a connection was made between drama and therapy by Peter Slade who, working in schools in the 1960s, encouraged his pupils to express themselves through the dramatic medium. Then as now, the theory that play is *the* natural expressive medium for children underpinned his practice and, in his own words showed 'how it can reveal our state of being and how it can heal' (Slade 1995, p.2). Play then may be said to be the free-flowing element within which the discipline of dramatherapy with children is embedded. By its very nature play is absorbing, unpredictable and amorphous. It cannot, nor should it, be curtailed. It is the outward expression of the sometimes turbulent, often chaotic inner life of the child. At the very least it offers a means of externalizing that inner life and obtaining some relief from feelings which threaten to engulf and submerge. Through play the dramatherapist can provide the safe setting within which the child can approach that which he had hitherto found unapproachable. He can learn to explore the complexities of life and reduce his world to a size that is both manageable and safe.

Since a feeling of safety is paramount for the child (and therapist) and a prerequisite of the trust-building process when working therapeutically, it would seem that schools (on the whole staffed by caring professionals) might provide a positive working environment. However, dramatherapy with children in schools has had an interesting, if somewhat difficult, start in life. It is only latterly that there has occurred a shift in thinking. Back in the 1980s and 1990s, the idea of arts therapy was regarded, in many schools, 'with as much suspicion as a two headed monster'; recently, however, it has become 'not only acceptable, but desirable' (Jennings and McFarlane 2015, p. 245). Perhaps one of the reasons why dramatherapy has become 'desirable' in schools is that it provides a means of accessing the voice of the child, especially the younger child who has not reached that stage of emotional development to be able to use words to explain their difficulties. It is not the aim of this chapter to highlight the need for this access but rather to explain subtle and intricate patterns of interrelationship between dramatherapist and child, which allows the child's voice to be heard.

As already mentioned, the dramatherapist may weave between 'directive' and 'non-directive' techniques to support the child. By 'non-directive' I mean that a variety of props and mediums are provided from which a child may choose to direct and organize his own play. It is the child who directs his own healing. Similarly it is the child who is still in control when so-called 'directive' methods are employed. The difference is merely that the therapist, having witnessed the themes that the child has presented, may select the props and set the stage. The child will *always* be in charge of the script, will *always* be in control of his own drama.

If working 'non-directively' with a child could be loosely likened to a 'going with the flow' scenario, then perhaps the 'ebb' component of the tidal rhythm might comprise the withdrawing, reflective stage of dramatherapy practice which precedes the more 'directive' approach as described above. In other words, a dramatherapist might feel, on reflection, that the child would benefit from the inclusion of specific props such as mother and baby tiger puppets for a child with attachment problems, or lengths of material suitable for 'safe space' den building for the traumatized child.

Seven-year-old Zoran was referred to me with the objective of helping him become more resilient in coping with the separation of his parents. Outside agencies were concerned that Zoran had been through a horrendous history of events which had involved his abduction from the UK and back again with all family parties 'at war' with one another. Although he was currently living with his father it was suggested that he must 'miss his mother dreadfully' and that efforts should be made to reunite the pair even though the mother had proved unreliable in the past. Zoran presented as a very happy little boy, bright, sociable, well organized, with good eye contact and capable of focused and sustained play. School staff informed me that although there had been problems at one time, the school had put in strict measures around boundaries and structure and had been, for some time, very pleased with him. Zoran's tendency to have angry episodes had decreased and he had begun to settle well into class.

After some sessions of 'non-directive' play during which we had, I felt, built up a relationship of mutual trust, I began to weave some more 'directive' elements into the work. Consequently, I introduced Samu, a baby tiger soft toy, who, I informed Zoran, 'was very sad this morning because he had lost his mother'. Zoran pounced on Samu and, for the next few sessions while I withdrew into observational 'non-directive' mode again, proceeded to act out his own story through Samu and the big 'mother tiger' soft toy.

During his play it emerged that, although Zoran was well aware that he had 'lost' his mother, there were other people there to care for him. At no time did his play present as 'hopeless' or 'without solution'. Although baby Samu had lost his mother in a big jungle, other kindly animals in the shape of dog and cat soft toys had come and helped him find his way out of the jungle. In our short weekly 'check ins' before the session he always announced that he was 'very happy' and gave reasons. These reasons mostly concerned the outings he had had with his dad and his partner who, he told me in our last session together and in a very grown up way, was 'technically' his mum.

In conversation with Zoran's father I realized the depth of the father's feelings for his son and his desire and efforts to provide a stable home for him. We explored the need to allow Zoran to express any emotion with regards to his mother and what had happened, and for this to be a shared experience between the father and son. I also explained that, although I did not feel that Zoran would benefit from any further therapeutic intervention at the moment, this situation might change in the future depending on external circumstances. This line of support could then become available again to the family.

I felt that, contrary to general expectations, Zoran had developed his own coping strategies with regards to his past experiences and that these had been strengthened by the supportive, safe and nurturing structure of the school and by the efforts of his father to provide a stable home. In view of the picture of his emotional status, which Zoran had shown me through his play, I concluded that it would be in Zoran's best interests for these arrangements to continue with the minimum amount of disruption.

In the case of Zoran, as with most children, a period of 'non-directive' play for the first few sessions – where the child can feel that he or she is 'in control' – is often necessary to establish not only a relationship of trust between therapist and child but also a 'safe space'. It is here that possibly, and if appropriate, more 'directive' elements can be introduced. With Zoran, I felt that we could have continued 'non-directive' play in a positive but limited manner for months, unless I supplied the specific props which served to focus the work. The production of a toy or puppet whose story is similar to the child's is a technique which has proved very effective whether the underlying issue is known or only speculated. In the case of speculation, if the toy or puppet's situation does not resonate with the child, then the child will simply ignore it or will quickly move on to something else. Very often, in these scenarios, the story will be met by a look of blankness, sometimes even some impatience, as if the therapist is wasting valuable playing time. Another toy will be picked up or the child will move away to another area of the room. The therapist will then obviously immediately respect the child's communication and follow his lead. Alternatively, a pre-written story which alludes to (but is not an exact representation of) the child's personal story might be brought into the therapeutic space and presented as a potential springboard for safe exploration, being that it is only in the 'as if' and not the child's own truth. For example, two siblings suffering from emotional abuse or neglect who are continually at war with one another might use the story of the 'Babes in the Wood' to rediscover their allegiance to one another in the face of third party threat.

Just as the tides ebb and flow so the 'directive' and 'non-directive' phases of the dramatherapist's work with children find a rhythm of their own. This rhythm corresponds to the differing needs of each child as their play changes.

As we have discussed, the nature of dramatherapeutic work with children, based as it is on play, tends to be fluid in nature. It is, therefore, in my opinion, an advantage to have a structure within which to practise. That is not to say that the play itself should be structured but that there is a need for a structure within which the play may be assessed. The structure that I have found to be most helpful is the Embodiment, Projection, Role (EPR) model as presented by Sue Jennings. Since the EPR paradigm correlates roughly to the cognitive developmental models of psychologist Jean Piaget (1970) and psychoanalyst Erik Erikson (1994), it has been a useful tool not only for assessment purposes but also to underpin explanations of dramatherapeutic practice to educationalists and other non-therapists.

The Embodiment stage can be said to correspond to those early months/ years when a child is only aware of his own body, his own needs. This is the pure sensory stage. As a child develops emotionally and cognitively, he becomes aware that there is a world outside his own bodily needs; he becomes able to project his needs onto another. It is this Projection that enables a distancing of experience – so it is his teddy bear that is sad or tired or happy, not him. The Role stage is when a child becomes conceptually aware that he can see himself as others see him. In other words he is playing a role. It is him, but not him. Usually this stage corresponds to the time when a child becomes capable of understanding abstract concepts. Until then the world needs to be interpreted through the concrete. As most teachers are acquainted with the theories of Piaget and Erikson, these theories can be used as a springboard to illustrate how a child may, due to trauma, disability, illness or neglect, become stuck in either the Embodiment or Projection stage.

The next section of this chapter goes on to explore dramatherapy with children who have suffered from trauma. We will look at models of working therapeutically with traumatized children, how these models work within dramatherapy, and use the EPR model to exemplify a way to assess change.

Robert and Jamie were brothers. They did not often play together but this time, on the weekend specially organized for children and their families in bereavement, it was different. Their play was hectic, disorganized and bordering on the frenzied. They had demanded all the black and red material in the big bag even though some of the other children had protested. Their play was difficult and disturbing to watch. It was fairly obvious that the red material on which the big teddy bear was lying was representative of the blood they had seen as their father lay dying of bowel cancer. The family had insisted, against professional advice, that the father remain at home and that the boys be included in the situation as it unfolded. Now they played over and over again this situation as they had witnessed it. The red material was taken away and the teddy bear wrapped up in the black first by Robert and then by Jamie. They took it in turns until the therapist present asked what else the teddy bear might need or want to happen. Eventually, having played through the scenario a couple more times they carried the teddy bear in its black covering to a corner of the room where a doll wrapped in some white cloth was positioned over it. 'It's the angel. She'll look after him now,' said Robert.

Robert and Jamie's behaviour did not improve immediately after this therapeutic weekend but slowly they both became less agitated, less hypervigilant, more able to concentrate in class. Robert's nightmares ceased and Jamie stopped wetting the bed. In a follow-up visit three months later they proudly showed off the memory boxes they had made about their father. It seemed as if, although not forgotten, the trauma of that time had at least retreated to a place where it was manageable.

Edna Foa, pioneer of treatment for Post Traumatic Stress Disorder recognised by NICE,[1] advocates as part of her intervention a prolonged and repeated revisiting of the trauma memories and process of this experience. During her rationale for using this 'Imaginal Exposure' procedure, she will typically say to a patient, 'repeatedly revisiting and recounting the memory that distresses you so much will help you process it', and 'repeatedly retelling your memory will help you organize the memory and get new perspective about what happened during and after the trauma' (Foa, Hembree and Rothbaum 2007, p.83).

Although this particular procedure, as it stands, may be restricted to adults and teenagers, the principle remains the same: *that on some level the traumatic memory must be accessed and acknowledged to be modified or erased.*

Children who have suffered some degree of trauma usually need no bidding to repeatedly revisit the source of their pain once a safe space and safe relationship with the therapist has been established. For Robert and Jamie this was exactly the case. A morning's worth of fun and games, plus the presence of therapists with whom they had already established a rapport during home visits, coupled with an awareness, conscious or unconscious, of why they were on this weekend, gave them permission to play through their trauma. For Robert and Jamie, the safety lay in the 'dramatic distancing' of creating the roles, and becoming in the play their father's carers. They became empowered in a situation where they had, hitherto, felt totally disempowered. Zoran, emotionally and chronologically younger, used Projection through a puppet and the invention of a story, which was his and not his. It is as if children like Robert, Jamie and Zoran somehow know deep down, without being told, the theory expounded by Dr Foa and others.

Some children (despite their chronological age, and unlike Robert and Jamie) have not reached that stage of emotional development where they are able to take on Role; they are incapable of seeing themselves as others see them or of showing empathy or compassion. 'He shows no remorse,' or, 'She doesn't seem to understand what she has done wrong,' is a statement which I have often heard uttered by school staff as they despairingly try to remonstrate with a difficult child. It is my contention that it is not that many of these children *won't* show remorse or *won't* understand but that they *can't*. According to Sunderland, 'There is a mass of scientific research showing that quality of life is dramatically affected by whether or not you established good stress-regulating systems in

---

1   National Institute for Health and Care Excellence

your brain in childhood' (Sunderland 2006, p.27), and that a lack of these means that the, 'legacy in later life is that [the children] do not develop the higher human capacities for concern, or the ability to reflect on their feelings in a self-aware way' (Sunderland 2006, p.25).

Of course it is easy to blame the parents but it must also be remembered that many of these parents received inadequate parenting themselves or were exposed to such potentially traumatic situations as domestic violence, alcoholism or drug abuse. In many inner city schools, as a team of dramatherapists we are now seeing children as young as four or five whose parents were referred to us as children in their turn.

With children such as these it is important to return to whichever stage the therapist feels is most appropriate, usually Embodiment or Projection, and supply the appropriate props (sensory items such as clay, soft toys or material in the case of Embodiment, or puppets, small figures, etc. in the case of Projection) to allow the child to play through his or her own particular version of their, often traumatic, story.

Edna Foa maintains that in order for traumatic memories to be erased or modified they first have to be activated along with the fear factor. It is this fear factor which 'must be activated, otherwise it is not available for modification' (Foa *et al.* 2007, p.13). The analogy of a computer is a useful one: errors in software can only be edited once they are visible on screen; they have to be clicked on and brought 'online' so that they can be altered and then correctly filed away. Any faulty thinking which has arisen as a result of the fear can then be replaced by new, helpful information, 'new information that is incompatible with the erroneous information embedded in the fear structure must be available and incorporated into the fear structure' (Foa *et al.* 2007, p.13).

The skill of the children's therapist in helping modify traumatic memory lies in appropriately responding and relating to the process of the child within the rhythms of 'directive' and 'non-directive' play. 'Non-directive' play where the child is re-enacting an abusive situation is not helpful and can be re-traumatizing. Nevertheless the child must be allowed to revisit the memory, but from an empowered place where she or he is in control, perhaps necessitating the more 'directive' skills of the therapist. The key concept here is 'control', since in the original scenario the child would most certainly *not* have been in control. In the case of Robert and Jamie in their dramatherapy, it was *they* and not the carers who cleaned up the blood and put their father into the body bag. Their 'dramatic distancing' gave them the safety to take control.

Robert and Jamie took further control when, responding to the therapist's suggestion, they activated what psychodramatists term 'surplus reality' by arranging for the angel to look after him. By 'surplus reality' we mean the actions which the victims of the trauma would have liked to perform but were not in a position to do *at that time*. Unlike in the original situation, and difficult as it was, it was Robert and Jamie who were in total control of the whole proceedings through their re-enactment.

It is this regaining one's power and/or control in a previously uncontrollable scenario, and the expending of the residual energy in escaping or changing the outcome of the situation, which dissipates the erroneous and typical cognitions of the trauma survivor, 'I am incompetent', 'I can't cope', 'I am to blame' or 'There is danger everywhere'.

Children who have experienced trauma or distress at a preverbal stage will not be able to use words to describe their memories. This is where a return to the Embodiment/sensory stage of development is appropriate. Here the therapist provides the child with the safety, stage and props to explore what they are feeling in their body. One of my supervisees brought to me the case of a nine-year-old child who wanted to cling onto the bars of a chair and rock backwards and forwards repeatedly every session. We discussed the possibility that this child, who had been adopted at 12 months because of severe domestic abuse in the family, may well have been acutely distressed at what he had witnessed at a preverbal stage and was actually returning in his memory to rocking the sides of his cot or playpen. With prolonged and careful support, following the smooth rhythm of inter-relatedness between directive and non-directive therapeutic intervention, the child was encouraged by the therapist to let go of the feeling of helplessness and take some control within the situation. By embodying the memory and allowing it to work its way through in the rocking, the child expiated the painful feelings of that time. He was able to move on, with the therapist as his companion to the next stage of his emotional development.

Additionally, in the case of preverbal or lost memory, the developing relationship between the therapist and child may provide clues as to the source of the original distressing experience. The child may create through transference, and then counter-transference on the part of the therapist, the dysfunctional relationship which was present at the preverbal period of trauma. These interchanges then mirror 'a process of rupture and repair that is fairly typical of work with early-trauma patients, where the early trauma cannot be remembered but, owing to dissociation, must be *repeated*, this time hopefully toward a new ending' (Kalsched 2013, p.68). During this process it is down to the skill of the therapist to recognize, assimilate and act on this paralleling. She may become aware, perhaps within her own body, of feelings which are at odds with the current relationship with the child. These feelings may relate instead to a relational situation from the past that the child is trying to re-create in order to heal. This requires on the part of the therapist a fine sense of the rhythmical pattern of relating and comes with the experience of acting from the heart rather than the head, of being aware, as Levine would term it, of the 'felt sense' (Levine 1997).

Another model of intervention, which I have found useful for assessment purposes alongside the EPR model, is that of Mooli Lahad's six-part story. This method has its roots in Lahad's work on identifying coping strategies in individuals at the Community Stress Prevention Centre in Northern Israel (Lahad 1992). It focuses on 'the coping resources and the language of the client' by asking 'the client to tell us a story according to six questions' (Lahad 2000, p.98). These questions concern the hero or heroine of the story, the task or mission of the hero or heroine, his or her helper, the obstacles to that mission, how the mission is undertaken and the final outcome. 'The six answers to these questions are [then] either drawn in a cartoon style or are told or written as a story' (Lahad 2000, p.98). In this way the 'assumption is that by telling a projected story based on elements of fairy tale and myth, we may be able to see the way that the self projects itself in organized reality in order to meet the world' (Lahad 2000, p.99).

In my work within mainstream education this model has proved particularly useful with groups. So far in this chapter I have focused on individual practice. However, due to increasing pressure from schools to address growing needs amongst disaffected or damaged children, time constraints often mean that group dramatherapy may be considered. One obvious advantage to group work is that the process and potential emotional growth of each child can have more witnesses than the therapist alone.

Eleven-year-old Martin was such a child. Since his parents' separation and mother's subsequent depression Martin's behaviour in school had been very difficult. Aggressive and confrontational in class, he acted as a catalyst to his peers, continually 'winding them up' and annoying them by showing off. Out of class Martin seemed to need to be the centre of attention, continually forcing himself on others but playing the victim when ignored. He had few social graces, was always in trouble and had been excluded twice already, although only in the first year of secondary school. He became part of a group of peers who were having difficulty settling in to their secondary school and were, therefore, offered weekly dramatherapy sessions.

Martin was, to say the least, not popular in the group. His continual boasting and need for attention, positive or negative, annoyed the other members. I decided to put more structure into the proceedings and we started on the six-part story technique. This, after a preliminary visualization to elicit the individual stories of hero/heroine, mission, helper, obstacles, final attainment and outcome, evolved into a weekly enactment of each child's story. The owner of the story performed the role of the hero but also directed the others in their play. To deepen the work, I made one addition to Lahad's model: each hero/heroine had a secret.

Martin's hero was Rodney, a circus clown who loved performing tricks. Unfortunately for Rodney the tricks that the audience loved best were those that involved fire and Rodney's secret was that he was afraid of fire. Consequently he made all his animals perform the fire tricks for him. One day, however, just as he was about to direct his animals on one of the fire tricks the crowd started calling, shouting out, 'Rod…*ney*, Rod…*ney*', and Rodney knew that they wanted *him* to do the tricks instead. He was very afraid. The trick involved jumping through a blazing hoop of fire and Rodney felt sick when he looked at it. But the crowd went on shouting and finally Rodney jumped. Afterwards he was over the moon about what he had done. He said the crowd had always put him down because he would never do the fire tricks himself. Now that he had plucked up enough courage to do them and the crowd loved him for it, he didn't need his animals any more.

Martin seemed to visibly grow when, to the applause of the rest of the group, he mimed jumping through the blazing hoop. Afterwards, the group, as initiated by another member, carried him round on their shoulders in a victor's salute. Martin was ecstatic. Having made a few friends from the group, he began to settle into class and, although not an angel, was not singled out as a troublemaker again. As time went on he blended into the background of his tutor group and only came to general attention again when he had the leading part in an end-of-term production – as a clown.

If play, whether 'directive' or 'non-directive', can be said to be the free-flowing element within which children explore their feelings, then metaphor is the anchor which steadies and stabilizes this play, providing a continuous and sustainable foundation to whatever is rippling above. That is to say, that metaphor provides *safety*. The child does not have to confront his or her traumatic story directly, but whilst remaining in the land of metaphor, can use his own creativity to present and explore his own personal version of that story, as Martin did here.

Metaphor is fundamental to Jungian thinking. The creative, expressive model of dramatherapy, as expounded by Sue Jennings, has many connections to the Jungian ways of working. Psychologist Carl Gustav Jung, having been a pupil of Sigmund Freud, formed his own psychoanalytic way of thinking in 1913. One of Jung's main premises was that life has meaning and that this meaning can be understood and experienced symbolically through a series of images arising spontaneously from the unconscious (Jung 1978). His contention was that these images and symbols arose out of a need for the psyche to counterbalance the standpoint of the ego and that they were part of a drive towards wholeness or 'self individuation'. Thus it is that a child, while endeavouring to explain the feelings of frustration and abandonment he feels when his severely depressed mother is unapproachable, may create the metaphor of a dragon, which prevents the baby cheetah from reaching the mummy cheetah.

No matter how difficult or 'big' the feelings, the metaphor will provide safety and containment. For very young children who have not yet learnt to think in the abstract, the verbal concepts of 'good' and 'bad' are intangible. Once personified through the good prince or the evil stepmother, as in fairy tales, they are more easily understood and dealt with. A young child, having problems with schoolwork will explain how he feels inferior to his more intelligent brother by telling a story about a snail and a hare. It is the therapist's job to explore with him the alternative, perhaps less obvious, qualities of the snail. In this way both 'non-directive' and 'directive' ways of working are successfully exploited through the same metaphorical content.

Expanding our own watery metaphor, I can openly say that the journey of establishing dramatherapy in schools has more often than not left me feeling 'all at sea'. As mentioned at the beginning of this chapter, the introduction of a qualitative way of working into organizations which pride themselves on quantitative appraisal was regarded with much suspicion. There was, and still is, an overriding need on the part of the therapist for consistency, calmness and above all flexibility, at least on the surface! The ability to work in any nook or cranny (I drew the line at the boys' cloakrooms!), the availability to talk to teachers and parents and walk the tightrope between concern and confidentiality were, and are, essential prerequisites for 'making it work'. Perhaps now that arts therapies in schools are beginning not only to be accepted but also regarded as the norm there is not such a need for the therapist (although some might disagree) to 'prove him- or herself'. The journey, however, continues with the need to establish a wider and more profound credibility for dramatherapy in schools by the foundation of more robust methods of assessment and evaluation. This may then I hope result in the acceptance of therapists into the body of education on a more formal contractual basis.

Although much powerful and effective work is being done by therapists working in schools, there is often a problem of sustainability in therapeutic progress. Part way along the journey of setting up dramatherapy in schools I became aware of the fact that, with some children, although seemingly more settled, more emotionally stable and more resilient at the end of the summer term, by the time they returned to school in the autumn we were back to stage one. I began to feel the limitations of working with the child alone without involving the family. To this end I began to include one or both parents (with the permission of the child) in our sessions and the results were such that I now continue to advise my supervisees to do the same.

When we relate to children with the desire to facilitate their healing we are working on a level which is not always quantifiable. There comes a moment, sometimes through role-play, sometimes through metaphor, when the quality of stillness in the room changes. It is intangible but nevertheless present. It is as if a numinous 'other' has entered the room and, in my experience, signals a shift in perception, in awareness and in healing. It is as if all the work that has been done has resulted in something, which is effective, sustainable and, more importantly, 'more than a sum of its parts'. For Marianna it was her water princess, for Zoran it was when he told me very seriously that he 'technically had a mum', with Martin the jump through the blazing hoop and for Robert and Jamie, their Dad's guardian angel.

Our individual rhythms of relating to children may seem at times insignificant, insubstantial and inadequate in this world, which can sometimes be cruel and violent. At times we may feel that we are doing battle with an indifferent society on so many different levels and that our efforts are like a drop in a limitless ocean. Sometimes it is hard to remain positive faced with so much negativity, but who knows, our caring approach may be the one that a child remembers many years from now.

And, in any case, what is any ocean but a whole host of drops?

References

Erikson, E. (1994 [1959]) *Identity and the Life Cycle*. New York, London: W.W. Norton.

Foa, E., Hembree, E. and Rothbaum, B. (2007) *Prolonged Exposure Therapy for PTDS: Emotional Processing of Traumatic Experiences. Therapist Guide*. New York: Oxford University Press.

Gersie, A. (1991) *Storymaking in Bereavement: Dragons Fight in the Meadow*. London: Jessica Kingsley Publishers.

Jennings, S. and McFarlane, P. (2015) 'Arts Education and Therapy. The Importance of Dramatherapy.' In M. Fleming, L. Bresler and J. O'Toole (eds) *The Routledge International Handbook of the Arts and Education*. London: Routledge.

Jennings, S., Cattanoch, A., Chesner, A., Mitchell, S. and Meldrum, B. (1994) *The Handbook of Dramatherapy*. London: Routledge.

Jung, C.G. (1978 [1964]) *Man and His Symbols*. London: Picador.

Kalsched, D. (2013) *Trauma and the Soul: A Psycho-Spiritual Approach to Human Development and Its Interruption*. Hove and New York: Routledge.

Levine, P. (1997) *Waking the Tiger: Healing Trauma*. Berkeley, CA: North Atlantic Books.

Lahad, M. (1992) 'Story-making in Assessment Method for Coping with Stress: Six-Piece Story Making and BASICPh.' In S. Jennings (ed.) *Dramatherapy: Theory and Practice 2*. London: Routledge.

Lahad, M. (2000) *Creative Supervision: The Use of Expressive Arts Methods in Supervision and Self-supervision*. London: Jessica Kingsley Publishers.

Piaget. J. (1970) 'Piaget's Theory.' In P.H. Mussen (ed.) *Carmichael's Manual of Child Psychology*. Volume 1. New York: John Wiley.

Slade, P. (1995) *Child Play: Its Importance for Human Development*. London: Jessica Kingsley Publishers.

Sunderland, M. (2006) *The Science of Parenting*. London: Dorling Kindersley.

17

ESTABLISHING RELATIONSHIPS WITH CHILDREN WITH AUTISM SPECTRUM DISORDERS THROUGH DANCE MOVEMENT PSYCHOTHERAPY

A Case Study Using Artistic Enquiry

FOTEINI ATHANASIADOU AND VICKY KARKOU

Patrick by the window

Patrick was referred for Dance Movement Psychotherapy (DMP) because he did not interact with his classmates and participated in classroom group activities only when he was requested to and only for small periods of time. His verbal abilities were limited and he usually spent his time on his own, wandering apparently without aim. Patrick has a diagnosis of Autism Spectrum Disorder (ASD).

When Patrick arrived in the therapy room he moved directly towards the window and started looking through it. The therapist felt that 'holding' Patrick's desire to stand by the window and watch through it (i.e. his immediate experience) could be the starting point of their in-between relationship. Just standing with him by the window and mirroring his light and quick hand movements helped them to connect with each other.

A different kind of method

This chapter describes a series of case studies in which we explore how DMP can support children with ASD to establish relationships. Here we use artistic enquiry, otherwise known as arts-based research, in an attempt to avoid an over-reliance on the use of numbers and words, and so come closer to the non-verbal language often preferred by children with ASD. Our explorations will rely heavily on the use of artistic means and movement-based means in particular.

Artistic enquiry is a new methodological genre in postmodern qualitative enquiry (Finley 2005; Leavy 2009). Here, researchers who attempt an exploration through artistic enquiry use artistic methods to gather, analyse and present data, follow a creative process for their overall design, and analyse and synthesize data through their 'aesthetic values' (Hervey 2000, p.78).

Artistic enquiry is underpinned by social constructionist ideas (Schwandt 2000) and, as such, is especially suited to small-scale detailed analysis of relationships. Social constructionism argues that knowledge is created through experience and within context, while the context (our developing relationships) remains open to multiple 'truths' and interpretations of meaning. In addition, artistic enquiry allows space for 'aesthetic values' including intuition, embodiment, creativity, kinaesthetic empathy, imagery, emotions and inspiration. Hervey (2000, 2004) distinguishes six phases of the creative process. However, the creative process does not follow a prescribed, linear sequence, but the researcher is immersed in a 'spiralic process' (Meekums 1993, p.132), going back to the data, finding new material, making new associations, until she is satisfied with the meanings that have emerged.

As an initial example (see Figure 17.1), here is an image which relates the therapist's experience of her meeting with Patrick as he stood by the window.

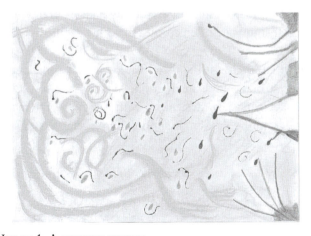

FIGURE 17.1 IMAGE 1: A JOURNEY IN TIME

The thick lines and the use of a warm yellow colour (that was used in the original drawing) depict my experience of wanting to provide attentive care and support to Patrick. The drop-like shapes (appearing pink in the original drawing) depict Patrick's initial hand movements, which became more distinct in the course of time. I felt like a mother who pays close attention to her infant and celebrates her infant's every single tiny effort to initiate action.

Interpersonal relatedness

Interpersonal relatedness is often seen as the core of human existence, enabling people to make sense of the world and acting as an important therapeutic agent within most forms of psychotherapy (Clarkson 2003; Yalom and Leszcz 2005). Humans are born with an innate ability and need to interact and share their experience with their significant others (Bowlby 1988; Hobson 1993; Kugiumutzakis 1993; Meltzoff 1990; Powers and Trevarthen 2009; Stern 1985). Within a meaningful relationship the infant slowly develops an experience (and then a sense) of self, gradually feeling (and then considering) herself as a separate entity from her parent/caregiver (Ciccone 2012; Stern 1985). The infant's self-regulatory, physical, emotional, cognitive and social skills all become integrated and further developed within a relational context (Greenspan and Wieder 2006; Stern 2012; Trevarthen *et al.* 1998; Wengrower 2010).

ASD and relationships

ASD is associated with impairments in social understanding and interaction, verbal and non-verbal communication, imagination, understanding another person's motives and thinking, and sharing experiences with other people (Hobson 1993; Wing 1996; Wing and Gould 1979; Trevarthen *et al.* 1998). Resistance to change, anxiety, stereotyped behaviour, lack of motivation and even depression and self-injury are often correlated with a diagnosis of ASD (Hobson 1993; Sigman and Capps 1997; Wing 1981). Deficits in social reciprocity have been observed in children with autistic features under three years old (Stone *et al.* 1999; Trevarthen and Daniel 2005; Wimpory *et al.* 2000). Children on the autistic spectrum have difficulties with reciprocal interactions, such as 'protodeclarative pointing',[1] 'joint attention'[2] and 'social referencing'[3] (Hobson

---

1   The baby's tendency to draw somebody's attention by pointing to an object or event in order to share interest in it or comment on it
2   The use of gestures and gaze, between an adult and a baby, in order to share a common interest or express intentions
3   The baby's ability to look at the adult in order to retrieve affective information about the adult's perception of an object or an event in the environment

1993; Trevarthen *et al.* 1998). In typical development it is these information-based reciprocal interactions through which a child learns how to respond to objects and events in practical, emotional and social ways. Deficits in symbolic representation, such as symbolic play (Baron-Cohen *et al.* 1996; Mundy *et al.* 1987), imitation (Rogers and Pennington 1991) and language (Hobson 1993; Trevarthen *et al.* 1998) are also often part of an autistic presentation.

All children with ASD have difficulties with interpersonal relatedness. But, there is evidence that suggests that children with ASD do form *basic* attachment relationships with their significant others (Hobson 1993; Trevarthen *et al.* 1998) and relate emotionally to other people (Cesaroni and Garber 1991). Children with ASD often lack the organized impulse and structured understanding of how they can respond and relate to other people, but not the desire to relate to others (Sigman and Capps 1997; Trevarthen *et al.* 1998).

Many interaction models (Alvarez, Reid and Hodges 1999; Burford 1991; Greenspan and Wieder 2006; Trevarthen *et al.* 1998 for an overview) suggest that child-led interactions (which follow the child's motives, interests and rhythms) are particularly effective when relating to children with ASD. Non-verbal modes of communication can support children with ASD to become more available to reciprocal experience (Trevarthen *et al.* 1998). Elements of 'proximal communication' (such as physical interaction with the child, minimum use of verbal language and following the child's lead) have been proved successful in developing social interaction skills in children with ASD (Whittaker 1996).

DMP, relationships and ASD

DMP acknowledges, builds and relies upon bridges of communication beyond the verbal (Karkou and Sanderson 2006). It works with the whole person. DMP practice is greatly influenced by our emerging understanding of innate infant intersubjectivity: the early impulses displayed by both carer and infant to share, explore and co-regulate mental and affective states through diverse verbal and non-verbal modes of communication, e.g. sound, gestures, words (Meltzoff and Brooks 2007; Stern 2005; Trevarthen 2005). True to the interactive ideas of Chace (Chaiklin and Schmais 1986), the DMP practitioner acknowledges therapy as the interchange between the therapist's and client's subjective experience and considers the collection of their in-between interactions in the present moment as a factor for therapeutic change and growth.

One significant aim when working with children with ASD is that of building a body image. Within a regular developmental trajectory, developing a body image supports the baby to distinguish herself from the environment (including other people). This functional distinction is integral to the ability to form relationships (Erfer 1995). Stern (1985) argues that an infant slowly builds a sense of core self from her birth until six months of age. During this period, an infant comes to understand that she is physically separate from the caregiver and therefore is able to start building a subjective experience. With felt subjectivity comes the possibility of entering the domain of 'intersubjective relatedness'.

Children with ASD can be supported in their development of their sense of physical self through sensorimotor-based activities. DMP can support children with ASD in sensory-motor integration (Scharoun *et al.* 2014). It is through sensorimotor activities that a child becomes able to build a body image and develop her self-concept (Erfer 1995). Dance movement psychotherapists working with children on the autism spectrum stress the importance for these children of experiencing their body as a whole first and later exploring different body parts (Sherborne 2001; Tortora 2006). Others describe how children with autism can become slowly more aware of themselves (and consequently more communicative) through touching their body parts (Adler 1970; Erfer 1995; Siegel 1963). In our case study, sensorimotor-based activities helped the children to explore their body, their body's possibilities and limitations and eventually build a stronger body image. It is important for us to note here that many children with ASD suffer from hypersensitivities including a hypersensitivity (sometimes aversion) to physical touch. This reality is given significant consideration by dance movement psychotherapists as it is specifically relevant to their practice. The therapist is always sensitive to, and led by the child – she accepts the child's choice in involvement in sensorimotor-based activities and follows the child's particular way, preferences and style. In addition, the therapist supports this involvement by the use of props and sensitive movement suggestions. The possibilities for sensorimotor-based activities are endless. There are a great many ways to support and empower a child in movement exploration.

Children with ASD can develop their social awareness and communication skills through imitation (Katagiri, Inada and Kamio 2010; Nadel and Peze 1993). However, dance movement psychotherapists do not simply imitate the other person's movements, but 'mirror'[4] the person's muscle tension, body shapes, movement rhythms and qualities using the same or different body parts. While the therapist is aware of not intruding into the individual's personal space and way of moving, she acquires valuable information about the other person's experience through 'kinaesthetic empathy', a term introduced by Berger (1972)

---

4   In DMP we use 'mirroring' as an umbrella term to include many aspects of the therapist's toolkit when communicating through the body in a responsive, dynamically communicative manner. Here the term would encompass classical therapeutic mirroring (or imitation), cross-modal attunement (Stern 2005) and any more-or-less abstracted movement pattern which encapsulates the underlying vitality of the child's energetic state (Stern 2010).

and cited in Fischman (2009). Adler (1970) offers a visual documentation of how two girls with ASD gradually become responsive to her through mirroring. Tortora (2006) describes how she progressively built a relationship with a boy on the autism spectrum through matching and attuning to the boy's actions and rhythms.

Through 'mirroring' the therapist acknowledges the child's way of being and accepts her unique way of expressing emotions, thoughts, needs and desires. The child, feeling accepted and confident, transfers her focus from inner reality to external environment and therefore is more likely to start interacting with people (Erfer 1995). Wengrower (2010), in a multiple case study with children diagnosed with ASD or PDD (Pervasive Developmental Disorder), describes how 'mirroring' led to mutual interactions between the therapist and the child and enabled the therapist to empathize better with the child.

Building a therapeutic relationship through 'mirroring' resonates with the intersubjective experiences between a caregiver and a baby in healthy development, described by Stern (1985) and Trevarthen (2005). From birth, the caregiver tunes into the baby's facial expressions, gestures, rhythms and sounds promoting reciprocal interaction and social dialogue. Once this type of relatedness is established, and their in-between relationship is enriched through quality interaction, caregiver and baby will be ready to share their attention towards an external object. This is the moment in development that Trevarthen *et al.* (1998) describe as the transition from primary intersubjectivity to secondary intersubjectivity.

Within our case study we incorporated play into our DMP interventions. For us here, this took the form of sensorimotor play using objects (e.g. throwing and catching the ball), embodied play (e.g. walking on all-fours and trying to catch each other) and symbolic play (e.g. the 'policeman game' described below). During these play activities the children seemed more active and involved in the group process. Play is a central feature of child development and the modality by which children express their emotions, concerns and construct their thinking (Axline 1971; Winnicott 2005). In their psychodynamic-informed intervention for children with ASD, Alvarez *et al.* (1999) involved play as they found it integral to each child's development and self-expression. Moore (2008) argues that children on the autism spectrum can find enjoyment, and gradually develop their social skills, through play.

Due to the fact that there is not sufficient literature regarding DMP and play, we searched for the use of play in dramatherapy and found the EPR model (Jennings 1999) informative and suitable for adapting for our case study. The EPR model outlines a developmental progression, a useful structure with which to assess and describe a child's pathway towards confident, skilful social interaction. The EPR model consists of three stages: 'Embodiment' – play includes physical exploration through the senses; 'Projection' – at this stage the child relates more to her external environment through toys and objects and starts using them symbolically; and 'Role' – at this stage the child plays with different roles and starts to identify more strongly with particular options.

Case study
Three children

Our study took place in a special school for children with ASD.[5] After a careful referral process, three classmates between six and seven years old were chosen to participate in the study.[6] We shall call them Patrick, Ben and Phillip. You have already been introduced to Patrick at the beginning of his first session.

The DMP intervention

The DMP intervention consisted of eight group sessions that took place once a week for 50 minutes. Each session was loosely structured around warm-up, mid-phase and closure.

The intervention was informed and inspired by a range of different movement approaches. including the Chace[7] interactive model of DMP (Chaiklin and Schmais 1986) and Sherborne Developmental Movement[8] (Sherborne 2001). The intervention was given support by intersubjectivity theory (Meltzoff and Brooks 2007; Stern 2005; Trevarthen 2005) and the developmental structure within the Embodiment-Projection-Role model (Jennings 1999). While interweaving these various influences and ideas, the intervention remained essentially person centred (Rogers 1967). Each session included spontaneous interactions and activities as suggested by the children and supported by the therapist.

---

5   The first author was completing her placement experience as a trainee dance movement psychotherapist and the second author was acting as her academic supervisor.

6   Consent forms regarding the participation of the children in the study and the video recording of the sessions were signed by the school's head teacher and the children's parents. Consent forms were signed by children.

7   The Chacian approach is underpinned by the following four basic principles: 1) the *therapeutic relationship* to promote trust, empathy and kinaesthetic awareness; 2) the *group rhythm* to develop vitality, group cohesion, and interaction between group members; 3) *bodily action* to strengthen body image and develop expressiveness through movement; and 4) *symbolism* to express inner reality and integrate emotions, thoughts and movements.

8   The Sherborne Developmental Movement approach is based on the principle that movement experiences are fundamental to the development of all children (Sherborne 2001) and aims to facilitate awareness of self and others through shared movement experiences.

Session 1: We introduced ourselves, explored the therapeutic space and familiarized ourselves with the camera.

Sessions 2–4: We explored ways of moving together. The children seemed interested in using props and interacting with me. From session 4 onwards, the children were more involved in the 'warm-up' phase than in previous sessions. Here, we played with shaping a circle and moving in or away from its centre.

Sessions 5 and 6: The children started to become involved in group activities. Moreover, a 'closure' phase became more apparent than earlier in the sessions, with all the children joining the relaxation play and sharing 'goodbye' movements.

Sessions 7 and 8: Group interactions became much lengthier than in previous sessions. The children seemed more aware and determined regarding what they wanted to do. Ben and Philip developed attentiveness towards Patrick and me.

Data generation, somatic response and the power of subjectivity

Data generation took place within and after the eight DMP group sessions. Three different methods were used for the generation of the data: 1) video recordings of the sessions; 2) multiple records of the therapist's somatic responses to the session-based interactions (including drawings of a body figure, and written and video recordings); and 3) written reflections based upon observations, feelings and ideas relating to our central study question: How can DMP support children with ASD to establish relationships? This led to the collection of multiple types of data (visual, kinaesthetic and text). Triangulation between these modes of data intended to increase the trustworthiness of the study (Batavia 2001). Text-based data was analysed using 'thematic analysis' (Braun and Clarke 2006). For the visual and kinaesthetic data the therapist/researcher engaged in 'dialoguing' with the data – as suggested by Hervey (2000). The findings of this case study were presented in the form of narratives and drawings (which are presented below) and through a recorded movement piece.

The first author was both the researcher and the therapist in this study, and was very aware that her emotions and personal experience would influence practice, data collection and reflection. This level of awareness is important when applying structure to subjective data. Within this structure, however, qualitative studies gain their power through researchers being encouraged to explore their personal experience in order to find meaning through it (Hervey 2000).

During the inner dialogue phase I was immersed in drawing and movement improvisations. I was responding to elements of each case study and connecting with the data gathered in and after the sessions. These dialogues began with an acceptance and openness to not knowing what would emerge and and how meaning would take form. I would let myself go through the gathered data, staying open until I felt somatic responses[9] emerge and the related urge to move and/or draw. This was a spiral process of creative improvisation in partnership with the data – developing improvisations apart from the data, recording and watching the improvisations, going back to the data, and starting the whole process again. While I was engaged in this process, certain patterns and themes started to emerge. These themes concerned how the three children were supported to establish relationships within the group's context. I continued moving and drawing to depict the themes and patterns in the form of movement sequences and on the paper. At this stage, I started to become aware of the personal meaning carried by the symbols and metaphors of my movement and drawings: drawing parallel lines resembled the mirroring activities with Philip; sitting on the floor in a closed body shape (head, arms and legs being together and not open to the space in front of me) and moving slightly resembled my initial contact with Patrick; drawing red angled-shapes resonated with my perception of Ben's vigorous and sometimes intrusive attitude at the beginning of the DMP intervention. Next, I started adding words and sentences that I later used to compose the narratives I share below (see 'Moving with the Children').

Focusing on my somatic responses within a free-flowing, creative, multi-sensory process enabled me to explore aspects of my perception that were not merely cognitive. This was invaluable. I no longer had to restrict myself to words and texts. Instead I had available other aspects of myself, including kinaesthetic and sensory awareness, intuition and emotions. In this way I felt I could conduct the case study with my full potential. The cross-modality of the sensory experience (movement and drawing) supported me to explore and be creative across two different mediums, become better aware of my somatic responses, and find links and patterns that the modality improvisations had in common. Dialoguing with the data was a long reflective process that took place on many different days.

9   Pallaro (2010) distinguishes these somatic response (sensations) into: 1) pure bodily sensations (such as dizziness); and 2) images that emerge from the somatic unconscious (e.g. a sudden desire to hold the infant-self of the patient.

This left me vulnerable to many moments of unknowing and confusion. But it was this process of inner dialogue which illuminated and informed me regarding my clinical skills and the ongoing development of the group.

Relationship themes

Within the group sessions, one-to-one relationships were formed with each one of the three children. Each of these relationships, between child and therapist, had a slightly different emphasis. As we will see in the following findings, with Patrick relationships were built primarily through sensorimotor interactions (Erfer 1995), with Ben through purposeful misattunement and embodiment play (Jennings 1999; Stern 1985), and with Phillip through the use of 'mirroring' (Erfer 1995; Wengrower 2010).

Moving with the children

Holding in time: Relationship between Patrick and therapist

We are back by the window with Patrick and his therapist in their first session (see Figure 17.1).

> I felt that 'holding' Patrick's desire to stand by the window and watch through it (i.e. his immediate experience) could be the starting point of our in-between relationship. Just standing with him by the window and mirroring his light and quick hand movements supported us to connect. I felt like a mother, who pays close attention to her infant and celebrates her infant's every single tiny effort to initiate action.

Here 'holding' resonates with the concept of a 'holding environment' (Winnicott 2005) – an environment of psychological and practical support, generated when a mother offers care and attentiveness to her baby. 'Holding' is a key feature in the baby's healthy development – it defines her early experiences in which her body becomes a secure place to in which to live (Winnicott 2005). Within a therapeutic context, 'holding' is given form through the therapist's attunement and adjustment to the client's experience, emotions and needs A therapeutic 'holding' relationship is one based on trust and acceptance (Barnes, Ernst and Hyde 1999).

That first session was defined by a developing sense of therapeutic holding and by connection through the therapist mirroring Patrick's actions alongside him. Slowly, in session 3, Patrick and the therapist moved towards a different quality of the mirroring experience – they moved into facing each other, having moments of brief eye contact.

I felt that this was a significant change both in our relationship and in Patrick's interest in interacting with people. In my reflective journal for session 4, I wrote: 'I find Patrick and myself somewhere between the state of being and the state of doing.' I depicted my somatic responses regarding this state with small dots (which were originally light blue). In accompaniment, I wrote, 'Movements in the air. Small, cute jumps in the air' (see Figure 17.2). This imagery with the small dots reflected the fleeting moments of interaction between Patrick and me (e.g. moments of brief, but significant, eye contact).

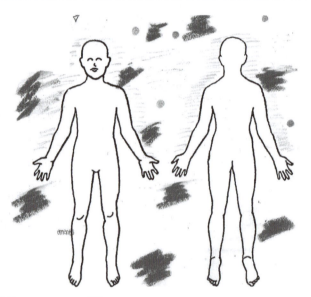

FIGURE 17.2 BODY DIAGRAM 1 [10]

Following Patrick's lead, the next few sessions were marked by shared sensorimotor explorations involving various props. Patrick and the therapist found ways to sense the texture and weight of beanbags, ribbons and small balls and to use these props to touch different parts of their bodies. For example, they put beanbags on heads, hands, arms, toes and knees, whilst exploring different ways of gesturing, posturing and moving. Patrick seemed to respond well to these sensory experiences. Sensorimotor activities have the potential to facilitate the development of a child's body image – defining that image and helping her to differentiate herself from other aspects of the environment and, as such, relate to other people (Erfer 1995). Multi-sensory games help an infant to

10 Each body diagram refers to a different session with the group, and not only to the particular relationship established between therapist and each child. This means that the qualities of different relationships can be found on the same body diagram, if they are linked to the same session.

integrate his sensory world – he learns that his visual world maps directly onto his auditory and haptic worlds, in one holistic experience (Stern 1985). Patrick was exploring his sense of self and finding meaning in his reality. He felt safe and confident enough to move away from the window. From session 4 onwards, Patrick and the therapist enjoyed jumping together, throwing balls in the air and throwing beanbags to each other in close synchrony. These activities supported Patrick and the therapist in finding and developing shared rhythms of movement. Moving in synchrony is of great therapeutic value as it supports bonding, interaction, communication and empathy. Throughout all of these experiences in process, Patrick would self-regulate by moving back to his known experience by the window. He could then engage again on his terms. Patrick's need to do this was always respected; the therapist's intention was to support him feel confident to express himself as and when he desired.

The therapist's somatic responses regarding her developing relationship with Patrick (up until session 5) were:

I had a strong need to rub my legs and the floor with my arms whilst sitting on the floor. This movement gradually led me to open my arms in the air, expand my kinesphere[11] (observing my arms and opening my gaze to the environment around me).

After session 5:

I had the desire to stand up and make some steps in the space. I felt that previously, rubbing legs and floor were as if Patrick was preparing himself to initiate more movements and interact more with me. Opening my arms in the air and making my kinesphere bigger (bringing more awareness of my environment) resonated with my experience when I observed Patrick walking away from the window, having eye contact with me and using the props. My somatic response to stand up and make steps resembled my belief that Patrick had acquired a stronger sense of self, was more aware of his desires and had enriched his movement repertoire.

From session 6 onwards, Patrick started to present with newly acquired movement and communication skills (some verbal). He was now moving far away from the window. He was moving in close with his peers, had started naming objects, and laughing, whilst continuing to maintain a close relationship with the therapist. Patrick, with the support of the therapist, appeared to have found a way into the world of this group.

---

11   The kinesphere: the three-dimensional space around the body which can be reached by extending limbs without making steps (Bartenieff and Lewis 2002).

'From chaos to containment': Relationship between Ben and the therapist

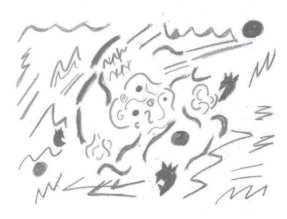

FIGURE 17.3 IMAGE 2: CREATING PATHWAYS

Ben displayed many social skills. He interacted with his classmates and teachers, used verbal language and suggested ideas for games to his classmates. However, Ben could not always regulate his emotions, especially his enthusiasm. This became intrusive when Ben tried to persuade other people to follow his suggestions and way of doing things. Ben was referred to the DMP group to give him a different type of exploration into social relating. The hope was that Ben might learn to interact more successfully with other people, including developing a respect for their desires and ways of doing things.

> My relationship with Ben started with an experience of chaos. Ben would run through the space, speaking in a loud voice, whilst I tried to hold all this vigorous way of being. Ben sometimes annoyed the other two children as he invaded their personal space and pushed them accidentally. This socially awkward connection was Ben's way of inviting me and the children to join him in his running. The sharp shapes in Figure 17.3 (originally red) represent my perceived feeling of Ben's way of being. I felt contradicted. I felt the need to handle Ben's experience (to control it to some degree) whilst still validating his willingness to initiate action and interact with the group members.

Reflecting on the following two interactions helped the therapist to understand how Ben might be supported to express himself in a more contained way and therefore be more able to build relationships. In session 2, the therapist invited the children to think of their favourite animal and embody it. Ben chose to move like a dog. He engaged in a 'run and fetch' activity with the therapist, which was repeated several times. Ben became more and more interested in this type of interaction with the therapist. As his interest and engagement deepened so, it seemed, did Ben's ability to regulate his own energy.

My somatic response came as an image of a shape with distinct pathways. The response was imbued with a feeling that embodied activity could support Ben to channel his forceful energy into creative play. So, I encouraged Ben to deepen his involvement with the 'run and fetch' game, by joining him in this play.

The in sync quality of this activity enabled a deepening of the connection between Ben and the therapist. In turn, this led to more sharing through further embodiment activities that developed spontaneously, such as pushing and pulling hands. There is literature mentioning that embodiment play supports the development of relationships (Tytherleigh and Karkou 2010) and offers the child skills to join the social world (Jennings 1999).

In session 3, Ben pretended to be a ghost by hiding himself under a big cloth. He then ran through space, approached other group members and made big and sudden movements and sounds to 'threaten' them. This seemed to irritate the other two children. The therapist decided to hide herself under the same cloth, pretending to be another ghost – connecting with Ben through his chosen symbol, while misattuning to his big and quick movements and loud voices. Stern (1985) discusses the concept of 'purposeful misattunement' when a mother intentionally over-matches or under-matches her baby's rhythms and intensity in order to change the baby's level of activity or affect. 'Purposeful misattunement' is one of a powerful range of tools that a mother will use to deepen experiences of emotional co-regulation for her child. The therapist misattuned to Ben's high-energy-level rhythms whenever she felt that Ben's level of activity did not support him to participate in the group. For example, the therapist purposefully misattuned to Ben's quick and abrupt movements by using same body parts and rhythm, but more gentle and softer movement qualities. Ben seemed to respond well to this type of interaction. His own movements and initiations became more contained (whilst his energy and intention remained empowered and positive) enabling more social potential.

My somatic experience, in relation to Ben's transition from a chaotic to a more contained way of being, was to move around and in front of piles of chairs. I had the need to have something concrete next to me in order not to move chaotically. The piles of chairs were acting as a point of reference in my mind that I could use in order to structure my movement away or near them and through the space. In my reflective journal I wrote: 'Interacting with Ben, through sound and embodied activities, supports our in-between relationship while feeling a sense of containment.' I depicted this experience in Figure 17.4 by making small shapes all around the body figures. To me, this represented my perception of a containing external somatic layer.

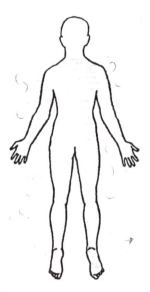

FIGURE 17.4 BODY DIAGRAM 2

Leading into, and including the last two sessions (7 and 8) Ben was more aware of personal boundaries and had clearly developed a degree of respect for other people's personal space.

The more gentle shapes in the centre of Figure 17.3 depict my experience in relation to Ben's more contained way of being.

'Following…': Relationship between Philip and the therapist

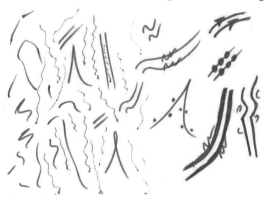

FIGURE 17.5 IMAGE 3: FINDING YOU

Philip used some verbal language, presenting echolalia, repetition and verbal content that was not relevant to the communicative context. Philip's movement patterns were also typical of an ASD presentation, including walking on his tiptoes, spinning and clapping his hands. He sometimes participated in classroom group activities but at other times appeared withdrawn, often talking to himself. On entering the therapeutic space, it was clear that Philip was able to make some eye contact with the members of the group and was confident enough to continue to maintain his level of verbal language. However, Philip did not interact with the therapist to any significant degree until after session 4.

> Philip seemed more interested in wandering in space, holding two small dolls in his hands, moving with his arms high in the air and talking to himself. I started mirroring his movement patterns, also moving my arms in the air whilst walking next to him, matching Philip's rhythms. Philip did not seem irritated or anxious by my close proximity, but neither did he seem to pay much attention. In my reflective journal for session 4 I noted, 'I feel disconnected and I don't know what to do.' I felt irritated by this. My somatic response regarding the lack of interaction between Philip and me was that of emptiness felt in my body. In my drawing I depicted this somatic experience by keeping the body figures blank (see Figure 17.2).

However, the therapist continued mirroring Philip, supporting his 'story' in the air, giving time to both of them to find how they could connect to each other. Eventually, in session 5, Philip showed overt interest in being mirrored by the therapist. The quality of their interaction shifted.

> Philip stopped wandering in space, stood opposite me and faced me directly. We sat down on the floor together and began a spontaneous movement interaction through touching and moving our hands. I wrote the following in my reflective journal: 'My interactions with Phillip are short, but, eventually, there is something happening between us'. The parallel (originally blue) lines in Figure 17.5 represent how our mirroring interactions supported Philip and me to find a way to relate to each other while being involved in movement. This type of interaction was repeated again in session 6.

Mirroring is a clinical tool that is widely used by dance movement psychotherapists when working with many different client groups. Mirroring can help a child with ASD to start noticing his external environment. Mirroring is a tool with which the therapist can communicate her empathy and develop a deep connection with the child (Erfer 1995; Wengrower 2010).

Interestingly, Philip's stereotyped movements (such as spinning) were less apparent when he was engaged in mirrored movement interactions with the therapist. It seemed that mirroring supported Philip to feel comfortable and self-aware of his way of moving and prompted him to create new gestures and movements. Through the mirroring process Philip appeared to have the opportunity to improvise with new movements and expand his movement vocabulary. This was a key factor in his interactions with the therapist. It seemed that the developing relationship with the therapist helped Philip to integrate his social skills and enabled him to enter the group relationship that followed.

'The window opened!': Group relationship

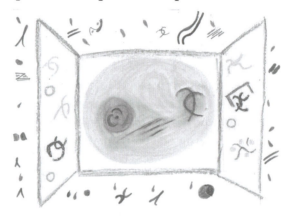

Figure 17.6 Image 4: Here we are!

Although brief group interactions occurred from the beginning of the therapeutic intervention, the development of a group relationship became apparent in the last two sessions (7 and 8). It was here that, for the first time, all the children became involved in the same role playing activity for a sustained period of time. During this interaction the children shared the same space, appeared aware of each other, laughed and shared similar rhythms of engagement and arousal.

My somatic response after session 7 was to make big shapes with my arms while running through the space. For me this movement resonated with my felt understanding that all the children had become more active, filling the space with creative activities. In my reflection on this session I filled a body diagram with clear shapes (originally drawn in vivid colours) (see Figure 17.7). It felt like all the previous sessions were preparing the way for the establishment of the group relationship. In my journal for session 6 I drew an image depicting this potential: a pink, vivid circle – I wrote, 'Something is floating amongst us (the children and me). It is warm.'

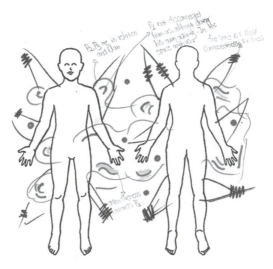

FIGURE 17.7 BODY DIAGRAM 3

It became apparent that role-playing was enabling group members to share emotions, ideas and personal motivations and, in doing so, expand the nature of their relationships. For example, the 'policeman game', a game that was created by the children and supported by the therapist in session 7, allowed them to take turns in playing the role of the 'policeman'. As each child took on the role he could share his contours of excitement and personal rhythms of engagement with the others. Together the children explored so many different social dynamics. Philip attempted to protect Patrick and the therapist from the 'policeman' played by Ben (who remained much more active and sometimes unaware of personal boundaries). But at the same time, Ben (who *had* progressed in *his* felt understanding of social limits) seemed more careful not to bump into the other children. Ben would shout warning instructions as a verbal reminder for the need to protect each group member's personal space. Although Patrick was less active compared to Ben and Philip, he did join in the group game and called the other children by their names. The shapes in the centre of Figure 17.7 illustrate the co-existence of the group members, whilst simultaneously portraying the differing levels of communication and cooperation in their in-between interactions. Each child brought various and different aspects of himself in the therapy – emotional, physical, verbal and relational – which are depicted as shapes all around the image's central theme. Validating, including and supporting each one of these aspects to evolve through interaction paved the way for the establishment of the one-to-one relationships and later for the development of the group relationship as a whole. We feel honoured having had the opportunity to explore all these relational dynamics and deepen our knowledge through our involvement in this case study.

Acknowledgements

We would like to express our gratitude to the children that participated in this study as well as to the school and the parents who gave their consent for the implementation of the study.

References

Adler, J. (1970) *Looking for Me.* DVD. Directed by Janet Adler. Berkeley, CA: Berkeley Media.

Alvarez, A., Reid, S. and Hodges, S. (1999) 'Autism and play: the work of the Tavistock autism workshop.' *Child Language Teaching and Therapy 15*, 1, 53–64.

Axline, V. (1971) *Dibs: In Search of Self. Personality Development in Play Therapy.* Harmondsworth: Penguin.

Barnes, B., Ernst, S. and Hyde, K. (1999) *An Introduction to Groupwork: A Group-Analytic Perspective.* New York: Palgrave.

Baron-Cohen, S., Cow, A., Baird, G., Swettenham, J. *et al.* (1996) 'Psychological markers in the detection of autism in infancy in a large population.' *British Journal of Psychiatry 168*, 2, 158–163.

Bartenieff, I. and Lewis, D. (2002) *Body Movement: Coping with the Environment.* New York and London: Routledge.

Batavia, M. (2001) *Clinical Research for Health Professionals: A User-Friendly Guide.* Boston, MA: Butterworth-Heinemann.

Bowlby, J. (1988) *A Secure Base: Parent–Child Attachment and Healthy Human Development.* London: Routledge.

Braun, V. and Clarke, V. (2006) 'Using thematic analysis in psychology.' *Qualitative Research in Psychology 3*, 2, 17–36.

Burford, B. (1991) 'Communicating Through Movement and Posture.' In W.I. Fraser, R.C. McGillivray and A.M. Green (eds) *Caring for People with Mental Handicaps.* (8th edn) Oxford: Butterworth-Heinemann.

Cesaroni, L. and Garber, M. (1991) 'Exploring the experiences of autism through first-hand accounts.' *Journal of Autism and Developmental Disorders 21*, 303–313.

Chaiklin, S. and Schmais, D. (1986) 'The Chace Approach to Dance Therapy.' In P. Lewis Bernstein (ed.) *Theoretical Approaches in Dance-Movement Therapy*, Vol. 1. Dubuque, IA: Kendall/Hunt.

Ciccone, A. (2012) 'L'eclosion de la vie psychique.' In A. Ciccone, Y. Gauthier, B. Golse and D. Stern (eds) *Naissance et développement de la vie Psychique.* Toulouse: eres.

Clarkson, P. (2003) *The Therapeutic Relationship.* London and Philadelphia, PA: Whurr Publishers.

Erfer, T. (1995) 'Treating Children with Autism in a Public School System.' In F.J. Levy (ed.) *Dance and Other Expressive Art Therapies: When Words are Not Enough.* New York: Routledge.

Finley, S. (2005) 'Arts-based Inquiry.' In N.K. Denzin and Y.S. Lincoln (eds) *The SAGE Handbook of Qualitative Research.* (3rd edn) London: Sage.

Fischman, D. (2009) 'Therapeutic Relationships and Kinesthetic Empathy'. In S. Chaiklin and H. Wengrower (eds) *The Art and Science of Dance/Movement Therapy: Life is Dance.* New York and Hove: Routledge.

Greenspan, S.I. and Wieder, S. (2006) *Engaging Autism: Using the Floortime Approach to Help Children Relate, Communicate, and Think.* Philadelphia, PA: Da Capo.

Hervey, L. (2000) *Artistic Inquiry in Dance/Movement Therapy.* Springfield, IL: Charles C. Thomas.

Hervey, L. (2004) 'Artistic Inquiry in Dance/Movement Therapy.' In R.F. Cruz and C.F. Berrol (eds) *Dance/Movement Therapists in Action: A Working Guide to Research Options.* Springfield, IL: Charles C. Thomas.

Hobson, R.P. (1993) *Autism and the Development of Mind.* Hove: Redwood Books.

Jennings, S. (1999) *Introduction to Developmental Playtherapy.* London: Jessica Kingsley Publishers.

Karkou, V. and Sanderson, P. (2006) *Arts Therapies: A Research-based Map of the Field.* London: Elsevier Churchill Livingstone.

Katagiri, M., Inada, N. and Kamio, Y. (2010) 'Mirroring effect in 2- and 3-year-olds with autism spectrum disorder.' *Research in Autism Spectrum Disorders 4,* 474–478.

Kugiumutzakis, J.E. (1993) 'Intersubjective Vocal Imitation in Early Mother–Infant Interaction.' In J. Nadel and L. Camaioni (eds) *New Perspectives in Early Communicative Development.* London: Routledge.

Leavy, P. (2009) *Method Meets Art: Arts-Based Research Practice.* New York: Guilford Press.

Meekums, B. (1993) 'Research as an Act of Creation.' In H. Payne (ed.) *Handbook of Inquiry in the Arts Therapies: One River, Many Currents.* London: Jessica Kingsley Publishers.

Meltzoff, A.N. (1990) 'Foundations for Developing a Concept of Self: The Role of Imitation in Relating Self to Other and the Value of Social Mirroring, Social Modeling, and Self Practice in Infancy.' In D. Cicchetti and M. Beeghley (eds) *The Self in Transition: Infancy to Childhood.* Chicago: University of Chicago Press.

Meltzoff, A.N. and Brooks, R. (2007) 'Intersubjectivity before Language: Three Windows on Preverbal Sharing.' In S. Braten (ed.) *On Being Moved: From Mirror Neurons to Empathy.* Philadelphia, PA: John Benjamins.

Moore, J. (2008) *Playing, Laughing and Learning with Children on the Autism Spectrum: A Practical Resource of Play Ideas for Parents and Carers.* (2nd edn) London: Jessica Kingsley Publishers.

Mundy, P., Sigman, M., Ungerer, J. and Sherman, T. (1987) 'Nonverbal communication and play correlates of language development in autistic children.' *Journal of Autism and Developmental Disorders 17,* 3, 349–364.

Nadel, J. and Peze, A. (1993) 'Immediate Imitation as a Basis for Primary Communication in Toddlers and Autistic Children.' In J. Nadel and L. Camioni (eds) *New Perspectives in Early Communication Development.* London: Routledge.

Pallaro, P. (2010) 'Somatic Countertransference: The Therapist in Relationship.' In P. Pallaro (ed.) *Authentic Movement: Moving the Body, Moving the Self, Being Moved. A Collection of Essays,* Vol. 2. London: Jessica Kingsley Publishers.

Powers, N. and Trevarthen, C. (2009) 'Voices of Shared Emotion and Meaning: Young Infants and Their Mothers in Scotland and Japan.' In S. Malloch and C. Trevarthen (eds) *Communicative Musicality: Exploring the Basis of Human Companionship.* New York: Oxford University Press.

Rogers, C.R. (1967) *On Becoming a Person: A Therapist's View of Psychotherapy.* London: Constable.

Rogers, S.J. and Pennington, B.F. (1991) 'A theoretical approach to the deficits in infantile autism.' *Development and Psychopathology 3,* 137–162.

Scharoun, S.M., Reinders, N.J, Bryden, P.J. and Fletcher, P.C. (2014) 'Dance/movement therapy as an intervention for children with autism spectrum disorders.' *American Journal of Dance Therapy 36,* 2, 209–228.

Schwandt, T.A. (2000) 'Three Epistemological Stances for Qualitative Inquiry.' In N.K. Denzin and Y.S. Lincoln (eds) *The Handbook of Qualitative Research.* (2nd edn) London, New Delhi: Sage.

Sherborne, V. (2001) *Developmental Movement for Children: Mainstream, Special Needs and Pre-school.* (2nd edn) London: Worth Publishing.

Siegel, E.V. (1963) 'Movement therapy with autistic children.' *Psychoanalytic Review 60,* 1, 141–149.

Sigman, M. and Capps, L. (1997) *Children with Autism: A Developmental Perspective.* Cambridge, MA: Harvard University Press.

Stern, D.N. (1985) *The Interpersonal World of the Infant.* New York: Basic Books.

Stern, D.N. (2005) 'Intersubjectivity.' In E.S. Person, A.M. Cooper and G.O. Gobbard (eds) *Textbook of Psychoanalysis.* Washington, DC: American Psychiatric Publishing.

Stern, D.N. (2012) 'Le processus de changement therapeutique.' In A. Ciccone, Y. Gauthier, B. Golse and D. Stern (eds) Naissance et développement de la vie Psychique. Toulouse: eres.

Stone, W.L., Lee, E.B., Ashford, L., Brissis, J. *et al.* (1999) 'Can autism be diagnosed accurately in children under 3 Years?' *Journal of Child Psychology and Psychiatry 40,* 2, 219–226.

Tortora, S. (2006) *The Dancing Dialogue: Using the Communicative Power of Movement with Young Children.* Baltimore, MD: Paul H. Brookes Publishing.

Trevarthen, C. (2005) 'Stepping Away from the Mirror: Pride and Shame in Adventures of Companionship. Reflections on the Nature and Emotional Needs of Infant Intersubjectivity.' In C.S. Carter, L. Ahnert, K.E. Grossman, S.B. Hardy *et al.* (eds) *Attachment and Bonding: A New Synthesis.* Boston, MA: The MIT Project.

Trevarthen, C. and Daniel, S. (2005) 'Disorganized rhythm and synchrony: early signs of autism and Rett syndrome.' *Brain and Development 27*, 25–34.

Trevarthen, C., Aitken, K., Papoudi, D. and Robarts, J. (1998) *Children with Autism: Diagnosis and Interventions to Meet Their Needs.* (2nd edn) London: Jessica Kingsley Publishers.

Tytherleigh, L. and Karkou, V. (2010) 'Dramatherapy, Autism and Relationship Building: A Case Study.' In V. Karkou (ed.) *Arts Therapies in School: Research and Practice.* London: Jessica Kingsley Publishers.

Wengrower, H. (2010) 'I Am Here to Move and Dance with You: Dance Movement Therapy with Children with Autism Spectrum Disorder and Pervasive Developmental Disorders.' In V. Karkou (ed.) *Arts Therapies in School: Research and Practice.* London: Jessica Kingsley Publishers.

Whittaker, C.A. (1996) 'Spontaneous Proximal Communication in Children with Autism and Severe Learning Disabilities: Issues for Therapeutic Intervention.' In *Therapeutic Intervention in Autism: Perspectives from Research and Practice. A Collection of Papers.* Durham: Autism Research Unit.

Wimpory, R., Hobson, R.P., Williams, M.G. and Nash, S. (2000) 'Are infants with autism socially engaged? A study of recent retrospective parental reports.' *Journal of Autism and Developmental Disorders 30*, 6, 525–536.

Wing, L. (1981) 'Language, Social, and Cognitive Impairments in Autism and Severe Mental Retardation.' *Journal of Autism and Developmental Disorders 11*, 1, 31–44.

Wing, L. (1996) *The Autistic Spectrum: A Guide for Parents and Professionals.* London: Constable.

Wing, L. and Gould, J. (1979) 'Severe impairments of social interaction and associated abnormalities in children: epidemiology and classification.' *Journal of Autism and Childhood Schizophrenia 9*, 11–29.

Winnicott, D.W. (2005) *Playing and Reality.* London: Routledge.

Yalom, I.D. and Leszcz, M. (2005) *The Theory and Practice of Group Psychotherapy.* (5th edn) New York: Basic Books.

18

COLLECTIVE MUSICALITY

Stories of Healing from Companhia de Música
Teatral and Other Musical Projects

HELENA RODRIGUES AND PAULO MARIA RODRIGUES

Overture: Defining the universes from where stories come

Music is an infinite universe: it is fruition, expression, communication, art, a
facet of the construction of self, an element of human development and so much
more. Music is inscribed in our biology and in the culture of all societies. It plays
a key role in the development of our individual and collective consciousness
and is one of the factors that contribute to the integral development of every
human being.

For Companhia de Música Teatral (CMT), the discovery of new ideas,
the search for relationships amongst different types of expression, the musical
development of people and the promotion of cooperation through music are
important and fertile territories to explore. CMT is an arts company based
in Portugal. At CMT, our love is to create artistic and educational projects
that develop and play with various techniques and languages of artistic
communication. In all our work, music is the basis for interaction.

Over the years, the manner in which we conceive our work at CMT has
changed. Deeply rooted in artistic experience, we came to realize that our
creative work has strong therapeutic and educational implications. We came to
conceive and nurture our work in a manner that would allow emphasis on the
creation, exploration and development of fruitful relationships. We proposed
the term 'artistic–educative constellations' to define a working model and
metaphor for our vision.[1] The metaphor provides us with a poetic sense of a

---

1   The 'artistic–educative constellations' model has deepened through cooperation with the
    Laboratory of Music and Infant Communication at the CESEM (Centro de Sociologia e Estética
    Musical) research unit at FCSH (Faculdade de Ciências Sociais e Humanas, Universidade NOVA
    de Lisboa) and at DeCA (Departamento de Comunicação e Arte, Universidade de Aveiro).

universe yet to be discovered, an objective and a strong analytical framework in which different 'bodies' interact through conceptual and aesthetic 'forces' or 'fields'.[2] We will expand on these ideas as we go on to explore the detail of our work with infants, children and parent–baby partnerships.

Our work with music in child development began in 1994 when we developed guided musical sessions for parent–baby partnerships, and for infants in a nursery.[3] The observations that came from these settings became the seeds for CMT's musical theater work – addressed to very young children and their families – including our first presentation of *Bebé Babá* in 2001. The *Bebé Babá* project[4] develops over five or six weeks, and involves a combination of parent–baby workshops and workshops for just the parents. This process culminates in a final festival on stage, allowing all the community to share the joy of making music together. The purposes of the project are: to enrich the musical and artistic life of the participants, to widen the artistic experiences of caregivers through exploring their expressive capacities in terms of voice and body, to share modalities of communication which foster parent–baby attachment, and to promote ongoing social relationships in the community through music. Even though the concept and structure of *Bebé Babá* remained constant throughout its several editions, its content changed according to the needs and the musical background of the participants. For example, when we presented *Bebé Babá* for mothers and their babies in a prison in 2008[5] this special edition included songs, mood tone and musical materials which reflected the ethnic origin of many of the participants.

The importance of early musical experiences has been emphasized in our work, and besides *Bebé Babá* we have created different types and formats of artistic interaction for infants and their caregivers. A good example is *AliBaBach*. This is a show for parents and babies, which explores the universe of J.S. Bach as an element of mediation for musical communication. *AliBaBach* was inspired by Bach's *Goldberg Variations* in a free exercise wherein elements of each variation gave rise to new tableaux that combine music, dance and theater. *AliBaBach* is grounded in rich, contrasting musical characteristics and explores the fundamental elements of musical speech and its comprehension (such as

---

2   This concept has emerged organically throughout our work over the years and has been consolidated more recently within the framework of Opus Tutti – a project supported by Fundação Calouste Gulbenkian that aims to develop good practice of an artistic nature that can contribute to a better quality of life in early infancy.

3   This work was inspired by our meeting with one of the most impressive music education leaders in the world, Edwin Gordon, and his book *Music Learning Theory for Newborns and Preschool Children* (1990). Our first presentation of *Bebé Babá* was dedicated to Edwin.

4   At the invitation of Colwyn Trevathen (another great source of inspiration to us) we reflected on the *Bebé Babá* experience in the book *Communicative Musicality* (Malloch and Trevarthen 2008). The *Bebé Babá* project has been unanimously recognized for its role in fostering very high levels of interaction and social impact (Rodrigues *et al.* 2010).

5   In collaboration with the Education Service of Casa da Música in Oporto.

tonal and rhythmic patterns). It is rooted in the voices of two interpreters, approached with plasticity through games based on musical elements and with clear references to various folk and cosmopolitan influences of vocal music. It is an invitation for parents and babies to enter into music (and that of Bach in particular) with ears and eyes wide open.

Bebé Babá and *AliBaBach* are productions that represent extremely different possibilities in the design of artistic creation for the early years. The first one results from a musical participatory process; the second one is mostly a contemplative action. Varied experiences such as these have led us to the belief that we are all born with the ability to process musical stimuli and that predispositions for music appear very early in infancy. Our observations along the way have shown us that, from birth, music is a very special channel of communication between human beings. Much of our early development as interacting, communicating beings is through processes that involve musical activity. We have been using the tools of 'musicality' (Malloch and Trevarthen 2008) to interpret the roots of connection, contact and community within our work.

A special type of community can emerge quite naturally within the context of shared musical experience (Barriga, Rodrigues and Rodrigues 2013). The implicit 'rules' of music (such as rhythm and pulse) are sensed by, and in, the bodies of listeners. These sensed 'rules', when uninhibited, translate spontaneously to impulse and musical action (as, for example, when a parent taps a baby's back according to a felt and/or heard pulse beat). That pulse and corresponding impulse flows from the single listener into the partnership (in our example, the parent–baby dyad). The baby then responds. But it is interesting to observe the extent to which the musical participation of babies is reinforced or limited according to models that their parents transmit: 'Is my father/mother singing? So, I'll sing too!' The potential flow of shared musical experience truly combines musical *and* social agreements.

The flow of musical experience from a single listener to the shared experience of community can be described metaphorically as a 'domino effect': music produces spontaneous responses in infants (such as body movements and vocalizations) that affect their caregivers and vice versa. The domino effect also moves naturally beyond the single partnership. When a caregiver and an infant are musically involved, their involvement easily spreads to other dyads. This effect is magnified when musical practice occurs in groups identifying strongly with a collective experience of parenthood – the conjunction of music and parenthood in shared experience is powerful in supporting the emergence of a special type of community (Barriga *et al.* 2013).

We also propose the same 'domino effect' to explain the catalytic effect that subtle communication seems to play in establishing a contemplative audience of parents and babies when they enjoy an arts performance together. We propose the ideas of 'listening engagement' and 'aesthetic appreciation' – as equivalents of 'joint attention' in dyadic learning (Stern 1985) – to describe transient states of empathy between the artistic discourse, the artists and the public. Music itself elicits a 'collective intersubjectivity' leading to 'perfect moments' in which an entire audience shares the passage of time in a mood of wonderment.

In several of our performances for parents and babies, external observers have felt a kind of magical atmosphere permeating the group (see Figure 18.1). Even though the specific feelings/emotions/thoughts of each person in the audience might not be clear, there is a palpable sense that the entire audience are in a shared energetic space. They are connected. This sense of being together in delight – accompanied by the pleasure of our bodies moving, hearing harmonious sound – could be interpreted as a social reinforcer or reward. The collective experience of sharing music clearly nurtures our impulse to cooperate and, as such, survive as a species. It looks as though the roots of musical expression define a matrix in belonging to the human 'tribe'. The impulse to cooperate musically and the need to belong to a group seem to be embodied – physically and spiritually – from a very early age.

In the next section we report and comment on a series of situations that have occurred in different projects over the years. This collection of short episodes is an attempt to illustrate how our beliefs and theory have been nurtured by direct observation of what happens when we work musically.

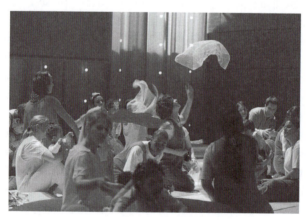

FIGURE 18.1 BEBÉ BABÁ – COMPANHIA DE MÚSICA TEATRAL

Stories about collective musicality in thirteen short episodes

Episode #1

During a session of *Orientações Musicais para a Infância* (music workshops for parents and babies), workshop leaders were improvising rhythmically, chanting with their voices. Infants were moving their torsos, their hands and their bodies. Unexpectedly, the workshop leaders moved into a patch of silence and created a long pause. Then, a 14-month-old child clapped and demanded, 'More!'

Comments

When we watch infants participating in a musical activity we can observe vocal production and body movement (physical expressions with hands, arms, torso and feet are impressive). Reigado, Rocha and Rodrigues (2011) have demonstrated that there are certain vocalizations that are *specifically* produced in response to musical stimuli. In addition to these observable behaviors it is evident, from an early age, that infants well integrated into a musical group demonstrate that they really want to be part of it. We have seen infants taking initiatives which animate the whole group. When they are familiar with the songs, for example, it is not uncommon that they 'lead the show'. The need to belong is probably one of the main impulses we are born with. Music provides an opportunity.

Episode #2

After attending 'Opus 2', one of a set of portable musical and theatrical pieces in the *Opus Tutti* project for presentation in daycare facilities and kindergartens (called *Portable Play to Play*[6]), a three-year-old child addressed the actress, saying, 'I liked it. I want to come again tomorrow.'

Comments

From a very early age children understand the meaning of mutual appreciation. A 'stage instinct' is revealed either when a baby presents something to be applauded or when he/she appreciates what someone else has presented. Even though spontaneous vocalizations and rhythmical movements can be interpreted as natural physiological reactions we have no doubt that, from a very early age, there is clear intentionality in their minds.

---

6   www.musicateatral.com/papi/en

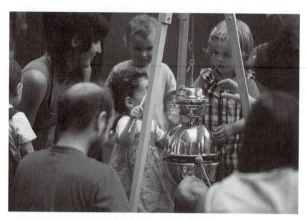

FIGURE 18.2 *Opus Tutti* – Companhia de Música Teatral

Episode #3

An infant born prematurely was participating in *Bebé Babá*. She was also undertaking physiotherapy sessions since she was facing difficulties with her motor development, particularly with standing up and walking. Surprisingly, she began to stand up at the general rehearsal and walked her first steps during the final show. Her mother came to us and, with raw emotion, said, 'Thank you! Bebé Babá has done much more for my daughter than ten sessions of physiotherapy.'

Comments

We certainly hadn't produced a miracle, and we do believe that the physiotherapy sessions were also valuable to this child. Perhaps the combination of the enjoyable and relaxing atmosphere of *Bebé Babá* and its movement activities were helpful stimuli for this child. Perhaps what this child had been lacking, up until this point, was the engaged impulse to move? We wonder if the collective musical experience held the child energetically and within this support also provided the movement momentum (the impulse) to initiate stepping. The felt pulse of the music draws out the pulse of stepping. Relating this idea to our 'artistic-educative-constellation' model in which different 'bodies' interact through conceptual and aesthetic 'forces' or 'fields', we could say that this child was held in a 'collective artistic field' and within this field she felt the integral 'pulse' of the shared music and was driven to move by it. In other words, the collective pulse became her individual impulse.

Episode #4

We have participated in an exploratory study of mother–infant group therapy in a residential Mother–Baby Unit for mothers with postnatal depression in Belgium.[7] We decided on a collective composition: a song whose lyrics included the nicknames that mothers would suggest for their own kids. At first there weren't any nicknames, just emptiness and silence. Step by step, we adopted physical theatre strategies with the mothers – for example, encouraging them to rock each other – facilitating a supportive group. Step by step, each mother created a nickname for her own baby, often inspired by other mothers' nicknames. Step by step, their voices filled the initial emptiness and silence. We modeled examples of playing with the infants, we sung and rocked for them. The mothers sung together, and sung for their babies and rocked them. At the end of the intervention, a participating mother said to us, 'Thank you! You showed me how to do it! I had no idea!'

Comments

It is difficult for a mother to feel how to connect with her baby, difficult for her to know how to take care if that mother missed out on receiving such experiences in her own infancy. But luckily that is not the end of the story. Taking care of someone can be learned in later life, simply through shared vivid experiences and human contact. Opportunities to observe, experience and to take the role of creating appropriate models for human interaction can be fostered. Some people are isolated; motherhood/parenthood is something that needs to be nurtured.

> Listening to someone singing a lullaby for a baby or observing someone rocking a baby is, somehow, a vicarious experience that can help to make up for missed lullabies and missed care. With proper guidance, getting involved in childcare can be a means to face one's own damaged childhood. To sing a lullaby for a baby evokes our deepest inner voices. (Rodrigues *et al.* 2010, p.79)

We have been observing the way that early bonds between parents and babies are established through musical interactions. Parents have 'intuitive propensities' to communicate musically with their babies (Malloch and Trevarthen 2008; Papousek 1996). Nevertheless, our contemporary lifestyle can neglect the intrinsic musical nature of human interaction and often inhibits the expression of our innermost 'intuitive' communication tools. Sometimes parents need help to restore those capacities. We can help parents to recover their inner voices and

---

7   For a detailed description of the study see Van Puyvelde *et al.* (2014).

their capacity to play with their infants. Here, musical improvisation is such a useful tool.

Episode #5

The first day we arrived in Santa Cruz do Bispo prison, ready to begin the *Bebé Babá* workshops, many of the mothers were very defensive and all the babies were crying. At a certain point the atmosphere palpably changed. One of the workshop leaders initiated a 'peekaboo game' with one of the babies. The baby smiled. The mother smiled. Then, the baby laughed. Then the mother laughed. The fun and relaxation spread quickly and within minutes the entire group became engaged in collective 'peekaboo'.

Comments

'Peekaboo' is an intrinsically rhythmical game and a great example of musicality in action. As that first baby responded with synchronous signs of joy to 'peekaboo', it was fascinating for us to notice how this responsivity had a knock-on effect on the 'affective tuning' (Stern 1985) and engagement of all the mothers in the room. We have played with this aspect of the 'domino effect' in many different ways – supporting the initial impetus of the infant's natural response with a musical scaffolding to help develop the mother–infant relationship. And again, what often follows is a movement from individual impetus, to dyadic connection and flourish, and on to a collective energy. *Baboushka, baboushka!*

The special edition of *Bebé Babá* in prison reinforced our conviction that through appropriate musical guidance and personal support it is possible to help incarcerated mothers to recover their inner resources for communication – their 'voices of motherhood' – in order to promote quality interaction with their children. Furthermore, by recovering functional communication skills in company with their own babies (who are an embodied metaphor for future life) these women can be helped to restructure themselves.

> Very often imprisoned women reproduce a cycle of violence as a response to a lack of affective and attached relationships in their own childhoods. So, it is important to help them to see their own baby as an opportunity to rebuild their lost daughterhood. Sensitive musicians and therapists can use music and voice as tools to simultaneously go back to the childhood of the mother and ahead into the childhood of the infant. (Rodrigues *et al.* 2010, p.79)

Episode #6

A nine-month-old girl was attending a performance of *AliBaBach*. Her eyes were completely focused on the performers. Her mother was also focused on the performers. Her mother caressed her torso in time with the music. After a while she was no longer interested in watching. Instead she danced with the upper part of her body, and her mother watched her as yet another participant in the performance.

Comments

We look at artistic performances for parents and babies as opportunities to share a focus, an opportunity to uncover intimacies. Brazelton (2013) has identified 'lack of time for family rituals' as one of the stressors for those who raise children. We believe that artistic performances for parents and babies are examples of rituals that offer time and unity to families. It looks like we humans are ready to appreciate musical events and a felt sense of sharing in ritual from a very early age. It is also interesting to note the girl's engagement was multi-modal: in the beginning she expressed her involvement through looking, but after a while her entire upper body was involved.

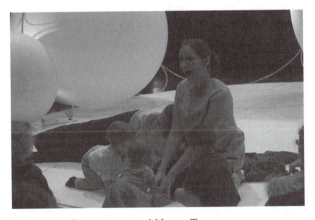

FIGURE 18.3 *AliBaBach* – COMPANHIA DE MÚSICA TEATRAL

Episode #7

'I was labeled tone deaf when I was a child. I come to these musical guidance sessions not just for my baby but also for myself,' said a father after a session of *Orientações Musicais para a Infância*.

Comments

Parents have found musical guidance sessions to be as good for themselves as for their babies. Besides nurturing babies musically and socially, musical guidance sessions are relaxed learning opportunities for parents: they often rediscover their own musicianship; they find new play resources and behavioral features in relationship with their children; and they share and develop their parental feelings through support from other members of the group.

Episode #8

'I decided to participate in the *Bebé Babá* project because I wanted to offer the best possible memories to my son during his last days [with me] in prison,' said one of the inmates. She would be separated from her child two weeks after the end of *Bebé Babá*, when he would turn four years old.

Comments

We did a follow-up interview with this participant mother. She told us that for the following year while she was alone in prison, and her son was living with her parents, she sang *Bebé Babá* songs to him whenever she phoned him. We hope that these memories will be a meaningful foundation for this boy and that music can awaken in him a strong connection with life and that he can find opportunities to participate musically with his community.

Episode #9

'You have to record the songs we have been learning during these workshops! My daughter, two and half years old, mixes up all the lyrics and melodies and I've been trying to correct her!' said a mother after a session of *Afinação do Ouvir* in the *Opus Tutti* Project. 'Your daughter is doing a good job. She is composing a "potpourri" song. Play with her and encourage her musical and language discoveries!' we replied.

Comments

Parents, like all of us, should be aware that human interaction is fundamental for learning. Papousek (1995) maintains that language acquisition and the development of musical skills can be indeterminately approached in early family interactions, as interrelated aspects of human communication in infancy. Singing, nursery rhymes, clapping, playing with dance and movement are all primary forms of communication that simultaneously incite the acquisition of maternal language and the development of musical competence. Pre-verbal communication established between parents and children is just as important linguistically as musically.

Episode #10

'I am no longer just the mother of my own son; I feel like a mother of all the children that are participating. I feel that other parents have the same feeling,' a mother told us at the end of the first edition of *Bebé Babá*.

Comments

It is interesting to observe how babies' spontaneous reactions to music stimulate parents to cooperate musically and socially. In our musical events it is very common for babies to vocalize or move to the music. These behaviors are rewards for the adult participants, recalling and restoring the fantasies of a magical childhood.

Babies open the gates of human kindness. And all agree that their own child is the best in the world!

Episode #11

During the special prison edition of *Bebé Babá*, some of the guards reported that mothers were studying together the lyrics of songs specifically composed for them. One of these songs included their names and the names of their babies; another included their babies' nicknames.

Comments

Mothers who were illiterate got help and support from their literate peers. Guards reported that during the project there were fewer conflicts and that the mothers were unified by the common goal of presenting a public performance. This seemed to be important for their self-esteem. As each mother was named in the songs they had a sense of becoming 'co-authors'. The opportunity to dance or sing alternating solos, with the musical support of the group, was one of the strategies that contributed to minimizing rivalry. Having their photo in a pamphlet, with their wishes for the future of their children, also reinforced their identity as mothers and emphasized hope for the future.

Episode #12

'And this way other people can see that we, people with cerebral palsy, can also make music. We might have difficulties walking and speaking, but we do know how to be on stage and perform,' says Joana at the close of a documentary directed by Pedro Sena Nunes about the *Icaro/Corpo Todo* project held at Casa da Música in 2008.

Comments

While coordinating the Educative Service at Casa da Música, the second author had the opportunity to develop a range of projects for people with physical and mental challenges. Throughout the year, these people would participate in many of the regular service events, frequently adapted or tailored to their specific needs. The festival *Ao Alcance de Todos* (Within Everyone's Reach) was a particularly important moment in the whole educational program, and many types of activities – from conferences and workshops to live performances (frequently involving music, dance and theater) – would be presented during that week. *Ícaro/Corpo Todo* was one of many projects in which children as well as adults were involved in creating and performing music. The quotation above is truly representative of the sense of satisfaction, pride, happiness and worthiness that was so often expressed by the participants.

Despite the vast potential of music to nurture communication among all people, music making and creating have evolved to be, to a great extent, activities dominated by people who have had intensive training on demanding instruments. A particular emphasis of the work at Casa da Música was to create and develop new approaches that would allow *everyone* to be involved in active musical relationships. And so people with certain disabilities, who may face many obstacles in their quest for self-expression through music, deserved special attention. We believe that music is an important aspect of everyone's development. This was exemplified many times by the role of musical experience in empowering disabled participants. So many positive, nurturing sentiments were expressed in a whole range of different manners: a 'sense of worth', 'belonging', 'connectedness', 'self-esteem', 'having a voice', 'being able to', 'achieving', as well as many non-verbal manifestations of deep emotional/psycho-sociological impact. We believe that through music it is possible to make a contribution to the general cause of empowering people with disabilities; fostering opportunities and access to activities that we believe contribute to happiness, dignity, wellbeing and human development. Making and creating music is a source of immense joy. People with disabilities have the right to access this experience.

Episode #13

Novas Linguagens is a project that is currently being implemented in three schools of Vila Nova de Famalicão, a municipality in the north of Portugal. Here, certain schools have dedicated rooms for children who need specialized help and whose mental or physical needs prevent their integration in a regular classroom. Each of these rooms is staffed by three or four professionals taking care of groups of up to six children, aged 6 to 12 years, diagnosed with syndromes as diverse as autism, cerebral palsy and non-specific cognitive deficit. The project aims to help these professionals to develop new ways to look at their daily routines and modes of interacting. It is grounded in the idea that non-verbal expression and artistic languages could be at the core of any successful intervention with children with these particular needs. We held music sessions in three facilities.

The experience of the sessions with the children was mixed. Some children engaged in attentive listening and gave positive feedback within the parameters of their experience, including body movements and the production of vocal sounds in clear attempts to engage in music making. Some showed a lot of interest in the Tibetan singing bowls that were used to produce sound, trying to feel the vibrations with their hands and other parts of their bodies including the tongue. Some, however, apparently ignored all musical initiations and a few showed occasional signs of distress and dislike. One situation was particularly striking. The following occurred within a session with four children with autism, all of whom displayed frequent challenging behaviors. One of the children, P., fully connected to the music and to one of the participating adults. After only a few initiations of close-proximity singing, P. spent the rest of the session embraced, gazing into the eyes of his adult partner, in a state of rapture. Two other children spent almost the entire session running erratically throughout the room. And another, J., was extremely disturbed by our presence and action, showing clear signs of anger and distress, to the point of becoming violent. At a certain stage, when all the adult participants were singing together, it was possible to engage J. in some moments of shared attention with one of the auxiliary staff cradling him against her body and moving his body with hers in a dance.

The following day we worked with educators from the three facilities as well as some young drama and dance artists about to begin a program of regular visits to the facilities. We followed the same strategies as in previous training sessions with educators and artists, fostering the discovery of personal abilities in the use of voice and body through creative exercises. These exercises gradually enable participants to express themselves through non-verbal means and build a sense of group. Simple informal games or improvisatory tasks are normally the starting point for further elaboration of voice and body discourses, which later reach the form of short performing tableaux combining music and movement. There were also moments for shared reflection about the work that had been done in their facilities the day before and, above all, about their normal routines, problems, expectations and their interest in finding new ways to work with the children. The lady who had worked so closely with P. in the example above told us that after we left P. was attached to her for the rest of the afternoon. When she went home and slept that night she had a dream in which P. started to speak. For the adult participants, a positive sense of achievement, relaxation and connection to the other people involved were the obvious results of this day of work. It is clear to us that the wellbeing of these adults is a major determinant of the wellbeing of the children they care for. Shared musical activities can certainly contribute to this wellbeing, as well as fostering changes in the perception these adults might have about child behavior and providing tools as modes of interaction.

Comments

> After many years of defending the idea that everyone is musical and having seen many times the positive effect that music has on people, the observation of some of these children's reactions, either absence or dislike, cast a shadow on my convictions… I also believe that the experience of deep communication I had with P., the child that got attached to me, was in essence musical, and by that I mean that it made me feel as in many musical situations when I am making music, playing or singing, with partner musicians. And, yet, that child could not sing or even speak. I therefore question what really is the essence of music and whether the presence of sound is a necessary condition. (Excerpt from 'Afterthoughts on Novas Linguagens'[8])

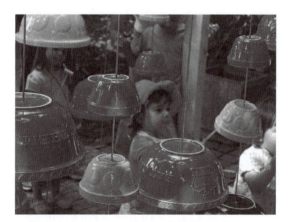

FIGURE 18.4 *Opus Tutti* – Companhia de Música Teatral

Coda: Redefining the universes where unfinished stories go

In short, Episodes from 1 through to 12 reinforced our belief that 'we are born musical' (Rodrigues and Rodrigues 2003, p.7[9]); so much of our early development as beings that communicate and interact occurs through processes

---

8   Part of the unpublished personal diary of Paulo Maria Rodrigues.
9   From the original foreword in English, by Colwyn Trevarthen.

that involve musicianship. We have been working with many people who are not only responsive to music but also able to integrate into a musical group, expressing some level of musical comprehension and participation.

Meanwhile, a question comes to our mind: how would the children described in Episode #13 have developed if they had been exposed to musical situations such as *Bebé Babá* and *AliBaBach* when they were babies? We brought our usual conception of music to our work reported in Episode 13. But, in certain children, we quickly observed a lack of common rhythmic sense and/ or a disruption of rhythmical synchronicity. We hypothesize that the type of listening required to facilitate musical interactions in a group was absent. Was it absent also when those children were infants?

Episode #13 pushed us to rethink what we mean by 'music', what is a 'musical being' and what our mission is as musicians trying to help people who might access music in ways different from our own. That short experience helped us to consider how difficult it can be to work under the conditions we observed at those particular facilities. The children seem to have very little in common. In fact, the only reason for them to be together is their apparent inability to be part of a group due to the disorders that severely impair their communication. And this applies to their relationship with music. Whereas with other groups of people, including those with physical disabilities, it is usually possible to rapidly 'tune in' to aspects of relationship through engagement in musical and movement activities. With some of the children we met in Episode #13 this seemed impossible. The musical means we used were chosen by instinct and experience, and we naively thought they would provide a 'universal key' to unlock the communication door that these children seem to have closed.

This particular experience powerfully challenged our convictions about the universality of music and its positive effect upon people. Perhaps for these children music is in some way innately inaccessible? Perhaps, as we wondered, developmental timing plays a crucial role in this potential? Or perhaps, in the case of these particular children, it is possible that we simply missed a fundamentally important aspect of music. In fact, we assumed that everyone would respond to the same sound material and we imposed that as a precondition to communication. In other words, we decided unilaterally that 'our music' would be the music that they would have to attend to. It was very effective with most of the children we met, it worked wonderfully with the educators the following day, but for the few who showed dislike, that choice was clearly a limitation. As musicians we are trained to think about music as a legacy. We learned music in order to perform music that someone had previously written or we had previously heard. Only later, and only for some of us, music became the expression of an inner creative voice. But we still 'speak' music the same way we learned it and we express ourselves within very precise and limited codes. We still have a lot to learn about listening. That is what allows us to communicate with others. And without listening maybe there is sound but not necessarily music.

Music, as we see it now, is a relational transient state with oneself and with others. It is mediated by movement, of which sound is the audible part. With listening it is possible that every sound may become music. But if there is no one to listen can there be music? Working musically with severely impaired children perhaps requires a shift in the way we think about music; maybe it is not about 'giving them' music but discovering what music they can express within themselves, and express themselves within. Once discovered, maybe from there we can build a relationship? It may be difficult or even impossible in a situation like the ones we faced in Episode #13. But it certainly can teach us a lot about ourselves and our calling.

Colwyn Trevarthen has suggested that 'because our communications are created musically, so too they can perhaps be "repaired" musically' (Miell, Macdonald and Hargreaves 2005, p.200). Maybe the first 'repairing' happens within our own capacity to listen? Perhaps healing is listening beyond physical sound?

Acknowledgements

We acknowledge Fundação Calouste Gulbenkian, Direcção-Geral das Artes da Secretaria de Estado da Cultura and Fundação para a Ciência e Tecnologia for supporting our work.

References

Barriga, M., Rodrigues, P. and Rodrigues, H. (2013) 'Giving Birth to Intergenerational Community Practices: The Music's "domino effect" in the Opus Tutti Project.' In J. Pitta and J. Retra (eds) *Proceedings of the 6th Conference of the European Network of Music Educators and Researchers of Young Children.* The Hague: Gehrels Muziekeducatie.

Brazelton, B. (2013) 'Valuing Baby and Family Passion: Towards a Science of Hapiness.' International conference, 7–8 May, Lisbon: Fundação Calouste Gulbenkian. Available at http://livestream. com/watch/search?q=valuing%20baby%20and%20family%20passion, accessed on 31 December 2015.

Gordon, E. (1990) *Music Learning Theory for Newborns and Preschool Children.* Chicago, IL: GIA Music.

Malloch, S. and Trevarthen, C. (eds) (2008) *Communicative Musicality: Exploring the Basis of Human Companionship.* Oxford: Oxford University Press.

Miell, D., Macdonald, R. and Hargreaves, D.J. (eds) (2005) *Musical Communication.* Oxford: Oxford University Press.

Papousek, H. (1995) 'No princípio é uma palavra – Uma palavra melodiosa.' ['In the Beginning was the Word – a Melodious Word.'] In J.G. Pedro and M.F. Patrício (eds) *Bebé XXI. Criança e família na viragem do século* [*The Child and the Family at the Turn of the Century*]. Lisboa: Fundação Calouste Gulbenkian.[10]

Papousek, M. (1996) 'Intuitive Parenting: A Hidden Source of Musical Stimulation in Infancy.' In I. Deliège and J. Sloboda (eds) *Musical Beginnings: Origins and Development of Musical Competence.* Oxford: Oxford University Press.

Reigado, J., Rocha A. and Rodrigues, H. (2011) 'Vocalizations of infants (9–11 months old) in response to musical and linguistic stimuli.' *International Journal of Music Education 29,* 3, 241–256.

Rodrigues, H. and Rodrigues, P. (2003) *BebéBabá – da musicalidade dos afectos à música com bebés.* Porto: Campo das Letras.

Rodrigues, H., Leite, A., Monteiro, I., Rodrigues, P. and Faria, C. (2010) 'Music for mothers and babies living in a prison: a report of a special production of BebéBabá.' *International Journal of Community Music 3,* 1, 77 – 90.

Stern, D. (1985) *The Interpersonal World of the Infant: A View from Psychoanalysis and Developmental Psychology.* New York: Basic Books.

Van Puyvelde, M., Rodrigues, H., Loots, G., De Coster, L. *et al.* (2014) 'Shall we dance? Music as a port of entrance to maternal–infant intersubjectivity in a context of postnatal depression.' *Infant Mental Health Journal 35,* 3, 220–232.

---

10 No translation has been published. However, for text that covers similar material, see Papousek H. and Papousek M. (2002) 'Parent Infant Speech Patterns.' In J. Gomes-Pedro, K. Nugent, G. Young and B. Brazelton (eds) *The Infant and Family in the Twenty-first Century.* New York and Hove: Brunner-Routledge.

19

MOVING FREELY TO MUSIC

Child-Centred Research Practice in Early Years

ANA ALMEIDA

Introduction

Some of my earliest memories as a child are those in which listening to music would make me burst into spontaneous dance. The intense feeling of being literally 'moved' by every single melodic or rhythmic nuance and the profound sense of immersion still resonates with me today. Music was movement and movement was music. Yet, this strong connection and creative expression would soon be challenged by my first formal music lessons. Not only was I invited to constrain the nature of my movement but also to reduce it to a conventional repertoire of gestures. Inevitably, I was *forced* to recognize the existence of two parallel musical universes in my life, the one that was internally driven and the other that dictated and externally structured my bodily experience. Whereas the first made me feel complete, the second often gave me a sense of physical disconnection with the music.

Many years later, while working with babies, toddlers and children in educational and artistic contexts, I gradually became aware of children's spontaneous choices of movement to music and of how that rich expressive information often passed unnoticed by educators. Parents and teachers also tended to predetermine the embodied musical experiences of the young movers by directly suggesting to them a set of actions that ought to be performed, even if they were not naturally selected by the little ones. Body movement was viewed as a functional tool (a means to an end) rather than as an expressive one.

These experiences led me to investigate the connection between young children's movements and music and, more specifically, their spontaneous embodied behaviour in response to particular structural musical features (e.g. rhythm). Despite my enthusiasm, I quickly became aware of certain key challenges that this type of research would involve. These were challenges of facilitation: first, children should be willing to move (voluntary action);

second, they must be fully engaged and confident in the act of moving in order to creatively explore different expressive possibilities for their actions; third, their participation must be experienced above all as fun and positive. Taking these priorities into consideration, I argue that investing in a more child-centred research practice can offer valuable opportunities for children to freely express their musicality through movement. An integrated approach based on these priorities will also provide a safe and trusting environment in which children's views and actions are valued and accepted without judgment.

This chapter explores the role of body movement in music perception and describes two approaches often used to study young children's embodied responses to music. The first is a functional-based approach focused on the accuracy of children's prescribed movements, and the second is an expressive-based approach interested in describing the repertoire of actions freely chosen by the young movers. The challenges identified in both approaches are discussed and child-centred strategies proposed, based on a study recently conducted with a group of preschoolers (Almeida 2015).

Perceiving as a way of acting

According to the theoretical framework of Embodied Music Cognition (Leman 2008), body movement influences the way we perceive and understand music. This proposition, strongly supported by neuroscience evidence (Bengtsson *et al.* 2009; Chen, Penhune and Zatorre 2008; Zatorre, Chen and Penhune 2007), shows that in a musical context, auditory and motor systems interact and are coupled (the principle of *perception-action coupling*). The two-way flow of information between perception and action implies that not only can music listening automatically elicit motor responses, but movements can also alter and shape perceptual processes (Maes *et al.* 2014). In practical terms this means that, through body movement, we are able to spontaneously articulate specific features of music, such as the beat, even at a very young age (Zentner and Eerola 2010). Furthermore, we can also shape and alter our music perception when making movement choices. For instance, Phillips-Silver and Trainor (2005) found that infants who were bounced rhythmically in a particular way (every two or three beats) would subsequently be more sensitive to the rhythmic stimuli that matched their bouncing experience.

Another related theory – Enactivism – suggests that our cognitive processing is deeply integrated with our sensorimotor capabilities, which enable us to interact with, and retrieve information from, the environment (Varela, Thompson and Rosch 1991). In other words, an enactive approach to cognition argues that instead of receiving this information passively, we actually shape our own understanding through skilful bodily interactions with the world.

Our unique bodies and the opportunities for action afforded by the environment will determine and constrain the way each one of us conceives the world. In this line of thought, Noë (2006) argues that '*What we perceive* is determined by *what we do* (or what we know how to do); it is determined by what we are *ready* to do' (p.1).

Noë's thinking suggests that our perceptual (musical) experience can be shaped by our unique repertoire of sensorimotor skills and by how we decide to employ them when interacting with specific structural features of the (musical) environment. It is highly likely that everyone perceives and understands music differently. Specifically for us here, children within the same age range may show differences in their music perception and meaning-making due to their unique motor development and distinct history of interactive experiences with the environment (Thelen and Smith 1994). This proposition implies that we can learn a great deal about each child's unique development from their individual preferences for certain movement patterns. These same patterns expressed will to some degree influence the type of musical partnership a child is able to develop with others. Both the enactivism and perception–action coupling principles suggest that effective therapeutic movement interventions may be customized for each child and each therapeutic partnership. The differences in how children move to music should be acknowledged, facilitated and celebrated.

The next section addresses the different ways in which young children's movement responses to music are often considered within music research.

Functional versus expressive-based approaches to movement

Body movement has been frequently used in research as a means to assess young children's musical behaviour. In some studies it is viewed as a functional tool to determine accuracy in task performance – for instance, to what degree can a child synchronize her response to an auditory beat (Provasi and Bobin-Bègue 2003). For control purposes, these movements are often prescribed, which means that the results are based on how well children use a specific set of actions to articulate certain features of the musical stimulus (e.g. *tapping* to the *beat*).

On the other hand, there are also more open approaches to facilitating movement for the purpose of describing children's creative responses to music. Sims (1985), for example, encouraged young children to move as they wish to three different musical pieces. The aim was to identify the children's spontaneous actions within the categories: movements exhibited, rhythmic characteristics and reactions to musical changes. According to Sims (1985), having a deeper understanding of the characteristics and capabilities of young children is important in planning successful movement activities within an early childhood music curriculum.

An expressive-based approach necessarily entails that the young movers are not only empowered to self-regulate their own body movements, but are also free to articulate their unique embodied experience of the music. The strengths of this more child-centred approach are, however, to be balanced with the challenges that researchers report regarding children's reluctance to participate in their move-as-you-wish tasks. The studies of Moog (1976) and Eerola, Luck and Toiviainen (2006) illustrate these challenges – in both cases a considerable number of children (three to five-year-olds) decided not to move at all and those who did tended to show, at times, some sort of inhibition. Moog (1976) was aware of this discomfort and even stated that children who promptly responded to his invitation 'were simply being obedient' (and therefore were constrained in their expression) whereas others had to be 'encouraged to make some sort of response' (p.126). Overall, the main reasons pointed out for children's unwillingness to move to music were the lack of familiarity with the setting and with the research team, and the child–adult power inequalities which tended to constrain children's experience and free choice of actions. I would add that the absence of a playful purpose or a clear engaging context for the movements could also have contributed to the young participants' inhibition.

Taking the above considerations into account, there is a need for more exploration and understanding of child-centred research practice; and practice which involves the facilitation of engaging, playful and trusting environments, and which encourages young children to move freely to music and explore their own expressive repertoire of actions.

In a recent study, conducted with a group of preschoolers in a Nursery and Primary school, I developed and analysed what I consider to be a child-centred method in music and movement research. In what follows I describe this method and my journey towards its development.

Developing a child-centred research practice

My recent study (Almeida 2015) aimed to identify and describe the free and individual movement choices of four- and five-year-olds in response to rhythmic music with a strong and steady beat presented at different tempi. In order to develop a child-friendly practice that could reposition children's actions at the centre of the research process, two distinct observational approaches were used in the study. The first consisted of naturalistic observations that took place during six visits to the Nursery and Primary School. The second approach – a video-based structured observation – was then used when the children participated in a *move-as-you-wish* musical activity.

Naturalistic observation: Building a trusting and play-oriented relationship

The weekly visits, over a period of three months, allowed me (as researcher) and the children to become familiar with each other and to gradually build trust. It was also a good chance to get to know the environment, the school routines, and the communication strategies normally used by the children and their teachers. This information was fundamental in helping me customize one of the particular musical activities for the young children participating in the study.

Once basic familiarity was established, I moved towards taking part more in group dynamics with the hope of becoming integrated and accepted. My presence was intentionally discreet and calm, but highly attentive to the needs of the children and teachers. I had the central aim of not wanting to impose myself on anyone – I decided that I would only join group activities if clearly invited to do so. This open, non-imposing approach paid off. When the invitations eventually happened they were authentic: eye contact, exchange of smiles and casual conversation occurred naturally between myself and the children.

One key moment (a significant sign of acceptance) happened in my second visit when I played 'duck duck goose', a traditional children's game in which one player walks around a circle tapping the top of each child's head and saying 'duck'. When one is finally chosen as the 'goose', he or she must chase the player to avoid becoming the next picker. After a considerable period of time without being chosen by anyone as the 'goose', one boy finally decided to take the risk and tap my head, which meant he was daring *me* to chase him. After this 'goose' moment many other signs of acceptance would follow. Certain children decided to include me in their role-play activities (e.g. cooking, cleaning, shopping, dressing, etc.). Others asked if they could comb my hair. Some were determined to draw my portrait. Some were eager to read me a story and to give me a goodbye hug at the end of each day.

Despite this evident closeness with most of the children, it was clear that some of them were more reluctant to interact with me. To build trust with these children, I decided to ask them courteously if I could join their group activities, especially when other children more accustomed to my presence were already involved. Gradually, confidence was built and spontaneous invitations to play started to emerge. Not surprisingly, the few children who frequently missed school, and thus my weekly visits, seemed to be less connected and less willing to engage with me. This lower level of familiarity would then affect, to some extent, their behaviour in the following stage of the study.

It was in the context of play, above all others, that my relationship with the children was evolving. The numerous playful and engaging interactive moments – facilitated further by the use of simple child-focused strategies, such as meeting each child at eye-level or wearing bright and colourful clothes as the four- and five-year-olds did – strongly contributed to minimizing child–adult power inequalities. These attempts to overcome disparities in power and status laid the foundations for our movement experiences. A child-centered relationship, as opposed to one which is authority centred, was fundamental in building confidence in each child – the confidence necessary to move freely to music when I later invited them to do so.

Video-based structured observation: Move-as-you-wish to music

Once we had developed trust and rapport, I invited four- and five-year-olds to participate in a very simple game. *Ana's Game* aimed to create a legitimate context and give the children a clear reason why they were being asked to move to music. This contextual game was absent in some previous studies (e.g. Moog 1976) that simply requested children to move to music without giving them a well-defined aim or reason for doing so. The use of a game was also intended to provide a playful and fun experience for the young participants.

Ana's Game was inspired by the traditional children's game *Musical Statues*, in which players have to *move to music* and *freeze to silence*. For each child the game lasted around two minutes, and consisted of five sections of music and four sections of silence. A square delineated on the floor (3m x 3m) defined the area where the game would take place. The aim of the square was to create a contained and safe space in the room for the children's movements, and so avoid them feeling overwhelmed by the amount of space available. Additionally, the square facilitated the use of a fixed camera and consequently freed me to interact with the players and to be more attentive to their needs. I chose one particular occasion, prior to playing the game, to invite the children to manipulate the camera (whilst turned off). This enabled the children to get accustomed to its presence in the room and helped considerably to minimize the reactivity effects during the game (e.g. looking at the camera or talking about it).

Before any of my visits to the Nursery, parental written consent for the children's participation was obtained. Children's verbal consent, on the other hand, was only intentionally sought before their participation in the musical game. This double consent meant that a child's willingness to participate never overrode their parents' decision for them not to take part in the study, and that a child's decision to withdraw always overrode their parents' consent.

When asked to play *Ana's Game* the four- and five-year-olds immediately responded with an enthusiastic, 'Yes!'. I explained to them what the game was about and what would happen next. Throughout this presentation I borrowed some of the communication strategies normally used by the teachers – e.g. seating the children in a circle, using extremely expressive vocal intonation, introducing surprising elements and using eye-catching props. My intention was to increase the positive impact of the message. Given that only one child at a time would be invited to play the game, it was fundamental to find an engaging way to inform the group about that process whilst randomly determining the order of the players. With the collaboration of the teachers, the children's names were pulled out of a *magical* box and immediately displayed on a colourful board. This performative and playful situation not only maintained the children's curiosity about *Ana's Game* but also gave them the information they needed to play it. However, of course, this did not avoid the insistent and enthusiastic questioning from some children, 'Is it my turn now?'.

At the beginning of each game I briefly reminded the children about the instructions of the game (*move to music* and *freeze to silence*). The open-ended nature of this instruction not only aimed to challenge children to move to music, but also to give them the opportunity to move freely and make their own movement choices. The game became the focus and so took their attention away from *how* each child was moving or what motor repertoire they were using and exploring. While the children were moving and playing *Ana's Game* I sat on the floor, near the square area, observing them. Throughout the game I encouraged and supported the children in their engagement by nodding and smiling. Often a child would respond by smiling back while maintaining their movements.

The music used in the game was carefully chosen with the purpose of encouraging movement responses in the young children. A groove-based music, defined by its power to make one want to move (Madison 2006), was considered during the stimulus selection process. Evidence shows that rhythmic features, such as beat salience and beat regularity, are consistently associated with the sensorimotor phenomenon of groove (Janata, Tomic and Haberman 2012; Madison 2006). Interestingly, even when people are instructed to stay still, high-groove music can still be 'especially powerful at activating the motor system via auditory–motor coupling' (Stupacher *et al.* 2013, p.134). With the aim of facilitating a tight link between music listening and children's spontaneous moving experience (perceiving as acting), I decided that a percussive rhythmic pattern with a strong and a steady beat would be used.

The chosen rhythmic pattern was presented in each section of the game with a different musical tempo (fast, moderate, slow and very slow). This was employed to assess whether children would adjust their movement responses to a new musical tempo, and if so, in what way. This information would then help me describe each child's perceptual embodied experience and identify potential differences across the group. With this information, we could shed some light on the principles of perception-action coupling and enactivism – that is, on the idea that the experienced (musical) world is characterized and determined by mutual interactions between the bodily features of the perceiver, their sensorimotor capacities and the (musical) environment.

After the end of the game each player was thanked for their cooperation and praised for their performance (e.g. 'Well done!', 'I really enjoyed your wonderful moves'). Their satisfaction and contentment were immense. As I accompanied each child back to the Nursery's main room I specifically asked them to not reveal the details of the game to the other children. I wanted the joy of surprise to be maintained. Every child immediately reassured me that they would keep this game a secret.

Ana's Game: Free movement responses to music

Level of engagement

Most of the preschoolers were clearly willing to participate in the game and showed no reluctance when moving freely to the music. They also exhibited signs of happy engagement, such as smiling, laughing, constant eye contact and making positive comments (e.g. 'This is fun' or 'Look at me'). Even though the majority of the young children were having fun playing the game, a very few participants were clearly self-conscious. This feeling of discomfort was usually evident in the avoidance of eye contact (e.g. looking down at the floor) and by very little movement. Two factors seemed critical in explaining this behaviour.

The irregular school attendance of some of the children inevitably reduced the time we spent together. Without this time to build our relationship, these children were less confident when it came to the time to move to music. Also, some of the children were naturally more introverted. This may have contributed to inhibited responses during the movement activity. To overcome this self-consciousness in future studies, redistributing the observation time differently could help ensure that 'hard to reach' participants have the necessary attention to overcome inhibition and to gradually develop a comfortable level of trust and familiarity with the researcher. In this way, observation time could involve creating moments in which the researcher quietly and calmly shares the same space and activities with these children (e.g. drawing or painting).

Movement repertoire

While being fully focused on the challenges of the game, most children were spontaneously exploring their repertoire of movements in response to the music. As a result, across the group of four- and five-year-olds, a great variety of rhythmic actions (e.g. jumping, bouncing, twisting, swaying, running, stepping, etc.) was observed (see Figure 19.1). Interestingly, despite this overall diversity of movements, each child tended to explore a fairly restricted repertoire and to show a clear preference for a specific action (Almeida 2015).

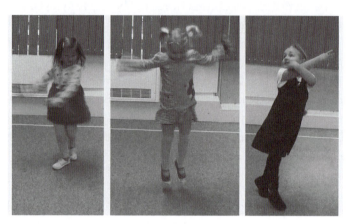

FIGURE 19.1 FOUR- AND FIVE-YEAR-OLDS MOVING FREELY TO RHYTHMIC MUSIC

These different movement preferences for the same music suggest that each child, with his or her unique body specificities and sensorimotor capabilities, recognizes different opportunities for action when interacting with the music stimulus, or more specifically, with its salient structural features (strong and steady beat). Even though the movements exhibited by the children reflected a regular accentuation, each child found their own unique way of spontaneously expressing it. For instance, while one child naturally engaged in a rhythmic stepping pattern, another child decided to tap her foot. This behavioural variability was also seen in each child's physical adjustments made to accommodate the new tempi. Most participants showed tempo flexibility in their responses but tended to move at a different speed from the one suggested by the music stimulus.

To illustrate these observations in more detail, I will describe a few strategies adopted by two children when moving freely in response to music. Andrew, a four-year-old boy, exhibited clear repetitive patterns reflecting the rhythmic nature of the stimulus and the regularity of the beat. Rather than just maintaining the same body action and simply adjusting his speed to the different tempi, Andrew decided to spontaneously change his type of movements and speed to better accommodate the new tempo. Whereas a moderate tempo encouraged the four-year-old to do a simple stepping pattern on the floor, the slower tempi prompted him to sway his body and a fast tempo to bounce energetically. For the duration of the five sections Andrew's whole-body movements were mostly done on the spot.

Lydia, a five-year-old girl, tended to maintain the same repetitive movement pattern throughout the game. Vertical jumping was her main choice. However, slight variations would often be added to help her cope with more challenging tempi. For instance, when the tempo became too slow, Lydia opted to use a star jump. This decision seemed to offer her the necessary stability to continue jumping at a slower speed and an opportunity to recuperate from the repetitive exertion of the dominant pattern.

Like Andrew, Lydia used whole-body movements that were often done on the spot and thus without accessing other areas in space. Based on these observations, we could suggest that the repetitive nature of the stimulus, its strong and steady beat and the different tempi involved had a distinct impact on the spontaneous decisions of the young participants.

Overall, my observations suggest that the rhythmic features of the stimulus were spontaneously embodied in unique ways by the four- and five-year-olds when playing the musical game, and that adjustments were promptly made in response to the tempo changes. We could therefore speculate that behavioural evidence has been provided to support the perception–action coupling claim and its two-way information flow. On the one hand, the stimulus selected encouraged each child to articulate the salient rhythmic features of the music and, on the other hand, children's individual movement choices seemed to reveal how each child shaped his or her rhythmic perception in real time.

We could speculate further and bring in the enactivism and the related concept of *body as constraint*. We could suggest that each child's use of different movements and strategies, while listening to the same stimulus, highlight the uniqueness of their physical characteristics, their sensorimotor capacities, their previous interactive musical experiences, and thus the specificity of their inner and outer rhythmic dialogue.

By giving children the opportunity to move freely to music and make their own choices rather than conform to other people's choices, researchers can enable children to find effective ways of physically expressing what they are perceiving in the music and acknowledge their body characteristics and sensorimotor capabilities.

Free movement to music can help young children to shape and develop their own perceptual experience and overcome unique challenges at their own pace. It seems that this method could become a valuable aspect of many therapeutic approaches. Embracing each child's creative rhythmic choices and unique sensorimotor skills may help therapists to regulate more effectively their embodied dialogue with the children. By focusing on each child's spontaneous movement patterns and on their preferred motor tempo a meaningful partnership can become possible. In this way, vulnerable children could be supported in the self-regulation of their emotional wellbeing, as well as in developing a strong connection with themselves and others.

Acknowledgements

I would like to thank all the children who took part in the study as well as their parents and teachers for their precious contribution. I would also like to express my gratitude to Dr Karen Ludke for her insightful comments on the chapter. Finally, I acknowledge the support of Fundação para a Ciência e a Tecnologia (FCT) through the doctoral grant SFRH/BD/78435/2011.

References

Almeida, A. (2015) 'Embodied Musical Experiences in Early Childhood.' (Unpublished doctoral dissertation). University of Edinburgh, UK.

Bengtsson, S.L., Ullén, F., Ehrsson, H.H., Hashimoto, T. *et al.* (2009) 'Listening to rhythms activates motor and premotor cortices.' *Cortex 45*, 1, 62–71.

Chen, J.L., Penhune, V.B. and Zatorre, R.J. (2008) 'Listening to musical rhythms recruits motor regions of the brain.' *Cerebral Cortex 18*, 12, 2844–2854.

Eerola, T., Luck, G. and Toiviainen, P. (2006) 'An Investigation of Pre-schoolers' Corporeal Synchronization with Music.' In M. Baroni, A.R. Addessi, R. Caterina and M. Costa (eds) *Proceedings of the 9th International Conference on Music Perception and Cognition (ICMPC9)*. Bologna: Alma Mater Studiorum, University of Bologna.

Janata, P., Tomic, S.T. and Haberman, J.M. (2012) 'Sensorimotor coupling in music and the psychology of the groove.' *Journal of Experimental Psychology: General 141*, 54–75.

Leman, M. (2008) *Embodied Music Cognition and Mediation Technology*. Cambridge, MA: MIT Press.

Madison, G. (2006) 'Experiencing groove induced by music: consistency and phenomenology.' *Music Perception 24*, 201–208.

Maes, P.J., Leman, M., Palmer, C. and Wanderley, M. (2014) 'Action-based effects on music perception.' *Frontiers in Psychology 4*, 1–14.

Moog, H. (1976) *The Musical Experience of the Pre-school Child*. London: Schott. (Original work published in German, 1968).

Noë, A. (2006) *Action in Perception*. Cambridge, MA: MIT Press.

Phillips-Silver, J. and Trainor, L.J. (2005) 'Feeling the beat: movement influences infant rhythm perception.' *Science 308*, 1430.

Provasi J. and Bobin-Bègue A. (2003) 'Spontaneous motor tempo and rhythmical synchronization in 2½- and 4 year-old children.' *International Journal of Behavioral Development 27*, 3, 220–231.

Sims, W.L. (1985) 'Young children's creative movement to music: categories of movement, rhythmic characteristics, and reactions to changes.' *Contributions to Music Education 12*, 42–50.

Stupacher, J., Hove, M.J., Novembre, G., Schütz-Bosbach, S. and Keller, P.E. (2013) 'Musical groove modulates motor cortex excitability: a TMS investigation.' *Brain and Cognition 82*, 127–136.

Thelen, E. and Smith, L. (1994) *A Dynamic Systems Approach to the Development of Cognition and Action*. Cambridge, MA: MIT Press.

Varela, F.J., Thompson, E. and Rosch, E. (1991) *The Embodied Mind: Cognitive Science and Human Experience*. Cambridge, MA: MIT Press.

Zatorre, R.J., Chen, J. and Penhume, V.B. (2007) 'When the brain plays music: auditory-motor interactions in music perception and production.' *Nature Reviews Neuroscience 8*, 7, 547–558.

Zentner, M. and Eerola, T. (2010) 'Rhythmic engagement with music in infancy.' *Proceedings of the National Academy of Sciences 107*, 5568–5573.

20

SEEING THE PLAY IN MUSIC THERAPY AND HEARING THE MUSIC IN PLAY THERAPY FOR CHILDREN RECEIVING MEDICAL TREATMENT

JANE EDWARDS AND JUDI PARSON

Introduction

Music therapy and play therapy at first glance seem closely related. They both involve playful, creative interactions between a child and a qualified therapist. Additionally, they are both *relational* therapies, emphasizing the interaction between the participants as a primary means by which positive changes occur for the client. Few publications have sought to examine or reflect on the similarities and potential for collaboration between these disciplines when providing ward-based services in healthcare. To redress the paucity of existing information, we present a discussion of the application of play therapy and music therapy for children in a medical setting. Within this context, we discuss the informative and practical potential in fostering working models based on shared insight from both disciplines.

The chapter presents the approaches taken in play therapy and music therapy in a paediatric hospital setting. Brian, a case study, is used to demonstrate how each professional would respond to, and work with, a child and his family.

The child in hospital: Understanding trauma risk and family distress

When a child is admitted to a hospital, it is a challenging time, for them and also for their family. If they are seriously ill they may not be able to understand everything that they are hearing or seeing. If they have been injured they will usually be experiencing pain and distress. There may also be uncertainty regarding their future physical functioning or mobility. If they have a chronic illness, their admission to hospital may mark a difficult development in their current treatment, leading to uncertainty about whether, or when, they will be able to normalize their routines, and how quickly they can return home. In all cases the child's everyday life is severely disrupted, along with those of their families. Exploration of the child's understanding of these circumstances is key to helping them to cope and adjust to their changed situation.

There is evidence that almost all medical procedures are experienced as aversive by children, and some procedures are undertaken in ways that can have traumatizing effects (Azeem *et al.* 2015). Aspects of medical procedures contain the basic ingredients of trauma, which are fear and inescapability, leading to recognition of the phenomenon of *paediatric medical traumatic stress* (Kazak *et al.* 2006), a type of iatrogenic trauma. As many as 30 per cent of medically ill children develop symptoms of posttraumatic stress, with a proportion of these children meeting the criteria for Post Traumatic Stress Disorder (Forgey and Bursch 2013).

It is increasingly acknowledged that the effects of a traumatic injury for a child, followed by hospitalization, can also have deleterious psychological effects for parents (Balluffi *et al.* 2004; Kent, King and Cochrane 2000). In a study of 107 parents in general wards, not including the intensive care speciality, it was shown that for these parents 'anxiety and uncertainty during hospitalization, and use of negative coping strategies, such as denial, venting and self-blame, were associated with higher post-traumatic stress symptoms scores at three months post-discharge' (Franck *et al.* 2015, p.10). Psychosocial care is therefore an essential part of safe, effective practice with children and their families in the hospital context. Careful work is needed to buffer the effects of stress and reduce the risk of trauma.

Working on the hospital ward

When offering services on a ward, music therapy and play therapy are provided in ways that are uniquely different to the classical psychological therapy services model. For example, there is rarely an opportunity to use a room space with a closed door. Treatment rooms can be busy, as staff may need to come and go.

The therapist might find themselves squeezing into a corner to be out of the way, but still be able to interact effectively with the child and other family members.

Bedside work necessitates a context that lacks privacy, and therefore confidentiality may need to be negotiated. Family members are often involved where possible. Sessions can sometimes be interrupted by other healthcare workers needing to perform tasks, or the child may need to be taken elsewhere for tests. The work can end abruptly if a child is transferred to a different treatment facility, or is discharged home on a day when the therapist is not at the hospital. Therefore the medical context, especially when using play therapy or music therapy to support medical procedures, requires a flexibility of approach in both disciplines. This is in contrast to more traditional approaches and techniques in these fields where clients are ideally seen at designated times, in purpose-built therapy spaces.

Music therapy and play therapy offer ways of being with children that are familiar to them, and to which they readily relate. Music and play provide ways for a child to express their needs and to process what is happening for them, ways to create meaning and safety. Therapists work with the knowledge that they must speak up to stop events occurring that could be dangerous for a child's wellbeing. This can be challenging within the hierarchical structures of a hospital. The practitioner is at once a diplomat and advocate for good practice in serving children's needs. It is challenging if one finds oneself 'conforming to oppressive and silencing practices' within healthcare (Edwards 2015, p.47). It is therefore necessary and helpful to attend regular supervision sessions with someone independent, familiar with the context, who brings a child rights perspective, whereby strategies to challenge ineffective practices can be explored and applied.

Family-centred care for hospitalized children is widely considered ethical and appropriate (Jolley and Shields 2009). Many hospitals now have facilities for parents to sleep in the child's room, or beside their bed on a ward (McLoone *et al.* 2013). Staff endeavour to engage the resources of the parent, and teams value the support parents can offer to their child. Increasingly, parental experiences of their child's hospitalization have been recorded in the professional literature (for example, Purdy 2014). There are multiple sources of evidence that healthcare treatment for children has come a long way since the days of keeping parents out of children's hospital environments (Davies 2010; Markel 2008). However, in spite of the intention to support families within the hospital environment, the authors have observed that this approach can sometimes be difficult to enact optimally for staff in busy medical-treatment-focused environments. Nonetheless, hospital charters and practices increasingly evidence the view that a child is no longer only a sick or injured body, but also a person with needs, rights and valuable connectedness to family and community.

Music therapy

Music has a long history of use in healthcare settings (Edwards 2008). Initially, music therapy services for children in hospital were considered an opportunity for *distraction* (Edwards 2005a). This language considered the child's boredom, pain or psychological distress as factors which could be ameliorated by simply switching their attention to something else. As music therapy work has developed into an allied health discipline in healthcare, more emphasis on *integration* has emerged. Therapies needed to *reframe* their approach towards an understanding that the child is experiencing themselves within a complexity of events and interactions, which includes their physical and mental state, their family context, and the hospital treatment team and other staff interactions. Therefore, contemporary music therapy can have multiple goals, addressing many needs directly and indirectly (Edwards 2005b).

Music therapy for children in a hospital is regularly offered within a family-centred care model of services (Edwards and Kennelly 2016). Where it is possible, and appropriate, family members are included in sessions, and are encouraged to take an interest in their child or sibling's music making and music listening needs outside of sessions within a stress and coping framework (Edwards and Kennelly 2016).

Music therapy's theoretical basis has been strengthened by the emergence of an understanding of *communicative musicality* (Malloch and Trevarthen 2009), which provides a basis for the relevance of musical work with families. The earliest interactions between infants and their caregivers are highly musical, contributing to deeply shared experiences, and developing the bonds of lifelong attachment (Edwards 2011, 2012; Malloch and Trevarthen 2000). Where these bonds have formed securely, the attachment theory developed by Ainsworth and Bowlby proposes that the child operates from what is considered a *secure base* (Ainsworth and Bowlby 1991; Bretherton 1992). When providing musical interactions, and supporting the resultant creativity, the music therapist is accessing, facilitating and building on existing collaborative structures of communication with which the child is highly familiar.

Play therapy

Play therapy focuses on the whole child within a developmentally sensitive, relational and systemic world view. And most importantly, play therapy is built on an understanding that the child's most natural way to communicate is through play (Landreth 2012). Hospital ward-based play therapy is very different from a traditional school- or community-based play therapy model. Out in the community, play therapy can ideally be based in a private consulting playroom, with the potential for long-term therapeutic input, consistency and confidentiality. On the ward the play therapist must adapt to the medical environment, often with limited space and resources. Here, the focus of therapy has additional acute dimensions in the form of acute illness, real-time worsening of the child's condition, and/or the current trauma of specific medical interventions. The child's physical condition, or the medical intervention, may either exacerbate the child's emotional responses or may be the source of distress. Given the constraints of the ward, the play therapist reflects on, and adapts as necessary, the basic essence of the therapeutic powers of play to optimize the therapeutic goal (Schaefer and Drewes 2013). The first step requires building rapport and a trusting relationship with the child and family.

The hospital-based play therapist is an allied health professional who is skilled in preparing children for procedures and the hospital experience. Our methods assist in reducing children's anxiety, pain and suffering. This in turn promotes the child's recovery both in the short and long term.

Finding links between music therapy and play therapy

Play therapy and music therapy share an emphasis on the quality, and qualities, of interaction between the therapist and the client. Although the focus of both therapies during procedures may be on vital concerns such as pain reduction, the relational dimensions of the interaction between therapist and client remain equally crucial. In both our approaches, the therapist provides a sense of safety through empathy, trust and comfort that support the child's psychological endurance of the procedure. In both worlds of practice, psychological safety is considered the polar opposite of trauma. The psychological safety of the child is therefore the goal of procedural support in both disciplines. The therapist's capacity to provide therapeutic presence that is *grounded, immersed* and *spacious* (Geller and Porges 2014) brings safety and certainty to the child's often unpredictable, and frequently distressing, responses during a procedure. The goal of building the therapeutic relationship is to decrease distress, increase coping, and build capacity for comprehension and control during hospitalization and treatments.

Brian: A case study

Brian[1] is a seven-year old boy who was transferred from a farm to a tertiary paediatric hospital. Brian's mother, Sally, travelled with Brian the thousand-kilometre-plus journey with the Royal Flying Doctors Service (RFDS). Brian was involved in a tractor accident. Brian's father, Andrew, was driving the tractor when it rolled onto its side. Andrew was able to jump clear, but he had not seen Brian running up to speak to him from the lower side of the paddock.

Andrew described events after the tractor rolled:

Brian was screaming, yelling out that he was stuck and couldn't move. Andrew quickly released the part of the harrow which had impaled Brian's leg. There was a lot of blood. He called for Sally; she had also heard the screams and was running over to see what had happened. Andrew put his shirt over the wound to reduce the bleeding and then called the emergency services. He ran to the house to get the first aid kit and told Sally to keep Brian still. Sally stayed with Brian throughout and tried to comfort him. Recently the family had relocated from New Zealand, and Andrew had completed a first-aid training course soon after they bought the farm.

The RFDS arrived within an hour of the call and noted that Brian's parents had been able to keep him reasonably still. The medical team ensured that his spine was immobilized for transfer to the hospital. The RFDS team administered pain medication and put up an intravenous line to start fluids. Brian had a compound fractured right femur and there was concern he had fractured his spine when the tractor rolled on to him.

When Brian arrived at the hospital, the emergency department was ready and assessed him. This was followed by x-rays, and CT and MRI scans. The operating theatre was alerted that Brian had arrived and would need an open reduction once the medical team had ascertained the extent of physical trauma.

Brian was observed as highly anxious, keeping a close eye on his mother. He protested when she was asked to leave him so he could have his tests. Brian was prepared for a number of procedures – staff introduced him to distraction techniques, to help him if he felt worried or in pain when a procedure was being carried out. Brian was passionate about playing football and all the while he kept asking if he would be able to play with his team on Saturday.

Sally was not familiar with the hospital environment or the specifics of the required medical procedures. She needed information and support regarding

---

1   The case is a *composite* case. Although there are intended similarities between Brian and patients we have both worked with in a hospital setting, we have never worked in the same team, nor with the same patient. Brian and his family, in the case material, does not exist. Any resemblance to an existing person, or similarities noted by any former patient or co-worker, are coincidental.

multiple aspects of Brian's admission, from Brian's prognosis down to the details of her accommodation while Brian was in hospital.

Music therapy response

Thoughts prior to meeting the family

The music therapy referral received was related to pain management and psychosocial support. Hearing what had happened, I was concerned for Brian, but also for the wellbeing of the whole family. I decided I would seek signs of family resilience and work to strengthen these. I considered how I might be able to feed back to the team, via the ward manager, any incidental comments or concerns from my observations and interactions which would help the team to provide optimal service. I also considered how I could encourage the family to be information seekers, helping them to understand the best person to approach if they had questions or concerns about what was happening. I sought to provide normalizing experiences within what can be a terrifying and exhausting round of medical procedures and treatments. However, I also cautioned myself that this input must be provided sensitively, with respect for the medical environment and the fatigue and pain levels not only of Brian but the other patients as well. For example, I needed to consider those in the surrounding rooms who may have been able to hear any music we made together. In musical terms, I wondered how I would connect with Brian's musical preferences and interests. What if he was a heavy metal fan, or only liked certain rap music that I could only play via pre-recorded materials, not live?

Meeting the family for the first time

A message from the ward manager indicated that Brian and his mum were on the ward with a window of about 20 minutes before he was to be picked up to go to an MRI. On my arrival at his bedside Sally looked exhausted. As I approached I could hear she was talking to Brian, trying to explain what the doctor had told them earlier. I was wearing regular street clothing with a hospital laminated identity badge that included my photo, my title, a big V for 'visitor', and the description 'music therapist'. I was carrying a guitar and a bag of instruments. I introduced myself and told them that the ward manager had asked me to come over to see how I could help.

For someone who is not a music therapist, it could be a little challenging to imagine the following scenario being a usual part of professional therapy practice. After introducing myself to Brian and Sally, I picked up my guitar, put the strap over my body and said something like, 'A lot of people like music and know a lot of songs. I wonder if there is some music you really like?' This is a regular opening line for me. Then the session gets started. I would never do this without being referred or without consent (or some kind of assent) from those present. Often a parent will look up and smile, and a child, if they can, will lift their head a little, or turn to me when they see the guitar. I take these as cues that I am welcome. If a parent sighs and looks at the door, or a child closes their eyes or turns their head away I take note of this. I might persist gently to ensure I have read their non-verbal signs correctly. If I do not feel welcome, I let them know when I am available, and indicate that they can ask the nurse manager any time, and I will come back when it suits them. In my experience most families welcome music therapy interactions. This was certainly the case for Brian and Sally.

Brian was listening to his mum with a frown on his face as I walked in. Now, as I lifted my guitar, he looked at her with a smile and said that he loved Slim Dusty songs. 'He gets that from his grandpa,' said Sally, rolling her eyes. I started quiet picking of some introductory chords and then sang, 'I'd love to have a hug with Grandpa, I'd love to have a hug right now.' We all smiled. I asked, 'Is there anyone else who needs a hug?' Brian said, 'Mum needs a hug.' We sang the words to the verse and I encouraged them to sing, 'coz Mum is my mum' instead of 'mate' at the end of the chorus. Brian started being quite playful. He mentioned his dog Rusty needing a hug, and then the rooster Bertie needed a hug. We sang together, and whenever I sang 'Bertie' or 'Rusty' Brian giggled and couldn't sing the word because he was laughing. We were trying to decide the next person or animal who needed a hug when the orderly arrived to take Brian to the MRI. I knew that Brian had been observed to be anxious on separation from his mum so I started singing, 'I'd love to have a hug with an MRI, I'd love to have a hug right now.' Brian reached out for his mum's hand and the orderly told her she could come down to the suite with them if she wanted to. I sang them out of the ward. The ward manager gave me a quick 'thumbs up' on my way back into the ward to look for my guitar case.

Session 2

I arrived for my regular session at the hospital to find a follow-up referral for Brian which indicated 'pain and anxiety during procedures'. After entering the ward I had to wait a while until the ward manager was free to update me. I read Brian's recent chart entries and noticed that dressing changes had been difficult. This was because Brian became upset and angry at the nursing staff, especially if either his mum or dad were not present. The ward manager told me that every time Brian heard that he had to go for a test, he started to protest, and this was disruptive to the calmness of the ward. I agreed to catch up with the family after the ward round.

As I entered the room I noticed there was a man sitting beside Brian's bed. He was unmistakably related to Brian, so I smiled and asked, 'Are you the dad?'

He nodded and put down the newspaper he was reading. I introduced myself again and reminded Brian that we had met the other day. In reply, Brian gave me a little wave and a glimmer of a smile. I asked where Brian's mum was and he told me that she was downstairs having some breakfast. I mentioned that I had been asked to see if I could find a way to help Brian feel more comfortable during procedures. I asked Brian whether he had a favourite Slim Dusty song. From there we discussed songs he had learned at school, and the sounds of instruments he knew and liked. I asked if he had any kind of music-listening device. Andrew held up his mobile phone and pointed to it. I said I wasn't sure if mobile phones were allowed in some of the treatment spaces. I indicated that I needed to check, and if mobile phones weren't allowed I would come back with an iPod or iPad to download some music for use when Brian is having a treatment.

Having tracked down the available gear, later on I sat and talked with Brian and his dad about how music listening can be very helpful before and during procedures. 'But,' I said, 'before starting to listen to the music it is a good idea to take some slow deep breaths and to count backwards from ten.' We all practised together. I put my hand on my chest to show that when my chest rises that means I am breathing deeply. Both Brian and his dad copied my hand-on-chest movement and we repeated the process of taking a deep breath. We softly counted backwards from ten.

We then spent time choosing half an hour of music that Brian knew well and liked, and with which he had positive associations. We chose one song that reminded him of Mum, and one song for his sister Chloe. He couldn't decide which one to choose for his dad. Andrew suggested a song that Brian's class sang at last year's Christmas concert, which they used to sing in the car sometimes. We discussed what to call the playlist, and decided it should be 'Brian takes it easy'. While we continued talking, I wrote out a list of the steps for music listening. It started with, 'Are you taking Brian to a procedure or about to do a procedure at bedside? If yes, please remember he loves using the iPod for support. The playlist to choose is *Brian takes it easy*. I included a reminder of the calming breathing techniques we practised. I drew a smiley face and an approximation of an iPod with headphones. After agreeing with Brian and Andrew that I couldn't draw, I pinned the list on the noticeboard above Brian's bed. I stood up, picked up my guitar and said, 'Take it easy, Brian,' and he smiled. I asked Andrew to let me know via their nurse if they wanted some more help with music for procedures. I turned and waved when I got to the ward entrance and said, 'Let me know how you get on.' Andrew held up his hand with fingers crossed.

Session 3

I asked the ward manager if she wanted me to see Brian and his family. She gave me an update, telling me that Brian was doing well with the iPod during procedures and that if the staff forgot to take it someone would have to run back for it, as Brian let them know he needed it. She told me that Brian's dad had returned to the farm to be with Chloe, and Sally was still at the hospital. There was now a discharge proposal in place over the next two weeks after which, barring any infections or untoward outcomes, Brian would be heading home. Brian would only be able to mobilize using a wheelchair for the next ten weeks once home. Therefore, the family were involved in intensive preparation from the allied health team to get used to what daily life would be like: having showers, keeping the wound sites dry, and getting in and out of bed. The ward manager advised me to see Brian to assess how he was adjusting to the news that it would be quite some time before he was able to go back to school or play with his friends.

From the doorway of the room I noticed Sally looked more awake and less tired. She was wearing make-up and her hair was brushed. Brian's mouth was tight, and he was frowning. 'Hey, good to see you. How are things?' I asked. They both looked up at me. 'We were wondering if we would see you again,' Sally said. I suggested if they would like to see me they could always ask their nurse who could page me or leave a note for me when I was on the ward next. I asked how the procedures had been going with the iPod. 'Oh, God forbid we forget the iPod,' Sally said with a wry smile. 'Good then?' I queried. 'Yeah it's a bit better now,' she said.

I sat down on a chair, took my guitar out of the case, and pulled the strap over my head and shoulder. 'Have you ever written a song?' I asked Brian. 'Nope,' he replied. I said if he wanted to we could try to make up a song together. I suggested we could make it about hospital, his school, the family or something else. Brian thought for a bit, and he decided to make it about hospital. I offered some options of tunes we could use. I demonstrated a bright major tune with a rock feel, and then a slower minor tune suitable for a ballad. He chose the major key. I asked him to tell me some things about hospital he could put in the song. He listed them one by one: everything hurts, sometimes it's boring, why aren't I allowed to eat, Dad had to go home, music helps me take it easy, it's hard to sleep.

Playing the rocking beat with major key I sang some opening close caption lyrics for each line and Brian chose the topic to include from the list we had made. We worked on the chorus together.

Verse 1

> *I had to come to hospital because my leg got hurt*
> *The hardest thing about it is everything hurts*
> *I have learned a lot about being bored*
> *And now I want to take it easy*

Chorus

> *Take it easy*
> *Take it easy*
> *Take it e-ea-sy*
> *You have one life and you never know what will happen*
> *Take it easy Brian, take it easy Mum*
> *Take it easy Dad and Chloe*
> *Take it easy, take it easy, you have time*

Verse 2

> *Now I want to make sure that children don't get hurt*
> *And that when they need to sleep they can*
> *The best thing about hospital is Mum is here*
> *But I really hope that Dad can be here too*

Chorus

After we had sung it a couple of times I wrote it out on a piece of paper using a child's crayon because, as sometimes happens, I forgot to bring a pen. We then sang it again, changing a few words, before I recorded us singing it on my iPad. In this final recorded version the ward manger dashed over and sang with us, playing the egg shaker (completely out of time) and dancing around, making us all laugh. As I pressed stop I looked at the time and realized I was minutes away from another engagement, so I scrambled to pack up. I let them know I would make a nicer print version of the lyrics on the computer and leave this for them.

In my reflections on this composite case of Brian and family, I am struck once again by the privilege of belonging to a profession in which music making brings fun, play and lightness into people's lives at times of great stress. Music can hold and reflect the emotional and psychological challenges of receiving medical care and treatment, contributing to coping and self-regulation. Music provides familiarity, control and enjoyment to families and provides an uplifting atmosphere to the ward.

Play therapy response

As we have already found out, the hospital environment is a unique therapeutic space. Therapeutic toys and expressive materials are limited to space availability and transportability, and must be used within the infection control guidelines. In offering support to Brian and his family my challenge was to maintain a therapeutically 'containing' environment in each and every unpredictable space and moment. My play therapy intervention would focus on facilitating communication and fostering emotional and psychological wellness within an overarching child-centred theoretical approach. The following response occurred concurrently with music therapy, and the treatment plan was flexibly prioritized according to Brian's day-to-day needs.

Our first session

I knocked on the door to Brian's room and introduced myself saying, 'Hi, my job is to play with some of the children on the ward, I wonder if I could come in?' I waited for a response. I saw Brian's eyes light up for a moment. He looked at his mum and then me and said, 'Play? Play what? I'm stuck here.' I acknowledged how he was feeling, saying, 'Stuck, huh? It seems like you are not sure what you can play while you are in here.' My statement helped Brian feel that I understood his feelings and concerns. It demonstrates both empathy and reflection, two of the core skills in child-centred therapy. I then explained to Brian that I had brought a few things with me to show him, basically a range of selected toys and craft material.

Brian told me he liked to play football and, when he spotted the twistable crayons and colourful paper, he added that drawing can also be fun. I reflected to him, 'You've worked out that there are things you can do even when you have to stay in bed.' I cleared a space for him to draw on his over-bed table, and placed the other toys at the bottom of his bed. Brian began to draw. As he did so, I focused my attention on what he was doing and how he was doing it – 'tracking' his actions and feelings. 'Tracking' is the act of reflecting play behaviours by verbalizing what the child is doing. I was communicating to Brian that I was interested in what he was doing and that I was concentrating on him. Brian drew a picture of a black coloured figure. He labelled it *monster-man* and told me that the monster-man was going to attack the tractor.

Brian then told the story of how the monster-man became friends with a boy, Luke, who was also seven years old. The monster-man defends Luke against the aliens from outer space. On the same page, and near the head of the monster-man, Brian drew a spaceship. I observed that it looked like the bright lights of the operating theatre, although I did not say this out loud. Brian said that Luke was really scared of the aliens. When I asked him what they looked like he told me that they are covered in green slime, and even have strange masks, hats, gloves and shoes to hide their hideous toad skin. If the toad skin touches you, you get in pain and you have to die. Staying with the child's metaphor is another important principle of child-centred play therapy – the symbolic distance of metaphor enables a degree of safety in exploration of difficult emotions. So I reflected how frightening it must be for Luke to see the aliens. Then I asked what Luke was going to do to next. Brian said, 'It's OK because monster-man will stop the aliens from hurting Luke.' However, I noted the ambivalent way Brian said this. After this he quickly finished his drawing and said, 'That's it!'

The abrupt ending of the drawing was a break in the play sequence that might indicate the story metaphor was evoking a traumatic memory. Under such circumstances it was important for me to go at Brian's pace, not to hurry the therapeutic process. I reflected by saying, 'You have decided that the story is finished.' I heard the loud silence of an unfinished and incomplete stanza to the story.

Brian had readily demonstrated his ability to use his vivid imagination to produce a dramatic story laden with metaphor. His story indicated many *potential* themes, such as worry and fear, power and control, need for protection and nurturance, as well as feelings of being stuck or trapped and in pain. In play therapy it is usual to hypothesize on the themes in the story, and to wait for their re-emergence in later sessions. At this point in time, it was clear that Brian was not ready to bring information to his conscious awareness as indicated by staying within the monster-man metaphor. A child's process in play therapy will flow through many different stages. An adaptive therapist will make decisions to sensitively employ different tools and emphases along the way – for instance, to be more, or less, directive. Yasenik and Gardner (2009) formulated the play therapy dimensions model (PTDM) to help integrate and facilitate this therapeutic decision making along two main continuums: the directiveness continuum and the consciousness continuum. These continuums are then cross-correlated and represented schematically, giving us four quadrants (types of appropriate response): 1) Active utilization; 2) Open discussion and exploration; 3) Non-intrusive responding; 4) Co-facilitation (Yasenik and Gardner 2009). Brian's communication within the above play sequence stayed in the unconscious and was non-directive in nature. Employing the PTDM model, I was pointed towards quadrant 3 (non-intrusive responding) as a helpful mode of response (Yasenik and Gardner 2009).

Session 2

The next day the nurse came into the ward to administer intravenous antibiotics. He asked to speak to me afterwards and said that Brian had had a difficult time with the cannulation the previous evening. Having a cannula (a port for intravenous access) inserted into the body is a painful and emotionally challenging experience for many children. The nurse asked if I could provide some psychoeducation to support further cannulation procedures.

When preparing a child for a procedure such as a cannula insertion, play therapists understand that information must to be offered within a developmentally appropriate frame of reference. This should include sensory information, in other words: what the child will see, hear, smell, touch and/or feel (Parson 2009). To do this the actual medical equipment is provided for the child to play with.

I brought in a special doll on which Brian could later explore a mock medical procedure if he wanted. Calico dolls, also called trauma dolls, are simple human-shaped dolls made with plain fabric and filled with polyester fibre stuffing. They are available in a range of skin tones. The child is able to select and draw on the fabric to create their own doll with a unique design and personality. I asked Brian if he would like to draw on the calico doll with special fabric markers and I explained that he could keep the doll afterwards. Brian said, 'Only my sister has dolls.' I reflected by saying, 'You think that dolls are just for girls, but this one can be for boys or girls.' Brian was OK with this and he decided he would draw some eyes, ears, mouth and clothes on it. Whilst Brian was drawing on the doll I explained to Sally some ways in which she could support Brian using the doll for any future procedures. These support strategies included sitting close to Brian and maintaining eye contact during the procedures, in conjunction with using the iPod music (as prepared by the music therapist) and related deep-breathing exercises. I also discussed 'comfort positioning', which refers to different ways to hug and hold a child undergoing procedures, as well as distraction strategies with toys, books and playful props. I reassured Sally that she and Brian would be supported by the staff as well.

Brian showed me the doll he personalized and I asked if he could give the doll a name. He called it Bob. I showed Brian and Bob some medical equipment (such as a tourniquet, a cannula to show how the needle part is removed, a syringe, bandage, tape and alcohol wipes) and demonstrated a cannulation procedure on Bob. I then supervised Brian in touching and feeling the equipment and provided an opportunity for him to explore the medical equipment and ask any questions. I introduced Brian to 'Buzzy', a little electronic device in the shape of a colourful bee which combines cold sensation and vibration to interrupt the sensation of pain (Inal and Kelleci 2012). As I observed Brian play, I noticed that he did not avoid the medical equipment. He was curious and played with the needle and syringe with the doll. Using Bob the doll gave Brian a safe distance from his personal worries. Here, in this safe place, I was able to facilitate an open discussion about procedures and potential coping mechanisms. In contrast to our first session, here Brian and I were involved in more directed play and communication. Employing the PTDM, this level of engagement suggested response from two quadrants: 4 Co-facilitation; and 2 Open discussion and exploration.

The role of the play therapist is to use specific skills such as tracking, empathic reflection, emotional congruence and attunement to build the therapeutic relationship. A trusting relationship helps the child feel safe even though potentially painful or frightening procedures are anticipated. During our procedural preparation session, I spoke to Brian about his likes and dislikes and noted this information for when distraction may be necessary during the next procedure. During such a session, I always let the child know what *they can* do, by saying for example, 'The most important job you have is to stay still, but you can cry and squeeze Mum's or my hand.'

As with all play therapy interventions, time to reflect on my own practice was paramount. I reflected on my trust in the child-centred model and on just how effective this approach is in quickly building the therapeutic relationship. My early relationship building with Brian and his family helped facilitate further opportunities to work within metaphor and to develop psychoeducational opportunities. Knowing that Brian had a creative and active imagination was helpful. I could use this information to inform our play and, in turn, to advance his coping skills. I also reflected on my role as a play translator in facilitating communication between Brian and his family, as well as with other members of the healthcare team. It is a privilege to work playfully with children like Brian, and to be in a position to optimize their medical experience for both the short and long term.

Conclusion

Music therapy and play therapy both strive to normalize hospital experiences by reducing the impact of the child's condition and subsequent treatment on their psychological and cognitive development. Both approaches operate from a creative and playful foundation, accessing the child's capacities and interests through the development of a therapeutic relationship. The service wraps around the family, seeking the resources of the parents to support the child, and helping the whole family feel secure and safe in spite of the accident and potential trauma.

We agree that if it were possible that both play therapy and music therapy were available to a child in a hospital setting, it might not be optimal to offer both at the same time. It can be difficult to coordinate contact with the family. Also, one psychotherapeutic service is often adequate in addressing each family's needs. However, we continue to be interested in what collaborative work might look like. Deciding which children would benefit most from play therapy and which from music therapy would require a consistent and fruitful decision-making process. We consider age to be a dynamic consideration in this thought process, a possible rule-of-thumb being that younger infants (perhaps before the age of three) should be considered as primarily good candidates for music therapy, and older children be referred to play therapy services.

Play therapy work in medical contexts continues to develop in Australia. At the time of writing, within medical care, music therapy has a more established presence than play therapy. However, it is concerning that many paediatric facilities have neither music therapy nor medical play therapy services. Knowledge of the need for trauma informed services is increasing, especially as the evidence for medical induced trauma continues to grow. Specialized music therapy and play therapy practitioners are urgently needed: specialized practitioners who can work quickly and effectively with children and families, developing rapport, building trust, providing psychological education, making therapeutic spaces and facilitating feelings of safety and security during the stress of hospitalization.

References

Ainsworth, M.S. and Bowlby, J. (1991) 'An ethological approach to personality development.' *American Psychologist 46*, 333–341.

Azeem, M.W., Reddy, B., Wudarsky, M., Carabetta, L., Gregory, F. and Sarofin, M. (2015) 'Restraint reduction at a pediatric psychiatric hospital: a ten-year journey.' *Journal of Child and Adolescent Psychiatric Nursing 28*, 4, 180–184.

Balluffi, A., Kassam-Adams, N., Kazak, A., Tucker, M., Dominguez, T. and Helfaer, M. (2004) 'Traumatic stress in parents of children admitted to the pediatric intensive care unit.' *Pediatric Critical Care Medicine 5*, 6, 547–553.

Bretherton, I. (1992) 'The origins of attachment theory: John Bowlby and Mary Ainsworth.' *Developmental Psychology 28*, 5, 759.

Davies, R. (2010) 'Marking the 50th anniversary of the Platt Report: from exclusion, to toleration and parental participation in the care of the hospitalized child. *Journal of Child Health Care 14*, 1–23. DOI: 10.1177/13 7493509347058

Edwards, J. (2005a) 'Developing Music Therapy Approaches to Pain Management in Hospitalized Children'. In C. Dileo and J. Loewy (eds) *Music Therapy at End of Life*. Cherry Hill, NJ: Jeffrey Books.

Edwards, J. (2005b) 'The role of the music therapist in working with hospitalized children.' *Music Therapy Perspectives 23*, 36–44.

Edwards, J. (2008) 'The use of music in healthcare contexts: a select review of writings from the 1890s to the 1940s.' *Voices: A World Forum for Music Therapy 8*, 2.

Edwards, J. (2011) 'The use of music therapy to promote attachment between parents and infants.' *The Arts in Psychotherapy 38*, 190–195.

Edwards, J. (2015) 'Paths of professional development in music therapy: training, professional identity and practice.' *Approaches 7*, 1, 44–53 (Special issue: Music therapy in Europe: Paths of professional development). Available at http://approaches.gr/wp-content/uploads/2015/08/5-Approaches_712015_Edwards_Article.pdf, accessed on 19 September 2016.

Edwards, J. (2012) 'We need to talk about epistemology: orientations, meaning, and interpretation within music therapy research.' *Journal of Music Therapy 49*, 372–394.

Edwards, J. and Kennelly, J. (2016) 'Music therapy for hospitalized children.' In J. Edwards (ed.) *The Oxford Handbook of Music Therapy*. Oxford: Oxford University Press.

Forgey, M. and Bursch, B. (2013) 'Assessment and management of pediatric iatrogenic medical trauma.' *Current Psychiatry Reports 15*, 2, 1–9.

Franck, L.S., Wray, J., Gay, C., Dearmun, A.K., Lee, K. and Cooper, B.A. (2015) 'Predictors of parent post-traumatic stress symptoms after child hospitalization on general pediatric wards: a prospective cohort study.' *International Journal of Nursing Studies 52*,1, 10–21.

Geller, S.M. and Porges, S.W. (2014) 'Therapeutic presence: neurophysiological mechanisms mediating feeling safe in therapeutic relationships.' *Journal of Psychotherapy Integration 24*, 3, 178.

Inal, S. and Kelleci, M. (2012) 'Relief of pain during blood specimen collection in pediatric patients.' *MCN: The American Journal of Maternal/Child Nursing 37*, 5, 339–345.

Jolley, J. and Shields, L. (2009) 'The evolution of family-centered care.' *Journal of Pediatric Nursing 24*, 2, 164–170.

Kazak, A.E., Kassam-Adams, N., Schneider, S., Zelikovsky, N., Alderfer, M.A. and Rourke, M. (2006) 'An integrative model of pediatric medical traumatic stress.' *Journal of Pediatric Psychology 31*, 4, 343–355.

Kent, L., King, H. and Cochrane, R. (2000) 'Maternal and child psychological sequelae in paediatric burn injuries.' *Burns 26*, 4, 317–322.

Landreth, G.L. (2012) *Play Therapy: The Art of the Relationship*. London: Routledge.

Malloch, S. and Trevarthen, C. (2000) 'The dance of wellbeing: defining the musical therapeutic effect.' *The Nordic Journal of Music Therapy 9*, 2, 3–17.

Malloch, S. and Trevarthen, C. (eds) (2009) *Communicative Musicality: Exploring the Basis of Human Companionship*. Oxford: Oxford University Press.

Markel, H. (2008) 'When Hospitals Kept Children from Parents.' *New York Times*, 1 January, F6.

McLoone, J.K., Wakefield, C.E., Yoong, S.L. and Cohn, R.J. (2013) 'Parental sleep experiences on the pediatric oncology ward.' *Supportive Care in Cancer 21*, 2, 557–564.

Parson, J. (2009) 'Play in the Hospital Environment.' In K. Stagnitti and R. Cooper (eds) *Play as Therapy: Assessment and Therapeutic Interventions*. London: Jessica Kingsley Publishers.

Purdy, J. (2014) 'Creating Partnerships for Life: One Family's Story of Paediatric Patient and Family-centred Paediatric Care.' In R. Zlotnik Shaul (ed.) *Paediatric Patient and Family-centred Care: Ethical and Legal Issues*. New York: Springer.

Schaefer, C.E. and Drewes, A.A. (2013) *The Therapeutic Powers of Play: 20 Core Agents of Change*. Hoboken, NJ: John Wiley & Sons.

Yasenik, L. and Gardner, K. (2009) *Play Therapy Dimensions Model: A Decision-making Guide for Integrative Play Therapists*. London: Jessica Kingsley Publishers.

21

AND THEN I BELONGED

Relational Communication Therapy in a Remote Tanzanian Orphanage

CHANTAL POLZIN, ULRIKE LÜDTKE, JOSEPHAT SEMKIWA AND BODO FRANK

From the very first moment I saw Radhia, I was moved by her condition. In the turmoil of the orphanage, she expressed this oppressive loneliness. She was all alone. The other children struggling for attention were the noise around this sad girl who remains isolated in her own world.[1]

We tell the story of a girl named Radhia who lives at a small orphanage in the Usambara Mountains in the northeast of Tanzania. It is a story about how a bicultural training, research and therapy project changed her life as a member of the orphanage community, rescuing her from isolation. In discussing the multi-layered impact of this project, we will be framing the input at the orphanage in terms of, 'performative' events of sensitive cooperation. We use the word 'performative', as first used by Austin (1962), to get a sense of the potential underlying our acts, gestures, facial expressions, speech, and so on, the potential to create social and communicative reality. To be clear, we are not referring to an actual organized performance on a theatre stage.

When you visit the orphanage for the first time, you come to an attractive, clean place with flowers in the garden and green grass in the playground. Some 35 children live here. Their ages range from immediately after birth up to two years old. When the weather is nice, you may see some of the older children outside the buildings. Usually a group of about eight children who are around the same age can be seen sitting in the shade, or crawling or walking on the grass. Most of the time they are supervised by one young woman, who, when you enter this place, will greet you with a friendly but very shy 'karibu', meaning

---

1   This is the first of several reflections from the German therapist concerned, conveying her emotions and experiences following therapy sessions.

'welcome' in Kiswahili. The younger children are usually inside. During 'playtime' they sit together in the hall in front of their dormitories, mostly alone, not wanting to play with each other. The orphans in this institution have usually lost their mother at birth, due to delivery complications. The father is not able to provide the basic care they need for the first two years. After the children have learned to walk, eat and go to the lavatory on their own, they are often reintegrated in their families.

To coordinate the work of the community, there is a head 'mama'[2] in charge. If she is free, she will welcome you in person. She is a passionate and warm woman who rules with a consistent and disciplined hand. She works closely with her deputy, who represents her and helps her with many of the day-to-day challenges. The mama and her deputy are both educated and experienced nurses who have been doing practical work caring for children for many years.

The young woman, who you met earlier as she watched the older orphans outdoors, is also living and learning in the orphanage. She is one of about 30 caretaker students who are being educated in early childhood care and housekeeping there. These students, who were unable to complete secondary school for various reasons, are between 19 and 21 years old. They are given a place to sleep in basic dormitories on the compound, and their meals. They are not paid for their work, but their parents who sent them to the orphanage pay small school fees.

The caring ratio, 31 caretakers[3] to 30 children, appears generous. But this is deceptive. Most of the time there is only one caretaker for each group of children, while the other students and staff are busy with a myriad of practical duties which consume time and energy. They wash the clothes and diapers by hand in water boiled on a fire, till and harvest the fields, and care for the livestock. They cook for children and staff on a wood fire, sell their vegetables at market, sell snacks in their own kiosk at the orphanage, and play host to the many visitors from various countries who might be potential donors. In addition to this hard work, there are a few hours of theoretical and practical teaching per week taught by the one of the two head mamas.

The compound, which was built in the 1960s by German missionary women, has started to decay. The hard work involved in maintaining it and keeping it a clean and healthy place is very apparent. The plain structure with its purity and discipline seems quite untypical of Tanzania with its dusty roads and, to the Western eye, rather chaotic townscapes. For a visitor aware of the colonial

---

2   'Mama' is the Kiswahili word for 'woman' and is used as a respectful title in Tanzania.
3   There are 30 caretaker students and one of seven female members of staff at any one time. The latter are in charge of monitoring and supporting daily work. These women were former students and they draw a small salary in the orphanage. They work in day and night shifts and live in town.

history, it feels as if the spirit of the European missionaries is still alive (Fiedler 1996). This is immediately obvious in the plainness and austerity of the caring environment, and also apparent in the hierarchical structure of the community. Everyone has a clearly defined role that is reflected in their 'costumes', how they are dressed. The caretaker students, with their closely cropped hair, wear light-blue dresses and dark-purple pullovers. Their look differs clearly from the female members of staff dressed in light-purple dresses who wear their hair long with creative and individual hairstyles. The head mama and her deputy wear the dark-blue dresses of nurses with a checkered pinafore.

If you had the opportunity to take part in everyday activities, you would experience how the missionary spirit is reflected in the way care is organized. The hygienic and sanitary care is the guarantee first and foremost of physically healthy children, and it will keep severe illness or death at bay for decades to come. But at the same time this style of care, with its disciplined rituals, has a direct impact on the way communication is established with the children and how their relationships grow.

Loss of companionship in early childhood

The story of loss of companionship in early childhood is as old as the story of the human community itself, and the two stories are inextricably woven together. By 'companionship' we are referring to the deeply connected relationship which develops between an infant and her caregiver, a relationship built on thousands of shared moments of play. Companionship begins in shared impulses of vitality and imaginative self-awareness before birth and, through companionship, meaning is discovered in playful 'dialogue' way before language. Companionship grows in the thousands of nursery rhymes, play songs, and lullabies that there are across all the different cultures. It has been described in detail by many researchers over the last decades (Malloch and Trevarthen 2010; Reddy 2008). As research has revealed the complex beauty of these early forms of companionship in mental life, the more evident it has become just how important the presence of an affectionate and imaginative partner is for the healthy development of the child's ingenious self.

Companionship in early childhood and its temporal organization

A child needs to engage with a meaningful other from birth, an innate need for which the developing infant is psychobiologically predisposed (Trevarthen 1998). From the first minute after birth a baby expects someone to be there who will respond contingently to what they do (Brazelton 1979). The infant's multimodal expressions are intentional and ready to be shared with a feeling of confidence right from the beginning. They are offered to provoke responses and do not just imitate (Nagy 2008). At around two months of age, children take a big step towards proto-conversation – the sharing of non-verbal information within the rudimentary structures of a 'conversation' (turn-taking, imitation, rhythm, etc.) (Trevarthen 2008). Gratier (2003) describes the delicate temporal structure of such early dialogues using the concepts of 'interactional synchrony' and 'expressive timing'. In interactional synchrony, both communicating partners synchronize their movements and vocalizations as they intuitively attune to a common 'pulse'. Expressive timing is the playful variation of this 'pulse'. These temporally structured dialogues can be described as coherent narratives of 'musicality' in which the partners are exchanging their emotional stories and felt experiences (Malloch and Trevarthen 2010). These narratives are characterized by a beginning, a process of building towards a climax, and a conclusion, just like the nursery rhymes, play songs, and lullabies found all over the world (see Delafield-Butt and Trevarthen 2015; Gratier and Trevarthen 2008).

Where there is a loss of companionship, both self-confidence and trust become fragile. This is evident in the examples of parental borderline personality disorder and neonatal depression (Gratier and Apter-Danon 2010; Gratier *et al.* 2015), or in cases of severe deprivation of intimate care (Bowlby 1988; Spitz 1946). The temporal structure of mother–infant communication was studied in immigrant Indian dyads (from Indian families migrating into the US) and compared with non-immigrant dyads at home in India, France, and the United States (Gratier 2003). It was found that the immigrant dyads displayed a reduction in expressive timing and interactional synchrony (Gratier 2003). This confirms that a stable, active, and responsive social environment, favorable economic conditions, and familiar cultural settings may all play a crucial role in the development of enjoyable interactional play from the early months of a child's life.

It is important to emphasize that the story of companionship happens not only at the dyadic level (i.e. between mother and baby). We need to consider the whole 'sociosphere'[4] of friendly relationships with shared interests, on which meaningful participation in a culture depends.

In the orphanage lack of time for spontaneous play affects the emotional expressiveness or availability of the caretakers, limiting the companionship they are able to give in intimacy with a child. The institutional character of this particular sociosphere (Frank and Trevarthen 2012) prevents the development of enjoyable musical games that otherwise might have become treasured memories of a special relationship (Gratier and Apter-Danon 2010; Trevarthen 2008).

---

4   Sociosphere is a term which brings Habermas's 'lifeworld' concept (1985) and Bourdieu's 'relational sociology' (1998) of the adult world into relation with the theory of innate intersubjectivity (Frank and Trevarthen 2012).

Companionship in communication and language development

Figure 21.1 shows a sketch illustrating a vivid multimodal proto-conversation between mother and child with intense mutual interest.

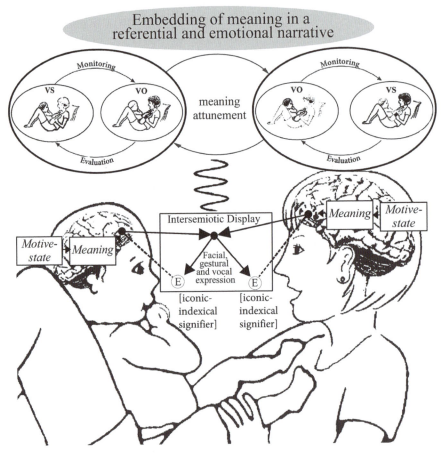

FIGURE 21.1 RELATIONAL EMOTIONS AS THE FOUNDATION OF COMMUNICATION AND LANGUAGE DEVELOPMENT (MODIFIED FROM FIGURE 11B IN LÜDTKE 2012, P.330)

Our exploration of this proto-conversation needs to encompass three levels. First, the proto-conversation starts with each participant expressing the relational motive to become 'meaningful' to the other. They smile in a teasing way, eagerly reach out for body contact, or curiously look each other in the eyes. Second, Figure 21.1 illustrates how meaning is created mutually and relationally, meaning is co-constructed (Bloom 2002). We will go into detail below about just how that meaning becomes embedded in narratives that are both emotional and referential. Meaning is understood here to be generated 'in process' (Kristeva 1998). Third, Figure 21.1 shows the process in which both communicating partners build an emotionally mediated and marked (hence relational) representation of the person or character of their partner (Bråten 2002). It follows that any 'meaning' in the dialogue is inseparable from the relational emotions felt in the 'present moment' (Stern 2004).

Mother and child monitor each other's expressions, or rather they monitor the idea they have in mind about their companion, here called the 'Virtual Other' or 'VO' (Bråten 2002, Figure 21.1). They also constantly evaluate how their own concepts of themselves – here called the 'Virtual Self' (Bråten 2002, Figure 21.1) or 'VS' – fit to their companion's expressions. This is our basic desire to feel validated by another, our desire to achieve a contingent 'match' with our partner's expressed view of us. This is one of the bases for a sense of satisfactory communication. Alternatively, a feeling of 'mismatch' creates emotional and communicative disturbance (Murray and Trevarthen 1985; Nadel and Han 2015). This disturbance can either initiate new communicative activities with each partner attempting to achieve a satisfying result, or cause distorted representations of self and/or other (Aitken and Trevarthen 1997; Trevarthen 2012).

The expressed elements of meaningful communication we refer to as shared 'signifiers'. In this early dialogue between mother and child (see Figure 21.1) signifiers could be an expression of mood or physical condition, such as a joyful squeak or a hungry sigh. These essential signifiers can be easily understood and 'answered' by persons of any age around the world.

As the infant–mother partnership develops in communicative sophistication, so does the nature of the iconic signifiers being shared. The most basic of signing, for instance, is the use of 'iconic' signifiers, 'images', or 'portraits' that refer directly to the appearance or form of an object of reference. We encode the 'meaning' of iconic signifiers with the help of our own felt experiences which, of course, are felt primarily within interaction.

Communicative development also involves the exchange and evolution of 'indexical' signifiers. Using this type of signifier, we can refer to something without naming it directly. Smoke, for example, is a typical index for fire. The earliest roots of this level of communication are found in gestures like pointing, or in vocalizations like reduplicated babbling.[5] In this way, infants and caregivers exchange indexical signifiers that refer to something not directly, but with a hint to the object of reference. To encode an indexical signifier you not only rely on your felt emotional experience, but you also need to refer to your knowledge of your environment. This is why indexical signifiers are a little less emotionally colored than iconic ones.

---

5   Reduplicated babbling is the first form of vocalization made by children aged about seven months and which involves the combination of a consonant and a vowel such as [ba] (Gerken 2009, p.70).

The last step in the development of communication and language is the use and exchange of symbolic signifiers. A child's first word (or attempt at a word) is the earliest of such signifiers, for example, a child's use of 'nana' for banana. To understand these signifiers, you need to have sound knowledge of conventionalized language symbols within specific countries and societies. As a child develops, the signifiers she uses and recognizes change, becoming increasingly more abstract and less emotionally colored (Lüdtke 2012).

Losing companionship in early childhood

With this evidence of how shared meaning develops in infancy in trusted and emotionally rich relationships, we come back to the story we want to tell about the little girl Radhia at the orphanage. We need to review what is known about the consequences of an early loss of loving companionship, a story that is deeply moving. First described by René A. Spitz (1946) and later shown in film documentaries (Spitz 1952), the developmental and communication problems caused by isolation and loss of maternal care in infancy became a major topic in pediatrics.

Spitz's studies in hospitals and orphanages presented a picture of children rocking steadily, absorbed in inspecting their own hands, staring in a depressed and unresponsive manner through the bars of their cots. Developmental disorders that followed this kind of institutionalization were later described in a number of studies from many different countries – for example, in England (Bowlby 1988), in India (Routray, Mahilary and Paul 2015), and in Romania (Nelson, Fox and Zeanah 2014).

In the case of Radhia, an unidentified developmental problem led to a cycle of neglect and withdrawn or so-called 'stereotypical' behavior. Her subdued attempts to communicate went unnoticed by the overburdened caretaker students, and their occasional somewhat 'clumsy' efforts at communication failed to stimulate responses from her. We became aware of her because she was not acting like the other children, who clung to us and struggled for attention whenever they saw us. She remained 'isolated in her own world'. The head mama was already keeping an eye on her, because she too was worried. At Radhia's age (22 months), most of the children in the institution could stand up and walk, but she did not seem to have any motivation to become mobile or to seek contact. First the staff thought she could be blind or deaf, but this suggestion was easily rejected by doctors.

In the orphanage, many institutional factors, (especially the pressure of the daily routine, and the lack of training for the caretaker students) could lead to situations where the infants' basic need for responsive intersubjective communication could not be met. When the head mama saw the videos of

Spitz's documentary during one of our presentations for the women staff at the orphanage, she said in front of everybody that this kind of distressed behavior was definitely part of their present reality, and that it must not be ignored. She said there was an urgent need to change their practice of care. The head mama's communication was one of the wider 'performative events' that started to change communication with the children and among the staff in the orphanage.

In our introduction we defined 'performative events' as acts of sensitive cooperation which create new social realities. In artful performance the reciprocal influence of performer and spectator creates momentary events that initiate change and generate *new meaning* for those who participate. We decided any therapeutic input for Radhia would need to be conceived as 'performative' within this wider, systemic emphasis. As the research team at the orphanage, we could only initiate change by acting with respect for the organizational and cultural habits of the institution. Only when referring to and accepting the staff's long-established culture could we bring about a new impetus through showing videos, doing workshops, and finally animating proto-conversation with a child who previously was perceived as not being able to communicate. In these moments of meeting, when everybody was present, we could share a world in which we could create a common social reality.

Establishing our 'Relational Communication Therapy' (RCT)

Out of the need to step into Radhia's world and to overcome the urgent feeling of being powerless, I took a step up to her bed and softly reached out my hand to Radhia. I slowly turned into her field of vision, imitated her introverted movements and while mirroring them carefully I slightly changed them. She recognized me; shortly her gaze met mine. She responded with a slightly changed movement. Slowly, and still not entirely believing what was happening, I felt a growing joy. I was relieved. She responds to me! Somehow she recognized me as someone who is able to 'understand' her movements. Even as these short mutual movements and touches and exact inspections of me climaxed in warm laughter, they always faded away. Her body and mind became absent again. After these short encounters, and despite the fragility of it, I was almost euphoric and highly motivated to build more bridges towards a shared world.

After this first encounter I had the chance to show this situation on video to the head mama. She was so excited and stated, 'I've never seen her like this before – she is so active!'

To begin the story of how a training and research project changed Radhia's life, we give a short outline of the project to implement our 'Relational Communication Therapy' for Radhia, and within the orphanage (Frank and Lüdtke 2012; Lüdtke 2012). The clear objective was to meet the needs of the orphanage through initiating the change for the children that the head mama wanted to implement after she saw Spitz's video (1952). To avoid a situation in which a therapist from abroad comes to the orphanage, conducts a therapy, and afterwards vanishes without any impact on their daily life, we pursued the approach of 'Participatory Action Research' (PAR; see Reason and Bradbury 2009). [6] All steps and methods used in this project were discussed, planned, carried out, reflected upon, and modified with the team. We had a firm foundation for such a close collaboration, because we had been working at the orphanage for many years. We could offer a training and research project with the RCT approach, which the head mama already knew was fruitful. [7] In our discussions it became clear that together we needed to implement a training program for the caretaker students which emphasized a relational way into establishing dialogue.

Our training program would need to encompass the sociosphere of the orphanage. In any attempt to support a change in the relational norms of the orphanage, it was important to take account of the sociological aspects, or institutional conditions, that affect Radhia's capabilities for development. Radhia needed to be freed from the present restrictions of this development. [8] A crucial step must be made towards overcoming the current and ongoing institutional habits, or 'looping processes' (Goffman 1961). These looping processes can cause staff or caretakers to become fixed in persistent communicative 'inabilities'. This background of institutional looping processes that handicap communication must be identified, discussed and corrected in joint efforts. In the case of Radhia, her therapy had to be continuously reflected upon as a co-constructing process. Everybody concerned needed to witness and feel Radhia's emotional development – these felt emotions would be the 'motor' for any dialogue to improve mutual understanding.

---

6   We name our activities 'Inclusive Scientific Research' (ISR; see Frank and Trevarthen 2015), which derives particularly from PAR, but also makes use of research methods from the science of infant intersubjectivity and their application in the field of special needs education.

7   Ulrike Lüdtke and Bodo Frank, both part time lecturers at SEKOMU, established practical work at the orphanage in close cooperation with the head mama and university students since 2008.

8   For this kind of 'shift' see Frank and Trevarthen's adaption of Habermas's term 'intersubjective claim of validity' (Frank and Trevarthen 2012).

Designing the training program in Relational Communication Therapy

Following the principles of intersubjective relating outlined above (see 'Companionship in communication and language development'), we established RCT with Radhia based on two fundamental assumptions: first that her communicative attempts may be guided by an inborn *relational motive*, and second by a feeling that she has become meaningful to other meaningful people. From this basis (i.e. with Radhia's help), she and her therapist will then be able to mutually create meaning in *emotionally relevant narratives*. This will assist her to acquire or build a *positive relational representation* of the therapist. The basic assumption is that the inner affective states of both Radhia and the therapist will be shown to one another in multimodal *emotionally colored expressions* (see Figure 21.1).

Our training program in the RCT approach aimed to develop the competences and self-confidence of the caretaker students in their care of children with developmental communication disorders. This level of care involves the caretaker student continuously triangulating three interconnected relational competences within the daily processes of interpersonal communication with the child (e.g. during nappy changing or feeding). These, defined as follows by Lüdtke (2012) and Schütte (forthcoming), are illustrated in Figure 21.3 (see p.351).

- *theoretical competence:* knowledge about theories concerning how infants communicate (e.g. Infant Intersubjectivity, or Communicative Musicality)

- *methodological competence:* the repertoire of methods the therapist is able to apply to initiate and 'guide' a dialogue (e.g. using subtle varieties of a smile to invite a response, exactly monitoring changes in movements, or picking up the rhythm of the child and playing with slightly breaking it)

- *dialogical competence:* the way the therapist invites and rewards the dialogue by emotional bonding and attunement (e.g. mirroring a warm smile, expressing sympathy for a mourning sigh, or sharing the pride of the child in managing a new task).

Delivering the training program – in the light of accessibility and cultural differences

These three competences were facilitated for the caretaker students through lectures in Kiswahili by trained Tanzanian university students (see Figure 21.2).

To explore the dialogical competences in a tangible way, we used videos that the caretaker students recorded on their own, using a feedback method adapted from Video Interaction Guidance (Kennedy, Landor and Todd 2011). The videos could be recorded in two different ways. First, our self-developed autonomous camera system,[9] which records three synchronous perspectives, was installed next to the nappy-changing table. The caretaker students simply had to press a button to start the recording. Second, they were introduced to a camcorder so that they could record themselves in everyday situations. They could choose those recordings that were most informative from their perspective. On the one hand, these videos provided a wonderful illustration for feedback concerning the dialogical competence. On the other hand, the videos were used to convey key theoretical insights by practical illustration.

We were aware that before we could teach the subtleties of the three *relational competences*, the proposed content had to be discussed in the light of pronounced cultural differences. For example, the communication style of African mothers and fathers is often described as involving more bodily expression and contact in contrast to the more vocal communication of Western families (Alcock and Alibhai 2013). The Tanzanian part of the project team could identify with this picture presented in the literature. For example, it is very common for them to touch children's faces as a greeting, something that is not common in Germany or in other Western cultures. But we also saw the cultural similarities. Despite the differences, the animating rhythm of 'Communicative Musicality' is always present in play with infants. This is what Rabain-Jamin notices when she refers to the way Wolof mothers from Senegal describe the synchrony of their rhythmic communications during the first few months: 'We say "ay" in their ears as we bounce them' (Rabain-Jamin and Sabeau-Jouannet 1997, p.429). After some enthusiastic discussions, the whole team could agree that the basic features of dialogue in early childhood communication (according to research on Infant Intersubjectivity in Europe and the US) also form the foundation for early communication in the Tanzanian culture.

---

9   The BabyLab INCLUDE at Leibniz University Hannover (LUH) follows an applied Intercultural Intersubjective In-vivo Research approach (III-R; Frank and Trevarthen 2015) to implement participatory research and interventions to support children with vulnerable communication and language development in institutionalized settings. In close collaboration with Professor Bodo Rosenhahn from TNT, Institute for Information Processing, Faculty of Electrical Engineering and Computer Science, Hannover, we are now on the way to refine this autonomous recording system.

Introducing the team

To implement our project, we brought six different individuals round one table: the head mama and her deputy, two Tanzanian research students from the local university, Sebastian Kolowa Memorial University (SEKOMU), and two German research students from Leibniz University Hannover (LUH). They were a highly heterogeneous group, whose differences included nationality, culture, ethnicity, socioeconomic status, religion, gender, and age.

But as in the African saying, 'It takes a whole village to raise a child', the whole team was much bigger than this small practice group. There were all the people who live and work at the orphanage. Their roles changed over the course of time from being spectators to performers. Also, more German and Tanzanian students became part of the team.[10] The Tanzanians were teachers; the Germans helped to coordinate and document. As support in the background, the research team could always rely on the help of the whole BabyLab INCLUDE Team from LUH.

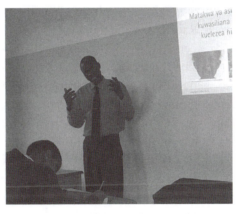

FIGURE 21.2 UNIVERSITY STUDENT TEACHING TOPICS IN INFANT INTERSUBJECTIVITY

From training, to therapy, to Radhia's happiness: An overview

For four weeks, ambitious university students acted as teachers for the caretaker students. The university students were highly motivated and expressed their appreciation of their task in elegant and even festive clothes and dresses. They implemented the teaching in a passionate, lively, and joyful way (see Figure 21.2). The caretaker students were moved by these charismatic teachers. The students were also often surprised at what children are capable of at a very young age. With the help of the self-recorded videos, they were even surprised by their own capabilities.

In the special case of Radhia, slow, sensitive, and non-intrusive steps were needed before we could include her in the intervention. In the months

---

10   The whole team consisted of 12 Tanzanian and 9 German students.

before any direct input we became familiar with the day-to-day running of the orphanage (we helped in daily activities such as feeding and nappy changing) and we became familiar to the children and staff. A crucial talk with the head mama about her worries concerning Radhia was a fruitful starting point for this relationship-based therapy.

Figure 21.3 gives a visual overview of the steps in Radhia's therapy. (Please note that the images in Figures 21.3 to 21.5 are stills from video recordings.)

First we gathered audiovisual data about Radhia's life. We saw her alone and absent most of the time (Figure 21.3, A). Then we began carefully building up short and fragile moments of companionship based on ideas resulting from these first recordings. We noticed, for example, that Radhia was awake during the midday nap and that she was inspecting her hands in these silent situations. The therapist used these opportunities to initiate fleeting dialogic moments with Radhia. In our example, the therapist sat with Radhia at her nap time and initiated gentle play in hand-to-hand physical contact.

As Radhia's therapy progressed, the whole team continued to be deeply involved via ongoing video feedback. We all saw the first mutual communications between Radhia and the therapist (Figure 21.3, B). And we all saw the relationship between Radhia and the therapist developing, saw them sharing truly meaningful time (Figure 22.3, C).

Afterwards, these extraordinary moments of companionship between Radhia and the therapist became part of the training. In this way the caretaker students could actually see Radhia developing from her initial isolation to gradually taking part in mutual exchanges with the therapist. The caretaker students started to show curiosity and sensitivity towards Radhia. In turn, Radhia began to recognize and accept the caretaker students into her personal world. At this point the therapist acted carefully as a bridge between different partners, carefully supporting the caretaker students into the role of therapist.

We continued to appreciate the progress between Radhia and her caretaker student/therapist through the ongoing video feedback. We all saw their shy steps towards companionship (Figure 21.3, D). In the end Radhia started to respond more and more to other people's communicative attempts. We all saw caretaker students and Radhia engaging in dialogue (Figure 21.3, E). Over time the increase in sympathetic engagement became clear to all. It warms our hearts to see the self-recorded video (made about one week after the workshop) in which Radhia laughs out loud with a caretaker student. We all saw them enjoying playful teasing (Figure 21.3, F).

What happens on these occasions? What defines the interactions that so benefit everyone involved? Let's have a closer look at an example of the individual therapeutic events that make up the whole story, that are part of the beginning of this change for Radhia.

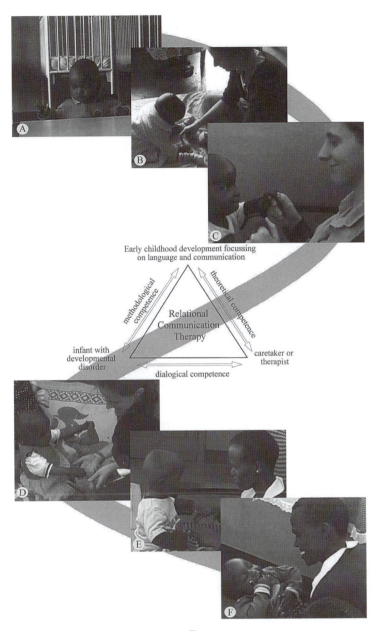

Inside the triangle diagram:

Early childhood development focussing
on language and communication

methodological
competence

theoretical competence

Relational
Communication
Therapy

infant with
developmental
disorder

caretaker or
therapist

dialogical competence

FIGURE 21.3 RELATIONAL COMMUNICATION THERAPY:
FROM ISOLATION TO COMPANIONSHIP

A: Radhia alone

B: First mutual communication between Radhia and the therapist

C: Radhia and the therapist sharing meaningful time

D: Shy steps towards companionship

E: Caretaker student and Radhia engaging in dialogue

F: Enjoying playful teasing

Radhia's progress: 'Performative' events in Relational Communication Therapy

After a long and exhausting day of project work with many small and large obstacles, a special moment occurred. It was in the late afternoon and we had just finished a session full of small dialogues, when I decided not to bring Radhia back to her room, which was full of the din of children. She should just have the opportunity to stay with me and the student who recorded the videos, on the couch and wait for our taxi to come. I was deeply exhausted, but Radhia was not. She sat on my lap and initiated a new 'dialogue'. She looked at me demandingly, but briefly. Then she vocalized with her mouth closed – humming, following a contour I already knew: rising – falling – shortly rising – short break – rising – falling – shortly rising again. She waved her hands in rolled fists in front of me, her whole body moved in sync with her humming. Radhia was communicating with me, addressing me directly with our personalized, very own and well-known, rhythm. It was the first time I felt addressed by her.

All the stress and tension fell away. In a blissful easing of tension, we shared some minutes of time. After this incident, I was surrounded by an infinite pride in Radhia and her change – a pride which the student and I could absolutely share.

During a joint video analysis, the head mamas at the orphanage were astonished by this scene; with a warm smile they said, 'She is very happy! You're singing together!'

In the scene described above, something beautiful happened which is not easy to grasp, but it was definitely felt by the people present.

On this occasion, Radhia initiated the dialogue by performing her 'very own and well-known rhythm' – a particular rhythmic expression that was already known to the therapist. Here, the therapist connected with this rhythm and began to alter it slightly, varying the repetition and, in doing so, created something new. This reveals the performativity of the mimetic play between Radhia and her therapist. They are co-creating meaning, through their combined performance, in a shared reality.

Radhia and her therapist shared time in their multimodal rhythms through many variations of intersubjective experience. Figures 21.4 and 21.5 give a detailed visual depiction of Radhia's transition between representational states – from a solitary self to an intersubjective, dynamic self/other representation.

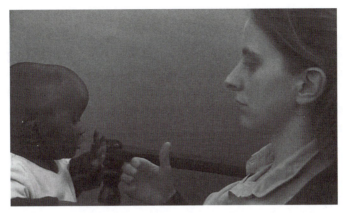

FIGURE 21.4 INTROVERTED AND SELF-DIRECTED MOVEMENTS BY RADHIA

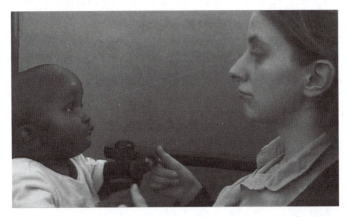

FIGURE 21.5 THE DANCE OF SHARED MEANING SHARED BY RADHIA AND THE THERAPIST

If you look closely at these encounters (Figures 21.4 and 21.5), you can see that the therapist sensitively invites Radhia by imitating her vocal, facial, and gestural signifiers again and again. The therapist is trying to become in tune with Radhia. Even if Radhia seems to be absent, the therapist remains connected alongside Radhia (Figure 21.4). This patient, open connection enables Radhia to recognize her therapist as a meaningful other, and then even joins her. In doing so, Radhia is beginning to create a positive representation of the therapist and their relational emotions of joyful play (Figure 21.5). In this way, Radhia's isolation within her close social environment was becoming more and more 'permeable' for social events, and the sympathetic bond between her and the therapist, and later on with her caretakers, was getting stronger.

Interestingly, the event described above (Figures 21.4 and 21.5) marked a turning point in Radhia's communication and language development. During the scene she vocalizes a combined consonant– vowel sound like /bɐ/ for the first time. Her vocal expressions change from only pure voiced humming to a more complex indexical articulation called reduplicated babbling. She took her first steps in climbing the ladder from iconic to more indexical signifiers (Lüdtke 2012). For Radhia, her relational impulses were finally being met by a real and responsive person (her therapist). In this meeting, her impulses could become a 'motor' of communication development precisely because this 'motor' is alive and vividly present in the form of an emotionally positive representation of the therapist as virtual other (Bråten 2002; Frank and Lüdtke 2012; Lüdtke 2012; Trevarthen 2012; and see Figure 21.1).[11]

Reflecting on the events with the head mama

Thanks to the benefits of using laptops and SD cards,[12] we could show the videos immediately to the head mama and her deputy (see Figure 21.6). In the first two weeks, this helped us establish a basis for trust. In this sharing, we were expressing our respect for their expertise, and we were receiving their trust, interest, and insight in return. They could see and hear on the video that something crucial was changing.

The videos, which showed the development in Radhia's extraordinarily beautiful communication – responding and calling for attention, smiling and laughing, 'singing and dancing' with the therapist, Radhia and a caretaker student playing a joyful intersubjective game – initiated a change in the mamas' view of Radhia's capabilities.

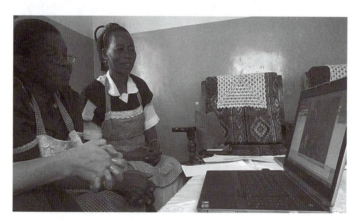

FIGURE 21.6 LEARNING FROM RADHIA: CO-CONSTRUCTING
RELATIONAL MOMENTS WITH THE HEAD MAMA AND HER DEPUTY

---

11   A detailed qualitative analysis of the performative events of this therapy will follow in Chantal Polzin's doctoral dissertation.

12   Secure Digital media storage cards.

In conclusion

All of us, as participants in this project, came away with a feeling of honor and pride because we had the chance to participate in something special and very intimate in those four weeks. Most of all, we experienced the importance of establishing relations across individual, institutional, and cultural levels in our implementation of RCT. The significance of this multilayered communication, epitomized by 'performative' events at many levels, became clearly evident in the developmental changes shown by Radhia. In communication therapy, the sharing of time and relational emotions, which has performative effects on every level, must be reflected upon and purposefully applied. We, as a research team, were able to experience the importance of relationships in a complex multicultural project, *and* the power of new relational emotions (from within the therapy) on everybody involved. The widely collaborative nature of the project gave a depth of support for the direct therapeutic work. As such, the therapy was truly meaningful, 'performative', and uplifting.

Acknowledgements

Our warm and sincere thanks first of all go out to the orphanage with all its children, students, and staff, especially to the head of the orphanage and her deputy, who opened their doors and hearts for this participatory project. Also we would like to thank our research fellows Ulrike Schütte and Afizai Vuliva for their tireless and irreplaceable work, as well as Colwyn Trevarthen and Stuart Daniel for their patience and editorial help. Last but not least, we thank our 'extended family' who made this wonderful project happen: the North-Eastern Diocese of the Evangelical Lutheran Church in Tanzania (NED-ELCT), Rev. Anneth Munga, Rev. James Mwinuka, all students who participated from SEKOMU and LUH, and the remaining BabyLab INCLUDE team at Hannover.

References

Aitken, K.J. and Trevarthen, C. (1997) 'Self/other organization in human psychological development.' *Development and Psychopathology 9*, 653–677.

Alcock, K. and Alibhai, N. (2013) 'Language Development in Sub Saharan Africa.' In M. J. Boivin and B. Giordani (eds) *Neuropsychology of Children in Africa: Perspectives on Risk and Resilience*. New York: Springer.

Austin, J. (1962) 'How to Do Things with Words.' In J.O. Urmson and M. Sbisà (eds) *How to Do Things with Words: The William James Lectures Delivered at Harvard University in 1955*. Oxford: Clarendon Press.

Bloom, L. (2002) *The Transition from Infancy to Language: Acquiring the Power of Expression*. Cambridge: Cambridge University Press.

Bourdieu, P. (1998) *Practical Reason*. Stanford: University Press. (Original work *Raisons pratiques* published in 1994.)

Bowlby, J. (1988) *A Secure Base: Parent–Child Attachment and Healthy Human Development.* New York: Basic Books.

Bråten, S. (2002) 'Altercentric Perception by Infants and Adults in Dialogue: Ego's Virtual Participation in Alter's Complementary Act.' In M. Stamenov and V. Gallese (eds) *Mirror Neurons and the Evolution of Brain and Language.* Amsterdam: John Benjamins.

Brazelton, T.B. (1979) 'Evidence of communication during neonatal behavioural assessment.' In M. Bullowa (ed.) *Before Speech: The Beginning of Human Communication.* Cambridge: Cambridge University Press.

Delafield-Butt, J.T. and Trevarthen, C. (2015) 'The ontogenesis of narrative: from moving to meaning.' *Frontiers in Psychology 6,* 1157, 1–16.

Fiedler, K. (1996) *Christianity and African Culture: Conservative German Protestant Missionaries in Tanzania, 1900–1940.* New York: Brill.

Frank, B. and Lüdtke, U. (2012) 'Förderschwerpunkt "Geistige Entwicklung".' In O. Braun and U. Lüdtke (eds) *Enzyklopädisches Handbuch der Behindertenpädagogik. Bd. 8: Sprache und Kommunikation.* Stuttgart: Kohlhammer.

Frank, B. and Trevarthen, C. (2012) 'Intuitive Meaning: Supporting Impulses for Interpersonal Life in the Sociosphere of Human Knowledge, Practice and Language.' In A. Foolen, U. Lüdtke, T. Racine and J. Zlatev (eds) *Moving Ourselves, Moving Others: Motion and Emotion in Intersubjectivity, Consciousness and Language.* Amsterdam: John Benjamins.

Frank, B. and Trevarthen, C. (2015) 'Epilogue: Emotion in Language Can Overcome Exclusion from Meaning.' In U. Lüdtke (ed.) *Emotion in Language: Theory – Research – Application.* Amsterdam: John Benjamins..

Gerken, L.A. (2009) *Language Development.* San Diego: Plural Publishing.

Goffman, E. (1961) *Asylums: Essays on the Social Situation of Mental Patients and Other Inmates.* New York: Anchor Books.

Gratier, M. (2003) 'Expressive timing and interactional synchrony between mothers and infants: cultural similarities, cultural differences, and the immigration experience.' *Cognitive Development 18,* 4, 533–554.

Gratier, M. and Apter-Danon, G. (2010) 'The Improvised Musicality of Belonging: Repetition and Variation in Mother–Infant Vocal Interaction.' In S. Malloch and C. Trevarthen (eds) *Communicative Musicality: Exploring the Basis of Human Companionship.* Oxford: Oxford University Press.

Gratier, M. and Trevarthen, C. (2008) 'Musical narrative and motives for culture in mother–infant vocal interaction.' *Journal of Consciousness Studies 15,* 10–11, 122–158.

Gratier, M., Dominguez, S., Devouche, E. and Apter, G. (2015) 'What Words Can't Tell: Emotion and Connection between "Borderline" Mothers and Infants.' In U. Lüdtke (ed.) *Emotion in Language: Theory – Research – Application.* Amsterdam: John Benjamins.

Habermas, J. (1985) *The Theory of Communicative Action, Volume 2: Lifeworld and System: A Critique of Functionalist Reason.* Boston, MA: Beacon. (Original work 'Theorie des kommunikativen Handelns' published in 1981.)

Habermas, J. (1985) *The Theory of Communicative Action, Volume 2. Lifeworld and System: A Critique of Functionalist Reason.* Boston, MA: Beacon. (Original work: 'Theorie des kommunikativen Handelns' published in 1981.)

Kennedy, H., Landor, M. and Todd, L. (2011) *Video Interaction Guidance: A Relationship-Based Intervention to Promote Attunement, Empathy and Wellbeing.* London: Jessica Kingsley Publishers.

Kristeva, J. (1998) 'The Subject in Process.' In P. French and R.-F. Lack (eds) *The Tel Quel Reader.* London: Routledge.

Lüdtke, U. (2012) 'Relational Emotions in Semiotic and Linguistic Development: Towards an Intersubjective Theory of Language Learning and Language Therapy.' In A. Foolen, U. Lüdtke, T. Racine and J. Zlatev (eds) *Moving Ourselves, Moving Others: Motion and Emotion in Intersubjectivity, Consciousness and Language.* Amsterdam: John Benjamins.

Malloch, S. and Trevarthen, C. (2010) *Communicative Musicality: Exploring the Basis of Human Companionship.* Oxford: Oxford University Press.

Murray, L. and Trevarthen, C. (1985) 'Emotional Regulation of Interactions between Two-month-olds and Their Mothers.' In T.M. Field and N.A. Fox (eds) *Social Perception in Infants*. Norwood, NJ: Ablex.

Nadel, J. and Han, B. (2015) 'Emotion on Board.' In U. Lüdtke (ed.) *Emotion in Language: Theory – Research – Application*. Amsterdam: John Benjamins.

Nagy, E. (2008) 'Innate intersubjectivity: newborns' sensitivity to communication disturbance.' *Developmental Psychology 44*, 6, 1779–1784.

Nelson, C.A., Fox, N.A. and Zeanah, C. (2014) *Romania's Abandoned Children: Deprivation, Brain Development, and the Struggle for Recovery*. Cambridge, MA: Harvard University Press.

Rabain-Jamin, J. and Sabeau-Jouannet, E. (1997) 'Maternal speech to 4-month-old infants in two cultures: Wolof and French.' *International Journal of Behavioral Development 20*, 425–451.

Reason, P. and Bradbury, H. (eds) (2009) *The SAGE Handbook of Action Research: Participative Inquiry and Practice*. London: Sage.

Reddy, V. (2008). *How Infants Know Minds*. Cambridge, MA: Harvard University Press.

Routray, S., Mahilary, N. and Paul, R. (2015) 'Effect of maternal deprivation on child development: A comparative study between orphanage and urban slum children in Odisha.' *International Journal of Bioassays 4*, 3, 3701–3703.

Schütte, U. (forthcoming) 'Culturally sensitive adaptation of the concept of relational communication: an exploratory study in therapy as a support to language development in collaboration with a Tanzanian orphanage.' *South African Journal of Communication Disorders, 63*, 1, a166.

Spitz, R.A. (1946) 'Anaclitic depression.' *Psychoanalytic Study of the Child 2*, 313–342.

Spitz, R.A. (1952) *Psychogenic Diseases in Infancy*. A film produced by the Psychoanalytic research project on problems of infancy. Available at www.youtube.com/watch?v=VvdOe10vrs4, accessed on 25 May 2016.

Stern, D.N. (2004) *The Present Moment in Psychotherapy and Everyday Life*. New York: Norton.

Trevarthen, C. (1998) 'The Concept and Foundations of Infant Intersubjectivity.' In S. Bråten (ed.) *Intersubjective Communication and Emotion in Early Ontogeny*. Cambridge: Cambridge University Press.

Trevarthen, C. (2008) 'The musical art of infant conversation: narrating in the time of sympathetic experience, without rational interpretation, before words.' *Musicae Scientiae 12*, 1, 15–46.

Trevarthen, C. (2012) 'Intersubjektivität und Kommunikation.' In O. Braun and U. Lüdtke (eds) *Enzyklopädisches Handbuch der Behindertenpädagogik. Bd. 8: Sprache und Kommunikation*. Stuttgart: Kohlhammer.

CONTRIBUTORS

Ana Almeida

Ana Almeida is a postdoctoral researcher at the Institute for Music in Human and Social Development, University of Edinburgh, currently working on a pilot trial of an interactive music programme for individuals living with dementia. Her research interests focus on embodied musical experiences across the lifespan, in particular on the spontaneous movement interaction of young children with music. As a performer, Ana is also involved in early years artistic, educational and community projects (e.g. in schools and refugee camps) across Europe.

Foteini Athanasiadou

Foteini Athanasiadou is a registered dance movement psychotherapist. Her clinical experience includes work with children, adults and elderly people in various settings, for example, special and mainstream schools, day centres and NHS settings. Foteini is experienced in facilitating movement-based personal development workshops with adults and well-being programmes with children. Currently, she works as a dance movement psychotherapist with people facing acute psychosis at the NHS Lambeth Hospital, South London and as a freelancer in Brighton.

Sarah Butler

Sarah Butler leads a Foundation Stage Unit in Newton Abbot, Devon. She has worked with and studied children under five years old for over 25 years. As a specialist leader in education (SLE) in Early Years, she has supported nursery settings and schools across the South West in finding ways to develop creative approaches to learning, ensuring the child's voice is central within each learning story.

Stuart Daniel

Stuart Daniel runs a therapeutic service based in a unit for children with emotional/behavioural difficulties in Devon, UK. He is qualified in play therapy, Dyadic Developmental Psychotherapy and Sherborne Developmental Movement. He has previously worked in many special education schools, for the Royal Hospital of Sick Children, Edinburgh, and even freelance in a shed! Having a passionate interest in early communication, severe learning difficulties and medical trauma, he has authored scientific and therapy articles in these areas.

Katy Dymoke

Katy is a dancer working in community, health and education contexts. A Body-Mind Centering® (BMC®) practitioner and teacher, she worked with BMC approaches as a DMP in the NHS learning disability services for nine years and undertook doctoral research on the impact of touch in her case work. Katy is a somatic movement therapist and program coordinator of the BMC training with Embody-Move. As director of Touchdown Dance, she delivers workshops, research projects and training for visually impaired and disabled people of all ages and ability.

Jane Edwards

Jane Edwards is Associate Professor in Mental Health at Deakin University, Australia. She is a qualified music therapist with expertise in the role of music therapy to promote optimal parent–infant relationships. She has championed the role of psychosocial care for children receiving medical care. She is currently a board director for the Association for the Wellbeing of Children in Healthcare, Australia. She is the former director of the Music & Health Research Group at the University of Limerick, Ireland.

Cochavit Elefant

Cochavit Elefant, PhD, is a music therapist and is Head of the Graduate School for Creative Arts Therapies, University of Haifa, Israel. Her clinical and research areas are music therapy, community music therapy, working with people with Parkinson's and early communication with children with Rett syndrome and autism. She has published several articles and two books on these topics. She is Associate Editor of the *Nordic Journal of Music Therapy*.

Bodo Frank

Bodo Frank is currently a postdoctoral researcher and director of the BabyLab INCLUDE at Leibniz University, Hannover. His scientific interest interweaves sociological, psychological and neuroscientific aspects of intersubjective dialogues in therapy for investigating the physical structure of mother--infant interactions. He cooperates closely with the Institut für Informationsverarbeitung: Computer Vision and Human Motion (TNT) for the development of modern and refined technologies for field research in participatory approaches, supporting inclusion for handicapped children and adults in Germany, East Africa, India and Mexico.

Carolyn Fresquez

Carolyn Fresquez, RDMP UK, earned her MSc in dance movement psychotherapy from Queen Margaret University in Scotland. She is a trained dancer, with experience as a performer, choreographer and movement teacher and consultant. Carolyn has worked with children and adults in a variety of settings in both creative and therapeutic capacities. She believes in the wisdom afforded when, with curiosity, playfulness and safety, we turn our attention to the many ways we move.

Daniel Hughes

Daniel Hughes, PhD, is a clinical psychologist with a limited practice in South Portland, Maine. He founded and developed Dyadic Developmental Psychotherapy (DDP), a treatment of children who demonstrate ongoing problems related to attachment and trauma. He has conducted seminars and spoken at conferences internationally and provides consultation to various agencies and professionals. He is president of the Dyadic Developmental Psychotherapy Institute (DDPI) which is responsible for the training, supervision and certification of professionals in DDP (see ddpnetwork.org). Dan is the author of many books and articles.

Stine Lindahl Jacobsen

Stine Lindahl Jacobsen is Associate Professor and Head of the MA Programme of Music Therapy at Aalborg University in Denmark. She teaches music therapy improvisation skills, group music therapy skills and music therapy assessment. She has published various books, articles and chapters in the area of working with children and families at risk and in the research area of standardized music therapy assessment tools. Jacobsen developed the music therapy assessment tool Assessment of Parent-Child Interaction (APCI).

Vicky Karkou

Professor Karkou is a qualified educator, researcher and dance movement psychotherapist, having worked with vulnerable children and adults in schools, voluntary organizations and the NHS. She holds the Chair of Dance at Edge Hill University. She is well published in national and international journals and acts as the co-editor for the international journal *Body, Movement and Dance in Psychotherapy*. She has co-written and co-edited three books including *Arts Therapies in Schools: Research and Practice* (Jessica Kingsley Publishers).

Peter A. Levine

Peter A. Levine, PhD, is the developer of Somatic Experiencing® and founder of the Somatic Experiencing® Trauma Institute, which conducts SE™ trainings throughout the world. He is currently a Senior Fellow and consultant at The Meadows Addiction and Trauma Treatment Center in Wickenburg, Arizona. Dr Levine has written several books about trauma. His books include the international bestseller, *Waking the Tiger: Healing Trauma*; *In an Unspoken Voice: How the Body Releases Trauma and Restores Goodness*; and *Trauma-Proofing Your Kids: A Parents' Guide for Instilling Confidence, Joy and Resilience*.

Ulrike Lüdtke

Ulrike Lüdtke is professor and head of department of Speech Language Pedagogy and Therapy at Leibniz University Hannover, Germany. She has authored and edited several books on the relation of language and emotion. Her research interest is dedicated to the influence of relational emotions on communication and language processes – be it language didactics, semiotics or early language development. This interest led her to establish the BabyLab INCLUDE Hannover that takes research as a relational process and focuses on in-vivo settings.

Stephen Malloch

Stephen Malloch works as a psychotherapist, executive coach, career coach, workshop designer and facilitator, and research academic in Sydney, Australia. His model of 'communicative musicality', co-created with Colwyn Trevarthen, informs his therapeutic and coaching practice, and is explored in numerous journal articles and book chapters. His commitment to individual and organizational wellbeing is further supported by his practice of mindfulness. He is founder/director of HeartMind, Principal Consultant at Audrey Page & Associates, and Researcher, Westmead Psychotherapy Program, University of Sydney.

Paulo Maria Rodrigues

Paulo Maria Rodrigues is a composer, performer, artistic director and educator. He founded the Companhia de Música Teatral and has developed many artistic and educational projects. Between 2006 and 2010, as Coordinator of Educational Services of the Casa da Música, he was responsible for conceiving and implementing a vast and eclectic programme of activities, including projects for the disabled, communities, schools and families. He is an assistant professor in the Departmento de Communicação e Arte at the Universidade de Aveiro, Portugal.

Dennis McCarthy

Dennis McCarthy is a licensed psychotherapist in New York. He has worked for 40 years with children using play therapy and with adults using dreams and bioenergetics. He has authored/edited several books and numerous articles in professional journals, including *A Manual of Dynamic Play Therapy: Helping Things Fall Apart, the Paradox of Play* published by Jessica Kingsley Publishers. He leads training workshops and supervises professionals. He also leads a biannual workshop in the Greek islands entitled 'The Heart Leaps Up…', which explores myth using the expressive arts.

Penny McFarlane

Penny McFarlane is a qualified dramatherapist and clinical supervisor in South Devon, UK having worked in education as a teacher and then a children's therapist for over 30 years. She founded a project bringing arts therapies into schools across an inner city and co-created a children's bereavement charity and therapeutic drama group. She has published books, chapters and articles about her lifetime's work on dramatherapy with children.

Hugh Nankivell

Hugh Nankivell is a curious composer and performer who plays in professional, community and educational settings. He has composed large-scale pieces for organizations including Opera North, Dartmoor National Park, UNESCO, The National Theatre of Scotland and on several Anglo-Japanese projects. Hugh is currently the Bournemouth Symphony Orchestra Music Associate for Devon, working on arts and health projects with early years, families and older people. He runs a creative community choir 'The Choral Engineers' and compulsively composes songs.

Nigel Osborne

Nigel Osborne MBE, FRCM is a British composer and Emeritus Professor in the College of Art at Edinburgh University, where he was Reid Professor of Music. His compositions have featured at major international festivals and have been performed by leading orchestras and ensembles around the world. He is interested in relating neurosciences and music and has pioneered the use of participation in creation of music as therapy and rehabilitation for children who are victims of conflict, his work being carried out in the Balkans, the Caucasus, Africa and the Middle East.

Judi Parson

Dr Judi Parson is a paediatric qualified Registered Nurse, play therapist and Lecturer in Mental Health and Course Co-Director for the Master of Child Play Therapy at Deakin University, Australia. As the past chair for the Australasia Pacific Play Therapy Association she plays an active role in developing play therapy in Australia and the Asia Pacific. She sits on the board of the Association for the Welfare of Children in Healthcare and has a special interest in medical play therapy.

Chantal Polzin

Chantal Polzin is a teacher for special needs education with a main area in speech and language pathology and arts. After her educational degree she joined a participatory research project at BabyLab INCLUDE Hannover at Leibniz University Hannover, Germany in cooperation with Sebastian Kolowa Memorial University, Tanzania. In this project she could follow her research interests in performativity, intercultural cooperation and early language and communication development. Currently she writes her doctoral thesis on performative moments of meeting in early dialogue.

Stephen Porges

Stephen W. Porges, PhD is Distinguished University Scientist at Indiana University, Professor of Psychiatry at the University of North Carolina and Professor Emeritus at the University of Illinois at Chicago and the University of Maryland. He is the former President of the Society for Psychophysiological Research and a recipient of a NIMH Research Scientist Development Award. He is the originator of the Polyvagal Theory and has published more than 250 peer-reviewed scientific papers across several disciplines.

Dee C. Ray

Dee C. Ray, PhD, LPC-S, NCC, RPT-S is Distinguished Teaching Professor in the Counseling Program and Director of the Child and Family Resource Clinic at the University of North Texas. Dr Ray has published over 100 articles, chapters and books on play therapy, specializing in research publications examining the effects of child centred play therapy. She is author of *A Therapist's Guide to Development: The Extraordinarily Normal Years* and *Advanced Play Therapy: Essential Conditions, Knowledge, and Skills for Child Practice.*

Helena Rodrigues

Helena Rodrigues is an assistant professor at the Faculdade de Ciências Sociais e Humanas, Universidade NOVA de Lisboa, Portugal and the artistic director of Companhia de Música Teatral. She introduced Gordon's music learning theory in Portugal. She has been searching for organic ways to communicate through vocal and gesture practices. She is often invited to give workshops and to design innovative approaches on training and on artistic practices related to infancy.

Josephat Semkiwa

Josephat Semkiwa is a lecturer for special needs education and researcher at Sebastian Kolowa Memorial University, Tanzania. His research interest is to deepen the knowledge on cultural specifics of communication and language development and to improve education of professionals dealing with vulnerable children in Tanzania. After his master studies at the Norwegian University of Science and Technology (NTNU) he joined the bi-national and participatory research project conducted by Sebastian Kolowa Memorial University and Leibniz University Hannover, Germany.

Colwyn Trevarthen

Colwyn Trevarthen is Emeritus Professor of Child Psychology and Psychobiology at the University of Edinburgh and is also a Fellow of the Royal Society of Edinburgh and a Vice President of the British Association for Early Childhood Education. He has authored many books and over 200 scientific articles on vision and movement, brain development, infant communication, infant learning and emotional health and well-being and the psychological aspects of musicality in communication.

Tim Webb

Tim Webb is co-founder and artistic director of Oily Cart, the London-based theatre company that for the past 35 years has been creating multi-sensory and interactive theatre for young people with profound and multiple learning disabilities and for those on the autism spectrum. In addition, each year they create an 'all-comers' show for children from two to five and their families. Their highly exploratory work has been performed in hydrotherapy pools, on trampolines and with their audiences suspended amongst the trapeze and bungie artists of a mini big top.

SUBJECT INDEX

AUTHOR INDEX